History of American Pediatrics

Thomas E. Cone, Jr., M.D.
Clinical Professor of Pediatrics, Harvard Medical School;
Senior Associate in Clinical Genetics and Medicine,
The Children's Hospital Medical Center, Boston

Foreword by Samuel X. Radbill, M.D.
Honorary Librarian of the College of Physicians
of Philadelphia

Little, Brown and Company   Boston

Published December 1979

Copyright © 1979 by Little, Brown and Company (Inc.)

First Edition

Library of Congress Catalog Card No. 79-91937

ISBN 0-316-152897

Printed in the United States of America

HAL

For Babbie
whose patience and understanding
made this book possible

Foreword

Thomas E. Cone, Jr., accomplished pediatrician, allured by the charms of seductive Clio Medica, has already regaled a wide reading audience for the past fourteen years with a series of historical vignettes in the official journal of the American Academy of Pediatrics. In addition he has prepared an attractive book, *200 Years of Feeding Infants in America,* in which we meet face to face with a procession of American pediatric pioneers who were not willingly submissive to the decrees of fate or ready to accept the preachments that the reason so many babies died was because it was the will of God, but instead strove to solve the mysteries of the nutritional needs of children, which were of such fundamental importance in pediatric care and so helped to deter the inflexible Atropos.

His historical diggings have unearthed the roots of our pediatric heritage, and not only have his historical papers and lectures provided pleasant literary fare for a wide circle of pediatric readers, but also his elucidation of the relevance of the past to the present has proved to be profitably pragmatic.

The year 1979 is the International Year of the Child, and 1980 will mark the golden anniversary of the American Academy of Pediatrics. Information about the history of American pediatrics helps us to carry out the Academy's charge for all pediatricians to "Speak up for Children." It places the lessons of the past in historical perspective and reveals the obstacle course which has stood in the path of pediatrics on its way toward reaching its goals for the welfare of children. The trail as outlined by Dr. Cone winds over treacherous paths through the seventeenth, eighteenth, and nineteenth centuries before the specialty of pediatrics emerged upon the high-speed road of the twentieth century.

During the seventeenth century the American colonies were like a fetus still attached to the mother country. The health and welfare of children depended upon European culture and tradition. The few English physicians here derived their pediatric lore from the medical teachings of the ancients and the novel ideas that filtered through from contemporary writings such as those of Pemmel and Harris on the diseases of children, and, above all, of that seventeenth-century English Hippocrates, Thomas Sydenham. The native Indian care of children, of which we vaguely learn from the inadequate hints in the writings of Josselyn and some of the other American voyagers, may have influenced colonial folk medicine to some slight degree, but it was the European connection that counted most of all.

The primary provider of care for the healthy child in all times has been the mother. Midwives, wet nurses, grandmothers, wise old women in general, all joined in to help mothers. Physicians were not much help in the seventeenth century; nor were the apothecaries, barber-surgeons, or other male health care providers who accompanied the early settlers.

The preacher-practitioners and the educated laymen like the Winthrops, father and son, were closer to the families and their medical advice was often more respected. Calvinistic colonials, convinced that the sins of the fathers were visited upon their children, believed that innocent babies were born full of sin and corruption, and so it is not surprising that devilish children had the devil beaten out of them, and when they were sick they were purged of their corruptions with tormenting purgatives, emetics, blisters, and bleedings. Now we do just the opposite. Instead of evacuating obnoxious humors by every corporeal outlet we pour doctored fluids into every available vein. But that was an age when pauperism was resented and foundlings as the fruits of sin had little chance of survival.

Infant mortality was heartrending. Doctors were unable to cope with devastating epidemics of the diseases like diphtheria, scarlet fever, or meningitis that periodically went on a rampage. Indeed, frustrated by their limitations, many of them shunned children and gladly relegated them to the care of the midwives

whom the people preferred anyway because they were cheaper. The rudimentary medical science of the early colonies is here presented in sharp contrast with our own science and technology. It must be borne in mind, however, that it formed the roots from which grew, feebly in the eighteenth century and at an accelerated pace in the nineteenth, the improvement of our knowledge and the resultant capabilities of today. But in the past, the only consolation left for desolate parents when the death of infants was inescapable was the faith that their innocent darlings made lovely angels. Thanks to a bountiful Providence, in spite of the rapacious claws of death, the fertile colonists expiated their sins with a high birthrate. Families of four, five and six were the rule, while even as many as ten or even twenty were not unknown. Some of the children did manage to survive without modern pediatric care.

The common ailments of children were worms, teething, and convulsions. Benjamin Rush once remarked that when he first commenced practice in Philadelphia he could not have retained the confidence of his patients when called upon to visit sick children unless he prescribed a worm medicine. It is hard for us today to realize the omnipresence of worms. Children then, like animals today, harbored all sorts of worms. Roundworms were passed in the stools singly and in wriggling masses; sometimes a tapeworm would protrude from the rectum in a strip a yard long or more, to the consternation of all who beheld it; and pinworms could be seen crawling about the anus as the child scratched to relieve the itch. Every imaginable disease might be attributed to worms whether or not they were visible.

So, too, from the time of Hippocrates, every undefinable disease in a child that occurred during the time of dentition could be ascribed to teething. Convulsions in particular were related to difficult dentition, as were fevers in general.

Fevers of all kinds were explained by the ancient theory of fermenting corruption. Equated with putrefaction, fever was visualized the same as rotting or putrefying organic material in which worms of all sorts were generated. A few of the fevers were already distinguished in one way or another by the seventeenth century: smallpox and measles since the time of Rhazes in the tenth century; intermittents, usually quartan or tertian malarias; continued fevers, often typhoid; hectic, often tuberculous, which had been differentiated even in the ancient days of Greece.

Then there was witchcraft. When no other cause of harm could be thought of, then the child was bewitched. The Massachusetts witchcraft trials were a sad blight in the history of American pediatrics. Yet the good doctor Sir Thomas Browne, loved and revered by all the English medical profession, as well as even more scientifically mature medical men of his period, accepted witchcraft as gospel truth. There is great risk in too much dependency on authority, so dear to the hearts of today's bureaucrats.

Throughout the ages, right up to the eighteenth century, in fact, childbirth and attendance on young infants were women's business. Thereafter an increasing galaxy of man-midwives invaded the lying-in rooms. To the midwives they were often considered interlopers. By the end of the eighteenth century they had captured a large portion of obstetrics. The midwives and wise old women, as a rule, were trained only by oral tradition and example; by the middle of the nineteenth century the male obstetricians instituted midwifery schools for men only, first privately and soon afterward in the medical schools. Midwives were thus an older breed of medical specialists. Among the functions of the midwife which the man-midwife usurped was included the care of young infants in health and in sickness. But the obstetricians, in contrast to the midwives of old, rendered only perfunctory service to children. They concentrated all their attention on the problems of labor and sadly neglected the infantile rewards of their labors. Nevertheless, another century passed by before the child could be wrenched free from the obstetrical hold and embraced within the care of the fledgling brood of pediatricians late in the nineteenth century.

Abraham Jacobi was among the first of these in America. He was a radical and was repeatedly slapped down when he first began to speak up for children. He exerted a powerful influence in this country and abroad along unconventional lines that raised many hackles in his time but enlisted many disciples.

Job Smith, his friend and colleague, shy bookworm that he was, through his research, teaching, and writing spoke up in his own way. Neither of these two trailblazers had the prestigious backing of a Harvard University like Rotch nor of a fabulously wealthy Rockefeller family like Holt, yet each in his own way was able to play effective roles in the advancement of pediatrics. In their day, children, like dolls, were to be seen and not heard. When Jacobi cried out in anguish against the plight of the dying waifs in his institution, the well-meaning benevolent ladies running the hospital fired him; and as for Smith in 1866, he had to worm his way into the Bellevue Hospital Medical College faculty at first as a lecturer in morbid anatomy in order to satisfy his teaching penchant and the eager appetite of the students for his instruction.

While the newborn and young infants traditionally came under the care of the midwives, the older children fell within the legitimate province of the physicians. This was true even in antiquity. There were, it is true, doctors in all times who had a special reputation of being good with children, but it was not until medical practice was fragmented into specialties late in the nineteenth century that children were released, reluctantly, by the internists to the pediatricians. Up until the middle of the nineteenth century there were no hospitals for children in America. Except for a few scattered orphan asylums (foundling hospitals were frowned upon in this predominantly Protestant nation), the almshouses offered the only haven for destitute, sick children. General hospitals were still few in number before the Civil War and these were geared to adults, accepting children only in case of emergency. The first hospital to devote all its attention to sick children opened as a benevolent institution in Boston in 1848 but had to close its doors within three or four years for lack of money. It was not until 1855 that the first hospital that limited its admissions strictly to sick children was established in this country. It was followed by a second in 1869. These institutions were decidedly a factor in the advancement of pediatrics as a specialty.

The succinct accounts of the important early pediatric texts are also informative in this regard. They show that American doctors were not only in step with their European colleagues, but also at times led the way, contributing their fair share to the advancement of pediatrics.

Research was mostly clinical. Children were readily available subjects for experimentation. When Nathaniel Chapman, during the first decade of the nineteenth century (when immunization against smallpox had achieved enthusiastic popular acceptance) experimented with measles immunization on children in his institution without success, God only knows what other diseases he transmitted to them. But no one thought of the ethics of using children for such research at that time. The need for more knowledge was more pressing then.

The transition of infant feeding from crude empiricism to a scientific footing began in the mid-nineteenth century with the chemical investigations of milk by Vincent Meigs. These were almost simultaneous with those by Biedert in Europe and were the basis of Rotch's efforts in this country to modify cow's milk so that it would more nearly resemble that of women. Evaporation of milk and canning methods for foodstuffs began also in the early nineteenth century and were likewise a part of the evolution of the commercial infant food preparations of today.

All these evolutionary steps in the development of pediatrics as a specialty may be discerned in Dr. Cone's story of American pediatrics. The diseases of children had to be unraveled and mastered; the hygienic and nutritional problems of infants and children had to be solved; social, economic, and environmental disadvantages had to be fathomed and corrected; and advancing scientific knowledge and technological skills had to be disseminated and applied to the health and welfare of children in order to stay the grim reaper's hand. All this, along with the outstanding spirits who led the way are graphically displayed by Dr. Cone in the light of his practical experience, historical acumen, and scholarly attainments.

Here again he has responded to the call of the American Academy of Pediatrics to "Speak up for Children."

Samuel X. Radbill, M.D.

Preface

For years I have thought of writing a history of American pediatrics but whenever I set my mind to it Ernest Caulfield's remark would discourage me. In 1952 he wrote: "Sometime someone will write the history of American pediatrics but not immediately, I hope, because it is much too soon to appraise properly many of the revolutionary changes of the past few decades."

Now, almost three decades after Caulfield's comment, I believe the time has come to prepare a historical survey of pediatrics as it has evolved in our country. Two reasons have persuaded me to attempt the task. The first and more compelling is that it will fill a wide gap in the history of medicine, because there is no published comprehensive history of American pediatrics. And my second reason is that my book may perhaps stimulate interest in the historical development of this branch of medicine.

It may come as a surprise that the best previously published history of pediatrics in the English language, *The History of Paediatrics* by Sir George Frederic Still, published in 1931, does not go beyond the eighteenth century and never mentions America.

In addition to Still's book, there are two histories of pediatrics written by Americans: Fielding H. Garrison's *History of Pediatrics* (1923) and John Ruhräh's *Pediatrics of the Past: An Anthology* (1925). Neither of these is concerned with American pediatrics. Garrison's history was written as an introductory chapter for Isaac Abt's multivolume *Pediatrics* (1923). It is an excellent review of pediatric history from prehistoric times to the beginning of the present century; however, American pediatrics is discussed only tangentially.

Ruhräh's text contains biographical sketches of the lives of some of the more important pediatricians of the past with a comprehensive selection of some of their published works. Ruhräh has thrown much light on the important contributions of long-forgotten writers (almost all non-American) by tracing the progress of pediatrics from ancient times to the nineteenth century.

My principal aim has been to write a history of American pediatrics encompassing the major contributions of American men and women in improving the care and management of sick children. I have not written the book primarily for the specialist in medical history, to whom most of the facts I have mentioned will already be well known. Rather, I had in mind the medical practitioner, the medical student, and all others who may have an interest in the evolution of contemporary medical care of children.

A story so broad as the history of American pediatrics covering almost four centuries must of necessity be incomplete. To those of my contemporaries whose names I may not have mentioned, my apologies. The omissions were not willful, but solely due to the constraints imposed in keeping this book within limits.

My obligations to many authors are indicated by the bibliographies at the end of each chapter. I have leaned especially on Faber and McIntosh's *History of the American Pediatric Society, 1887–1965*, Parish's *A History of Immunization*, Paul's *A History of Poliomyelitis*, Dowling's *Fighting Infections*, Garrison and Morton's *A Medical Bibliography*, Viets's *A Brief History of Medicine in Massachusetts*, Clarke's *A Century of American Medicine, 1776–1876*, and Packard's *History of Medicine in the United States*.

I am deeply indebted to Dr. Samuel X. Radbill for his continued and generous guidance over many years and for his willingness to read every page of my manuscript. However, if there are factual errors in the book, the fault is entirely mine. I wish to thank Mr. Richard J. Wolfe, Rare Books Librarian in the Francis A. Countway Library of Medicine, and his entire staff for helping me to locate many hard-to-find references.

My sincerest thanks to Miss Annette Cardillo for her unstinting willingness to type and then to retype the entire manuscript not once but several times.

For permission to use some of the material on infant feeding that originally appeared in *200 Years of Feeding Infants in America*, published in 1976, I wish to thank Ross Laboratories.

The publication of this book was made possible by a grant from the Johnson and Johnson Institute for Pediatric Service, New Brunswick, New Jersey. I take this opportunity to express my sincerest appreciation to Steven Sawchuk, M.D., Chairman, and to the other members of the Institute's Board of Trustees for their financial support. I hope this book will be considered worthy of their faith in me.

T. E. C., Jr.
Boston

Contents

Foreword by Samuel X. Radbill   *vii*

Preface   *xi*

The Colonial Period

1 Pastor- and Governor-Physicians   5
Immigration to the New World   Medical Training and Practice
Who Cared for the Children?   Colonial Infants Delivered by Mid-
wives   Birth Defects in Colonial America   Common Accidents and
Diseases of Seventeenth-Century Colonial Children   Seventeenth-
Century Medical Doctrines and Practice   Child Care and Child
Rearing   Seventeenth-Century Vital Statistics

2 Children Discovered   29
Medical Training and Practice   Epidemic Diseases   Benjamin Rush
and Pediatrics   Sources of Pediatric Information for Colonial Parents
Accidents and Common Diseases of Eighteenth-Century American
Children   Eighteenth-Century American Pediatric Publications

3 Feeding Colonial Infants   55
Breast-Feeding   Wet-Nursing   Artificial Feeding   Alexander
Hamilton on Infant Feeding   Hugh Smith on Infant Feeding   Lionel
Chalmers on Infant Feeding   Pap and Panada   Seventeenth- and
Eighteenth-Century Views on Weaning

The Nineteenth Century

4 "Perplexing Obscurity and Embarrassing Uncertainty"   69
Medical Education   Medical Practice   Infant Mortality   Care of
Dependent Children   American Pediatric Texts, 1800–1850   Some
Significant American Contributions to Pediatrics, 1800–1850   Chil-
dren Treated with Heroic or Drastic Measures   Child Labor

5 "Explorers in an Almost Unknown Country"   99
Emerging Interest in Child Health   Medical Practice and the Impor-
tance of the German School of Pediatrics   Pediatrics Emerges as a
Specialty   Health Problems of Infants and Children   Common and
Epidemic Diseases   American Pediatric Texts (1850–1900)   Ameri-
can Pediatric Journals (1850–1900)

6   *Infant Feeding of Paramount Concern*   131
    Advocacy of Breast-Feeding   Nineteenth-Century Rules for the
    Selection of a Wet Nurse   Artificially Fed Infants   Early Steps in
    Scientific Milk Modification for Bottle-Fed Infants   The Doctors
    Meigs of Philadelphia and Their Contributions to Infant Feeding
    Thomas Morgan Rotch and the Percentage Method of Infant Feeding
    Abraham Jacobi and Infant Feeding   The Calorimetric Method of
    Infant Feeding   The Amount and Frequency of Feeding the Infant
    Sanitary Milk Supply   Henry L. Coit and the Fight for Clean Milk
    Nathan Straus and Milk Stations for the Poor   Proprietary (Artifi-
    cial) Infant Foods   Introduction to Solid Foods   Nineteenth-Century
    Views on Weaning

The Twentieth Century

7   *Pediatrics Comes of Age*   151
    The Milk Problem   The Infant and Child Welfare Movement
    Pediatrics and the Child Welfare Movement   The Emergence of Bio-
    chemical Research in Pediatrics   Rickets   Scurvy   Supportive Ther-
    apy   Infectious Diseases   The Newborn Infant   Diatheses and the
    Thymus   Endocrine Disorders   Allergy   New Publications

8   *Antibiotics and Electrolytes*   201
    The Founding of the American Academy of Pediatrics   Fluid and
    Electrolyte Therapy   Hematology   Infectious Diseases   Nutrition
    and Nutritional Disorders   The Newborn Infant   Some New
    Pediatric Diseases   New Discoveries in Some Established Pediatric
    Diseases   Endocrine Disturbances   New Publications

9   *The Changing Face of Pediatrics*   229
    Federal Support of Pediatric Research   Sudden Infant Death Syn-
    drome   Battered Child Syndrome   Childhood Accidents   Some Re-
    cent Clinical Advances in Pediatrics   Some Newer Viral Diseases
    The Newborn   New Publications   The "New" Pediatric Morbidity

10 *From Complexity to Simplicity*   245
    Infant Feeding in Twentieth-Century America   Milk and Milk-Free
    Products Introduced for Infant Feeding Since 1900   Some Current
    Trends in Infant Feeding Practices   What Do American Parents
    Now Feed Their Infants?

Indexes

Name Index   263

Subject Index   271

The Colonial Period

Pastor- and Governor-Physicians *1*

Pediatrics is a modern specialty, and the practitioner or investigator devoting his whole time and energy to children is inclined to think our knowledge of the subject a thing belonging to the end of the nineteenth century and to the twentieth. . . . It is interesting, therefore, to look backward over the centuries and try to see what medical men of other times thought or knew about morbid manifestations in the young.

John Ruhräh (1919)

As the seventeenth century began there was no permanent English settlement or even a trading post in America. The thought of venturing out into the vast Atlantic Ocean was viewed with terror by the ordinary people of England, and yet within a few decades thousands of them would leave their homes, some alone and some as families with young children, to cross the mysterious emptiness of the Atlantic to settle in a strange and far-distant New World. They were spurred on by a new spirit of adventure engendered by the long reign of Elizabeth I, from 1558 to 1603, during which England had embarked on a course of expansion, spiritual and material, such as few nations had ever experienced. In the opening years of the century this spirit was to see a swarming of Englishmen and women being drawn to the New World to create a new life in the wilderness.

When the rest of medicine started to advance in the middle of the seventeenth century, pediatrics lagged far behind. A glance through the English pediatric texts of the period is disappointing. Some have the unmistakable flavor of charlatanry, which suggests, according to a modern medical historian, that "they were written with an eye to being sold to midwives rather than to physicians."[33] This was so because, as a rule, British physicians in the seventeenth century treated only children of the nobility and upper classes, and then only on occasion. If a physician did condescend to see a child, or to write about pediatrics, it was with the fascination of illness that he was principally concerned, not with the unexciting routine of infant management. It is small wonder that in the care of young children "the med-

5

ical profession at large had left nurses and mothers to deal with the worrisome little nuisances" who would then treat them with "kitchen physic." The doctor was called—if at all—only when all family remedies had failed.

As the seventeenth century ended, great strides had been made in medicine. William Harvey (1578–1657) had revolutionized medicine by the discovery of the circulation of the blood (1628), Francis Glisson (1597–1677) by his classic study of rickets, *De Rachitide* (1650), and Thomas Sydenham (1624–1689) by his descriptions of many diseases, notably scarlet fever (1676), measles (1676), hysteria (1682), and chorea (1686). From the pediatric point of view the most widely read contributions were made by Walter Harris (1647–1732).[38] His book *Acute Diseases of Infancy* (1689) was referred to by Sydenham as one that "may be of more Service to the Public, than all my own writings."

Harris's book was the popular pediatric treatise from his time until it was supplanted almost a century later by Michael Underwood's *A Treatise on the Diseases of Children* (1784). The difficulties and discouragements of pediatric practice in the seventeenth century made a deep impression on Harris and he let it be known:

I know very well in how unbeaten and almost unknown a Path, I am treading; for sick Children, and especially Infants, give no other light into the Knowledge of their Diseases, than what we are able to discover from their uneasy Cries, and the uncertain Tokens of their Crossness; for which Reason several Physicians of first Rank have openly declared to me, that they go very unwillingly to take care of the Diseases of Children, especially as such as are newly born as if they were to unravel some strange Mystery, or cure some incurable Distemper.

Immigration to the New World

Between 1620 and 1642 about eighty thousand, or 2 percent of all Englishmen, left Britain in quest of a better life.[6] Social and economic conditions were a propelling force, persuading many to leave their homeland for the New World. Life at home was made insecure by recurring economic depressions, by plague years, and by occasional bad harvests, but in themselves they may not have been sufficiently intolerable to make so many leave home in so short a period of time. Success stories about colonists in America and the lure of promotional literature gave new hope for a better life for the first time to ordinary English people. Within a period of fifty years, the east coast of North America was settled and colonized by about two hundred thousand colonists and a new and larger New England had sprung up beyond the Atlantic. A century later the population would swell to more than two million.

The First and Second Virginia Colonies

Even before 1620, Sir Walter Raleigh (?1552–1618) had attempted in 1585 to found an English colony on Roanoke Island in what he called "Virginia." However, these first English settlers, all men, abandoned the colony in 1586. The following year another group, the second Virginia Colony (1587–?), consisting of fourteen families which, with the unattached individuals, amounted to eighty-nine men, seventeen women, and eleven children, with the artist John White (fl. 1585–1593) as Governor, landed on Roanoke Island on July 22, 1587. These were the first English families with children to settle in America.

Two months earlier, on June 22, 1587, this second and ill-fated Virginia Colony had arrived at St. Croix, in the Virgin Islands, after having been at sea for eight weeks. Governor White[49] in his *Journal* described a painful episode that happened to some on shore.

As soon as we landed on this island some of our men and women were made ill by eating small fruits that looked like green apples. Their mouths began to burn, and their tongues swelled to such a size that many of them could not speak. Even a child nursing at the breast of one of these women was affected, its mouth so painfully burned that it was pitiful to see the infant's sufferings. But after twenty-four hours, the discomforts of the sickness disappeared.

These symptoms were undoubtedly caused by eating the poisonous manchineel(*Hippomane mancinella* L.) whose fruit looks like a small green crabapple, and is pleasantly aromatic to smell (Fig. 1–1).[30] According to Samuel Eliot Morison (1887–1976),[34] every navigator to the West Indies, starting with Columbus, had warned against this tree, but apparently this was not known to Governor White.

I believe that this is the first reference to a pediatric illness encountered by English colonists in the New World. In spite of the manchineels one can still imagine how delighted the English children must have been to be allowed to go ashore and to run up and down the beach after two months of being cooped up in a crowded little ship.

On August 18, 1587, White[49] wrote that "a daughter was born [on Roanoke Island] to Elinor, daughter of the Governor and the Wife of Ananias Dare, one of the Assistants." The child was christened by her grandfather on the following Sunday, and "because this childe was the first Christian borne in Virginia, she was named Virginia." A few days later, Virginia was provided with a little playmate when the wife of Dyonis Harvie was delivered of a child (name unknown), whom the Governor duly christened.

Virginia Dare was not the first white child born in America. This honor belongs to a boy named Snorri, the son of Gudrid, the handsome and intelligent widow of Thorstein Ericson, Leif's brother. Snorri

Figure 1–1. *Manchineel plant* (Hippomane mancinella, L.). *(Reprinted, by permission of the authors, K. E. Lampe and R. Fagerström, from* Plant Toxicology and Dermatitis. *{Baltimore: Williams & Wilkins, 1968}.)*

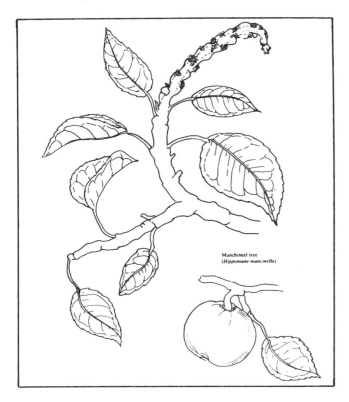

was born in the autumn of 1009 at Belle Isle or Great Sacred Isle off L'Anse aux Meadows at the northern tip of Newfoundland, almost six centuries before the birth of Virginia Dare.

Just what happened to Virginia and the Harvie child is unknown. Governor White went back to England for supplies nine days after Virginia's birth. It was not an opportune time for him to seek help from home because a Spanish Armada was about to invade England; and nobody could spare the effort to bring help to a tiny colony in Virginia. Even though the Armada was defeated in 1588, another two years passed before anything was done about Virginia. Finally, Raleigh arranged for three ships to carry supplies to the Virginia colony. As is well known, when the ships arrived there was no trace of the entire colony.

Nobody knows what became of the "Lost Colony." Most believe that some starved to death and others were killed by the Indians, who may, however, have adopted the surviving children. Although the Indians usually slaughtered children in warfare without compunction, those that they spared were adopted and treated as kindly as their own. Morison[34] noted that "to this day the Croatoan (now called Lumbee Indians) of Robeson County, North Carolina, maintain that the blood of Raleigh's colonists runs in their veins."

Jamestown Colony

On December 20, 1606, nineteen years later, one hundred twenty colonists, made up of men and boys, but no families with children, sailed from London in three little ships to settle in Virginia. On May 14, 1607, after almost five months at sea, the colonists went ashore on a low, swampy island that they named Jamestown. This was the first permanent English colony in America. Within six months, 51 died of disease and starvation and the mortality rate continued to be appalling, often reaching more than 20 percent per year. The swamps brought malaria and fevers with all the alarming concomitants of "fluxes" and debility.[3]

There were no women in the colony at first, but the next year two plucky women arrived; these two were followed by many more a few years later. Unfortunately, they stood the hardships even less well than the men and young boys, and few women were alive in 1620. The Virginia Company on several occasions undertook to recruit "young and uncorrupt maids" and to ship them to Jamestown, where a planter who wanted a wife paid the company 20 pounds of the best leaf tobacco for her.[5] Although the mortality continued to be high, marriages took place and children were born.

In 1619 the company sent out to Virginia one hundred boys to be apprenticed as servants for seven years. To meet the increasing demands for labor this practice would continue for many years.

A high death rate remained constant in Jamestown. Between 1606 and 1623 about five thousand immigrants came to Virginia and had attempted to raise families. Yet at the end of that period only a thousand were left.[3] The chances that any infant would survive were distressingly low, even after the early and most rigorous years. Unfortunately, we have little information about these infants, nor do we know what they died of.

Plymouth Plantation

The second permanent English colony was established at Plymouth, Massachusetts, in the fall of 1620 when the *Mayflower*, with sixty-nine adults and thirty-four children aboard, anchored off Cape Cod at dawn on November 9, 1620, after a rough voyage of sixty-seven days.[9] The first glimpse of the New World must have evoked strange sensations in the minds of the Pilgrims, many of them probably far from favorable. One wonders what thoughts went through the minds of the children as they gazed at the strange land, a silent, empty, and barren vista in the chill, thin air of a November dawn.

On November 27, 1620, Mistress White, a sister to Deacon-Physician Samuel Fuller (1580–1633), gave birth to a son, named Peregrine, the first English child born in New England, who eventually lived to be eighty-three years old. There was another child born on the *Mayflower* on December 22, 1620, while the ship was anchored in Plymouth Harbor, the stillborn son of Isaac and Mary Allerton; Mrs. Allerton died on the *Mayflower* several days later at the height of a winter gale.

There appears to have been little illness, other than seasickness, among the *Mayflower* passengers during their long and trying voyage.[7] No mention was ever made of how the children fared during the crossing. But scarcely had the *Mayflower* anchored in

Cape Cod Harbor before sickness and death began their cruel work. Including the thirty-five days' stay in Cape Cod Harbor, the passengers had been a hundred and two days en route from Plymouth, England. After they reached New England, their sickness ("the General Sickness") and formidable mortality were vividly described by William Bradford (1590–1657)[4], in his *History of Plymouth Plantation* (1620–1647) probably the greatest book of seventeenth-century America, although it was not published until two hundred years after his death.

But that which was most sad and lamentable was that in two or three months' time half of their company died, especially in January and February, being the depth of winter, and wanting houses and other comforts; being infected with the scurvy and other diseases which this long voyage and their inaccommodate condition had brought upon them. So as there died sometimes two or three a day in the foresaid time, that of 100 and odd persons [104], scarce fifty remained.

The "other diseases," besides scurvy, were not described by Bradford, but they must have included a combination of pneumonia, dysentery, and perhaps tuberculosis, brought on by months of bad diet, cramped and unsanitary quarters, exposure, and overexertion in all kinds of weather. Subsisting on salt meat and ship's biscuits, and probably little of either, the colonists died like flies.

When the worst was over, only three married couples remained intact. Mortality was highest among the wives, only five of eighteen surviving. More than half the heads of households perished. Only the very young escaped to bring down the overall mortality rate. Of seven daughters, none died; and of thirteen sons, only three.[50] Only fifty-four persons, twenty-one of them under sixteen, were left after the first winter to start the process that created the United States. Only five separatist family men survived—Carver, Bradford, Winslow, Brewster, and Allerton.[50]

Bradford[4] tells why the Pilgrims felt it necessary to leave Holland, where they lived in relative comfort, and to expose their children to the enormous dangers of the transatlantic crossing: "Of all the sorrows most heavy to be borne was that many of their children . . . [by] the great licentiousness of youth in that country and the manifold temptations of the place, were drawn away by evil examples into extravagant and dangerous courses, getting the reins off their necks and departing from their parents. . . . So that they saw their posterity would be in danger to degenerate and be corrupted."

The Massachusetts Bay Colony

The Puritans who founded the Massachusetts Bay Colony in 1630, like the Pilgrims in 1620, characteristically came to America as families. Passenger lists of vessels bound for New England chiefly consisted of entire families or of a portion leading the way for others temporarily left behind. Many of the settlers, headed by John Winthrop, Sr. (1588–1649), were men of landed estates, farmers from Lincolnshire, lawyers, scholars, and clergymen. They were mostly people who took religion seriously and who embraced the Bible and the predestinarian theology of Calvinism. Soon after the founding of the Massachusetts Bay Colony, serious and sincere efforts were made by the municipal authorities of England to send orphaned and abandoned children to the colony as a far better alternative than allowing them to grow up in almshouses or the Bridewell house of correction. Also, the Bay Colony's reputation for piety encouraged some English "gentlemen of quality, and others," to exile unruly sons there in the hope of reform.

Philanthropic efforts of both a private and a religious nature were also instituted to pay for the transportation of poor children to New England. For example, in 1639 James Parker,[6] a rich and charitable haberdasher of London, provided in his will that three hundred pounds be set aside "for taking up or out of the streets or out of Bridewell twelve orphaned boys and girls seven or eight years old, and paying their passages to New England where they might be bound apprentices to such persons as will be careful to bring them up in the feare of God and to maintain themselves another daie."

In seventeenth-century English society the family was of pivotal importance in the social order. The only colonists to preserve it from the very beginning were the planters of New England; elsewhere it had to be reconstructed. Carl Bridenbaugh,[6] a twentieth-century American historian, claims that "it was the transfer of Puritan families, whole and intact, that explains the uniqueness of New England." Entire families could not always migrate together. Sometimes the father, either out of caution or more likely because of lack of funds, went on ahead and then sent for his wife and children or returned to get them. The presence of both children and the aged in most families also differentiated the Puritans from the settlers of the other colonies, where the ages usually ranged from sixteen to thirty years.

The Middle Atlantic Colonies

The early Middle Atlantic colonies, for a variety of reasons, were settled mainly by individuals instead of families. Organized groups came to Virginia and Maryland, but rarely entire families. Individual indentured servants (often young boys) or farmers usually made up the passenger lists. The municipal authorities of England, who had responsibility under the Poor Law for the care of orphans and abandoned children, were a source of supply. Some were "spirited" for transfer by agents of merchants. Spirits were men commissioned by merchants and shipowners to recruit emigrants, frequently children and youths, often against the consent of either their parents or friends, and by dubious means such as bounties, bribes and even kidnapping.[5]

Transportation of idle and needy children from crowded England to labor-starved Virginia was regarded both as a boon to the Virginia planters and as a kindness to the children. From the early days of the colony, children were sent to Virginia as servants or apprentices. Efforts were made to put the importation of children on a systematic basis, as is evident by the Privy Council's granting to the Virginia Company[5] in 1620 authority to coerce children to be sent to Virginia, which read: "And if any of them [children] shall be found obstinate to resist or otherwise disobey such directions as shall be given in this behalf, we do likewise hereby authorize such as shall have the charge of this service to imprison, punish, and dispose any of those children, upon any disorder by them—and so to ship them for Virginia with as much expedition as may stand with conveniency."

Some of the colonies, such as Maryland and the Carolinas, passed legislation to encourage immigration by offering either land grants or bounties for each child, amounting in Maryland to "fifty acres for every child under the age of sixteen years."[5]

The Corporation of London also occasionally made vagrant children available for apprenticing in

Barbados and Virginia instead of binding them out at home. Winchester officials paid sixty shillings for the appareling of six poor boys destined for the Old Dominion. Hundreds of children were said in a letter of 1627 to have been "gathered up in divers places" and shipped to Virginia. Ship lists during the 1630's and 1640's reveal that many young boys aged fourteen were transported to the colonies.[6]

When orphan children were sent to the colonies, they were indentured to anyone who would pay their passages and were customarily bound until they attained majority. In 1628 Governor Harvey of Virginia asked the city of London to send over one hundred poor boys and girls to be bound out as servants upon reaching the plantation.[6]

New Netherland

The Dutch colonists who settled on Manhattan and Long Island and up the Hudson River were followers of Calvin, but unlike their New England neighbors, they had not come to the New World in search of religious freedom, for they had had that at home. They came with the simple worldly desire to better themselves.[23] Dutch ways with children were traditionally rather permissive—as the Pilgrims had so disapprovingly observed during their stay in Holland. Like Virginia, New Netherland became a refuge for children from the mother country's almshouses and orphan asylums. For example, the burgomasters of Amsterdam, mindful of the vast number of poor people in the almshouses, arranged to send over twenty-seven or twenty-eight boys and girls to ease the burden on the almshouses. The burgomasters also noted that if the population of New Netherland "could be advanced by sending over such persons, we shall on being informed, lose no time to have more forwarded."[5] Children from Dutch almshouses continued to be sent over to New Netherland for many years to be bound out as servants for a period of two to four years. Tax exemptions were also granted to colonists who would bring children to New Netherland or beget children after settling there.[5]

Medical Training and Practice

In the seventeenth century (and somewhat less so in the eighteenth), almost all young Americans who wanted to study medicine undertook an apprentice-ship with an established physician, usually for a term of five to seven years.[45] Any practitioner might act as a preceptor and the quality of instruction was subject to little or no supervision. By this arrangement an apprentice had the use of his master's library, whose shelves generally held a few medical books. Opportunities for clinical study consisted in witnessing and often assisting in the office practice of his master. There, or at the actual bedside of the patient, the apprenticed student pulled his first tooth, opened his first abscess, performed his first venesection, applied his first blister and learned cupping, and administered his first emetic; and there he also first learned the various manipulations of medicine and minor surgery.[13] The system of apprenticeship lasted well into the nineteenth century.[36]

The only bona fide medical publication in the colonies before 1700 was a single-page broadside. For this reason it is difficult to know what the physician thought about the causes of disease. As we shall see, it is largely in the writings of the preacher-physicians and governor-physicians that the medical theories of the age were expressed.

There was no eminent physician in New England before 1720 and no scientific work of importance was accomplished during this era. There was no hospital in the colonies before 1751, when the Pennsylvania Hospital was founded.

The few physicians who came to America were forced by the environment to serve as bedside doctors in a hard-bitten country without any of the European refinements rather than in teaching and debating the various theories of disease as did their confreres in England. There were no academies of medicine or Royal Society to publish their studies and not even a pharmacopoeia or a textbook. At least, the physician, whether pastor, governor, or educator, learned medicine by actual bedside instruction. From the very beginning, therefore, there was an eminently practical tendency toward empiric medicine in America.

Who Cared for the Children?

In colonial America the care of the child was largely in the hands of women; only sick children, as a rule, came in contact with physicians. Indeed, as previously mentioned, most physicians shunned infants, feeling unprepared to cope with their high morbidity and mortality and also feeling incompetent to diagnose or cure them. There were no hospitals—or hospital beds—for children. Neither the Anglican Church nor the nonconformist ones were involved with the hospital care of the ill.[13] Of necessity most colonists doctored themselves and their children by drawing upon recollections of folk wisdom, or upon homemade nostrums compiled by trial and error out of available roots and herbs and often written down in a commonplace book.[13] Even as late as the middle of the nineteenth century, it was unusual for the physician to care for the newborn infant, and not until the child was weaned did his medical care become the province of the physician. Older neighbors and grandmothers knew a little about herbs but much more about how to comfort the sick child.

Because of the dearth of physicians in the seventeenth century, children were often treated, as we shall see, by preacher-physicians like Samuel Fuller,[24] a *Mayflower* passenger, and Thomas Thacher (1620–1678),[46] author of the first medical publication in the colonies, or by correspondence with governor-physicians such as John Winthrop, Sr., Governor of the Massachusetts Bay Colony and John Winthrop, Jr. (1606–1676), Governor of Connecticut.[42] A medical career in the colonies during the seventeenth century and most of the eighteenth held little appeal to a European doctor. Only a very few came and still fewer stayed, and so the colonists were forced to help themselves as best they could. How fortunate they were to have had such capable men of the church and the law to assist them and to care for them in time of illness.

Pastor-Physicians

The relationship between medicine and theology developed naturally among English university students in the early decades of the seventeenth century. This was particularly so during the supremacy of William Laud (1573–1645), Bishop of London in 1628 and Archbishop of Canterbury after 1633.[6] Young divinity students of a nonconformist bent knew they had no chance of obtaining an appointment as a minister in the Established Church, but medical practice would still be open to them. The universities, anticipating the difficulties lying ahead for the nonconformist clergy, incorporated the study of physic in the curriculum for the divinity student. A part of this education consisted in the study of the ancient medical authors such as Hippocrates, Galen and Celsus. It was for this reason that some clergymen were well-read medical practitioners before they crossed the Atlantic and necessity often forced the two duties into one.

Of the many pastor-physicians in seventeenth-century New England, Samuel Fuller and Thomas Thacher are the best known.

Samuel Fuller was the earliest practitioner of medicine in New England. He was baptized at Redenhall Parish Church in the County of Norfolk, England, January 20, 1580, and he joined the Scrooby band of Pilgrims at Leyden in 1609. Fuller completed his theological studies at the University of Leyden, which was also the great medical center of the day. Undoubtedly, he acquired his medical knowledge at Leyden, for when he came to America, the list of the passengers sailing on the *Mayflower* gave his occupation as physician and not minister.[24] Fuller was frequently called to neighboring communities of the Massachusetts Bay Colony because of his willingness to give his services, even to the Indians. His third wife, Bridget Lee, whom he met and married in Leyden, was a highly respected midwife. When Fuller died of smallpox during the epidemic of 1633, he left a gap which was hard to fill. No detailed record of his medical practice has survived, though it was he who cared for the medical needs of the colonists and all of their children by treating them with herbs and bleeding during their first decade in Plymouth. We know little about the manner of medicine he practiced. His inventory records many "physike books," but their names are not given.[24]

Thomas Thacher,[46] the outstanding Puritan preacher-physician of his time, was born in Somersetshire, England, May 1, 1620 (Fig. 1–2). His father, the Reverend Peter Thacher, was rector of St. Edmunds at Salisbury, Wiltshire. When Thomas was fifteen, his uncle, who was about to sail for New England, proposed taking the boy with him; his father and mother planned to follow this uncle shortly. To leave England was a natural step taken by many dissenting ministers and their families in the early seventeenth century, but the death of Thomas's mother prevented his father from ever leaving England.

A few years after his arrival in New England, Thacher was put under the tutelage of Charles Chauncy (1592–1672), who came to New England

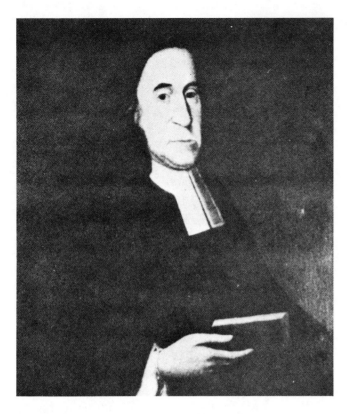

Figure 1–2. Thomas Thacher (1620–1678), the outstanding Puritan preacher-physician of his time. (Courtesy of the Countway Library of Medicine.)

tions for its control. The imprint of his broadside read, "Boston, Printed and Sold by John Foster 1677," and it was entitled *A Brief Rule to Guide the Common People of New-England How to Order Themselves and Theirs in the Small Pocks, or Measels* (Fig. 1–3). This is the earliest medical document to be printed in America, north of Mexico.[22] Just as in Europe the first medical incunabulum in 1456 was also a single sheet describing the procedure of bloodletting, so the first medical incunabulum of America was also a single printed page of practical direction.

The use of the term "smallpox or measles" in the title of *A Brief Rule* was the common practice of Thacher's day. Rhazes (?850–?923) only partly differentiated the two diseases and treated them similarly. He also used both names in the title of his book *A Treatise on the Small-Pox and Measles*. Among the contents of European treatises on diseases of

Figure 1–3. Broadside by Thomas Thacher, A Brief Rule to Guide the Common-People of New-England How to Order Themselves and Theirs in the Small Pocks, or Measels (Boston, 1677), the first medical publication in the English colonies of North America.

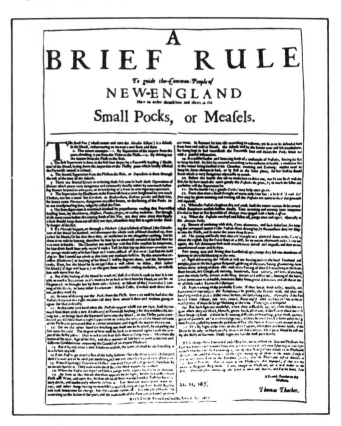

in 1638 and was later to serve as the second president of Harvard College. According to Cotton Mather (1663–1728),[35] "under the Conduct of the Eminent Scholar, he [Thacher] became such as one himself." The "angelical conjunction" between the offices of minister and physician, referred to later by Cotton Mather,[35] was truly exemplified by Thomas Thacher.

After his apprenticeship with Chauncy, Thacher was ordained as a minister at Weymouth in 1644 at the age of twenty-four. He moved to Boston in 1669 when he was chosen pastor of Old South Church. In this position he devoted much time to the practice of medicine, and his fellow colonists considered him one of the most skillful physicians in Boston. He died October 15, 1678, presumably from fever, following "a visit to a sick person."[46]

Near the end of his life Thacher had written a broadside, measuring 17 by 12 5/16 inches and dated "21.11.1677" (i.e., January 21, 1677/8), of a severe epidemic of smallpox in Boston, explaining the nature of smallpox to the people and giving instruc-

children from the fifteenth century onwards, it was the usual custom to include a chapter "On Smallpox and Measles." Sydenham in his first publication of 1666, *Methodus Curandi Febres*, did not advance beyond Rhazes, but by 1676, after he had studied an epidemic of measles in 1670, he clearly defined that disease and set it off from smallpox, although he continued to treat both diseases in a similar manner. Thacher, using Sydenham's work as a basis for his broadside, thus considered both diseases together.

Thacher's broadside followed Sydenham closely but unfortunately, was published without any recognition of Sydenham as its proper author. Thacher warned against overheating, excessive sweating, a weakening diet, and medication in the capacity of one who "though no physician means well with the sick." In a time when widespread bloodletting, purging, and sweating characterized medical practice, Thacher's suggestions were unusually perceptive. Sydenham's treatment of fevers with fresh air and cooling drinks—adopted by Thacher—was an improvement on the prolonged sweating regimens previously employed.

Thacher died the next year (1678) and no one else in America saw the advantage of publishing broadsides as a means of giving medical instruction in the years before the appearance of the first colonial newspaper (1690).

These pastor-physicians, besides keeping their congregations in spiritual health, also added another dimension to the minister's role in colonial life by easing pain, curing a sick child, and saving a life. They added little to advance the cause of medicine but they ministered to the sick when they were needed, and here and there among them one finds a man of memorable stature.[26]

Governor-Physicians

The outstanding members of the governing class who were acknowledged as physicians were the two John Winthrops, father and son. Governor John Winthrop, the founder of Boston, was actively engaged for a number of years in caring for patients. Winthrop's son, the Governor of Connecticut, was as much physician as magistrate. The two Winthrops served as the medical as well as the political advisers to the citizens of Massachusetts and Connecticut for two successive generations. The records

we have of their medical experience, which have fortunately been saved, offer a good idea of the manner in which patients were treated when they fell, in Oliver Wendell Holmes's (1809–1894)[26] words, "into intelligent and somewhat educated hands, a little after the middle of the seventeenth century."

As there were very few medical books for reference in the early colonial years, John Winthrop, Sr., sought the advice of Edward Stafford (1617–1651), a physician friend in England, who was probably the son-in-law of Elias Ashmole (1617–1692), the great Oxford antiquary. A long letter in reply to Winthrop dated May 6, 1643, containing a collection of prescriptions and therapeutic directions is still extant; on it appears the notation "Prepared for the benefit of Governor Winthrop here in New England."[53] In this letter of only four sheets of coarse paper about 6 by 7 inches, Stafford lists a number of "Receipts to cure various Disorders" such as would be needed and useful in the opinion of well-known physicians of that day. This manuscript is of tremendous interest because it may be considered the standard medical "text" in the colony for several decades. About 1860 Oliver Wendell Holmes found that the remedies were of three kinds: "herbs, or simples, such as hypericum (St. John's wort), elder, clown's all-heal, parsley, maidenhair, mineral such as lime, saltpeter, antimony; and thaumaturgic or mystical," the chief one of the latter being "My black powder against the plague, small pox; purples, all sorts of feavers; Poyson; either by Way of Prevention or after Infection." Holmes[26] also believed that Stafford's "practical directions to so considerable a person as Governor Winthrop in a strange land—might be taken as a fair example of a better sort of practice of the time."

A few of Stafford's "receipts" are of pediatric importance because they are the first written pediatric prescriptions prepared for use in the Massachusetts Bay Colony.

I. "For the *Falling sicknesse* Purge first with the extract of Hellebore (black hellebore I meane) and instead of St. John's Wort use pentaphyllon, (or meadow Cinquefoile). Use it [boiled in water] and God Willing he shall be perfectly cured in short or longer tyme, according as the disease hath taken root.

II. "For the *Bloodie Flix* [Flux]: Purge first with Rhubarbe torrified; and give the partie to drinke twice a day a pint of this caudle following: Take a dragme of the best Bole-Armoniak [a soft clayey earth of bright red color], and dragme of Sanguis draconis*; and a dragme of the best terra Sigillata† of a yellow colour seal'd with a Castle; Make these into a fine powder, and with a quart of red stiptick Wine, then adding the yolks of halfe a dozen eggs & a quantitie of sugar, make a Caudle, boyling the powder in [a] pipkin with the Wine, then adding the yolks of the eggs beaten, and lastly ye Sugar.

III. *For a broken bone, or a joynt dislocated, to knit them:* Take the barke of Elme, or Whitch-hazzle; cut away the Outward part, and cutt the Inward redd barke small, and boyle it in Water, till it be thick that it Will rope; pound well, and lay of it hott, barke and all upon the Bone or Joynt, and tye it on: or with the Mussilage of it, and bole Armoniack make a playster and lay it on.

IV. *For the yellow Jaundise or Jaunders*—Boyle a quart of sweet milke, dissolve therein as much bay-salt, or fine Salpeter, as shall make it brackish in taste and putting Saffron in a fine linen clout, rubb it into the Milke, until the Milke be very yellow; and give it the patient to drink. [A good example of the doctrine of signatures, described later in this chapter (pp. 24–25)]

V. *A Panacea—My Black powder against the plague, small pox; purples {purpura}, all sorts of feavers; Poyson; either by Way of prevention, or after Infection.* In the Moneth of March take Toades, as many as you will, alive; putt them into a Earthern pott, so it will be halfe full; Cover it with a broad tyle or Iron plate; then overwhelme the pott, so that the bottome may be uppermost; putt charcoales round about it, and in the open ayre, not in an house [probably at Mrs. Stafford's insistence], sett it in fire and lett it burne out and extinguish of itself; When it is cold, take out the toades and in an Iron-Morter pound them very well and searce them: then in a Crucible calcine them so againe; pound and searce them againe. The first time they will be browne powder, the next time black. Of this you may give a dragme in a Vehiculum (or drinke) Inwardly in any Infection taken; and let them sweat upon it in their beddes; but lett them not cover their heads; especially in the Small pox. For prevention, half a dragme will suffice; moderate the dose according to the strength of the partie; for I have sett down the greatest that is needful. There is no danger in it. Let them neither eate nor drinke during their sweat, except now and then a spoonefull of Warme posset-drinke to wash their mouthes. Keep warm and close, (for a child of 5 years, 10 graynes is enough in

---

* *Sanguis draconis* (dragon's blood) is a dark reddish-brown resinous substance obtained from the fruit of small palm trees that grow in the East Indies. It was formerly used as an astringent.
† *Terra sigillata* (sealed earth), a form of argillaceous earth, was once so highly valued as to be formed into small masses and impressed with a seal, hence the name. It was also prescribed for its astringent properties.

infection, for prevention 4 or 5 graynes) till they be perfectly well; and eate but little and that according to rules of physicke.

Most of Stafford's material was taken from John Gerarde's (1545–1612) *Herball*, first published in 1597, the most popular of all the English herbals. That the patients both young and old had the fortitude to withstand the assault of Stafford's remedies speaks well for the hardihood of the Massachusetts Bay colonists.

The first description of congenital syphilis in the colonies was given by Winthrop senior[36] in 1646.

There fell out a loathsome disease at Boston, which raised a scandal upon the town and country, though without just cause. One of the town—, having gone cooper in a ship into—, at his return his wife was infected with Lues Venerea, which appeared thus; being delivered of a child and nothing then appearing, but the midwife a skilful woman, finding the body sound as any other, after her delivery she had a sore breast, whereupon divers neighbors resorting to her, some of them drew her breast, and others suffered their children to draw her, and others let the child suck them, (no such disease being suspected by any,) by occasion whereof about sixteen persons, men, women and children, were infected, whereby it came at length to be discovered by such in the town as had skill in physic and surgery, but there was not any in the country who had been practised in that cure. But (see the good providence of God) at that very season there came by accident a young surgeon out of the West Indies, who had had experience of the right way of the cure of that disease. He took them in hand and through the Lord's blessing recovered them all in a short time. And it was observed that though many did eat and drink and lodge in bed with those who were infected and had sores, etc., yet none took it of them but by copulation or sucking. It was very doubtful how this disease came at first. The magistrate examined the husband and wife, but could find no dishonesty in either, nor any probable occasion how they should take it by any other, (and the husband was found free of it). So as it was concluded by some, that the woman was infected by the mixture of many spirits of men and women as drew her breast (for thence it began). But this is a question to be decided by physicians.

Governor John Winthrop, Jr.,[42] was born in Groton, Suffolk, England, in 1606, the oldest son of the elder John Winthrop (Fig. 1–4). He was educated at Trinity College, Dublin, studied law at the Inner

Temple, and after having been admitted to the bar in London in 1625, spent the next five years in travel and adventure. He visited Padua, Venice, Constantinople, and many other cities. It was during these years that he formed an acquaintance with many of the scientists and scholars with whom in later years he corresponded in Latin. He sailed in 1631 for Boston, which his father had founded the previous year. He was commissioned Governor of the new colony at Saybrook, Connecticut, in 1665. In 1646 he founded New London, and in 1657 and annually from 1659 to his death in 1676 he was elected Governor of Connecticut.

Winthrop gathered a considerable library and by his interest in the sciences helped to promote scientific study in the colonies. He was made a fellow of the Royal Society in 1663 and became the first member resident in America. He greatly surpassed his father in the extent of his medical activities. Many consider him the outstanding figure in the history of science in America during the seventeenth century. Mather wrote of the junior Winthrop that "wherever he came, still the *Diseased* flocked about him as if the Healing Angel of Bethesda had appeared in the place."

Among his published papers, which consist mostly of letters addressed to him, there are a number of significant pediatric interest. Winthrop would receive letters from people in all walks of life petitioning him for medical advice and offers for medication.[42] I believe no document gives a more vivid insight into the medical conditions of the early colonies than the letters written to Winthrop by his patients.

He accepted the iatrochemical theory of practice and his pharmacopoeia was largely a chemical one. His chief remedies were nitre and antimony, tartar, copperas, white vitriol, sulfur, iron, and occasionally a little calomel, although he also used biologicals such as human excreta, and even the occult powers of a unicorn's horn. In addition to the above, Winthrop also prescribed red coral, powdered ivory, resin, saffron, aloes, balsam, rhubarb, and various "simples" of the Galenists such as wormwood and anise. Most of the other early New England practitioners maintained the Galenic tradition of botanical remedies ("simples"), in opposition to the chemical —a contrast which reflected the European controversies of the time. The Galenic tradition lived on in

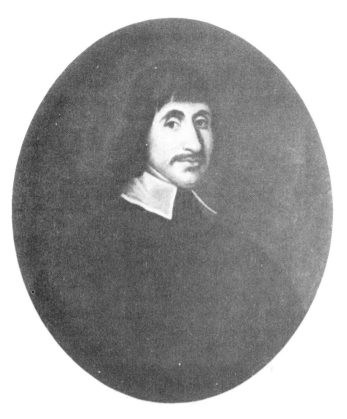

Figure 1–4. John Winthrop, Jr. (1606–1676), considered by many the outstanding figure in the history of science in America during the seventeenth century, and possibly America's earliest pediatrician. (Courtesy of the Countway Library of Medicine.)

popular American medicine to influence a major nineteenth-century sect—the Thomsonian or "botanic system." To this day, indeed, some proprietary remedies appeal on the ground that they contain "only vegetable compounds."

Theophilus Eaton (1590–1658),[42] the first Governor of the New Haven colony, in one of his letters to Winthrop described an early American case of child abuse. Eaton wrote that his second wife "pinched Mary, the governor's young daughter—until she was black and blue and knocked her head against the dresser, which made her nose bleed much."

In 1658, William Leete (1613–1683),[42] also a Governor of the New Haven Colony, and later of Connecticut, wrote to Winthrop:

Our youngest childe, about 9 weekes old, having ever since it was 3 or 4 dayes old, hath appeared full of red spots or pimples, somewhat like to measles & seemed allwayes to be bigg, and to hang over on the eye browes &

lids; but now of late the eye lids have swelled & look very red, burning exceedingly, & now at last they are so sweld up that the sight is utterly closed in, that he could not see, nor for severall dayes, nor yet doth, & the verges [edges] of the lids, where they close, have a white seame, like the white heads of wheales, wherein is matter; it is somewhat extraordinary, such as none of our women can tell that they have ever seene the like.

This child, named Peregrine, was the cause of much parental anxiety. Leete[42] later wrote of "his starting, & sometimes almost strangling ffitts, like convulsions, which have more frequently afflicted the infant of late than formerly." We are apt to conceive it probably," he wrote, "to proceed from more than ordinary painful breeding teeth." His eyes seemed to be somewhat better to Peregrine's father from the use of a "glasse of eye water" which was also used on the other children so that "a little further recruit" of the same was desired. Peregrine did not take up all the family's time, for his sister, Graciana was described as being a weakly puny thing. Her diagnosis today would probably be failure to thrive. Winthrop's treatment, whatever it was, must have caused an improvement, because shortly thereafter she began "to slide a chaire before her & walke after it, after her ffeeble manner." Like most children, Graciana would not readily take her medicine and her father asked Winthrop for directions "to make her willing & apt to take it; for though it seemes very pleasant of itselfe, yet is she grown marvailous awkward and averse from taking it in beer. Wherefore I would entreat you to prescribe to us the varyety of wayes in which it may be given soe effectually; wee doubt els it may doe much lesse good, being given by force onely." Other letters written by Leete to Winthrop concerned his son Andrew's "starting fits" as well as a "distemper which my son William's wife can best explain." Leete also wrote about a weak back which afflicted a neighbor's child.

Robert Bond[53] of Easthampton, Long Island, magistrate of the town as well as gospel minister, sought Winthrop's help for a neighbor whose children were "destempered with some disease of their heads. It appears to have been a whitish scabb—dry for the most part only uppon their takeinge coullde it have run exceedingly." The duration of the affection was two and a half years and "on the first risinge of it it came in spots like the forme allmost of A ring worme." The scabs gradually increased in thickness and sometimes could be removed by the application of "butter and beare." A violent itching of their heads also troubled the children, "most commonly about bed time." (?favus ?psoriasis).

John Pynchon (c.1626–1702/3),[53] of Springfield, wrote to Winthrop in July, 1663, about his daughter's diarrhea (?summer complaint). She was "about or neere one yeare and three quarters old. She hath not bin very well these 3 or 4 days but especially yesterday morning was taken with a greate looseness and vomiting which doth continue much and exceedingly weakens her. She is very restless and unquiet, and sleepes little and is exceeding dry craving for drink." Pynchon concluded his letter with these words of resignation: "How the Lord may deale with her & us we know not, but desire in the use of meanes to submit to his good pleasure." I believe this is the first documented case report of dehydration in colonial America and, to my knowledge, it has never before been published.

Samuel Stone (1600–1663), the assistant minister of the First Church of Christ in Hartford, wrote to Winthrop on February 28, 1652, for his help in treating his twenty-three-week-old infant son's jaundice. Stone was worried:

The child . . . hath been somewhat ill 3 or 4 weeks, unquiet his eyes looking yellow, having a cough especially when he takes his victuals. Wee thought he might have been breeding teeth: but about a week past we perceived that he had the yellow Jaundise. By Mrs. Hooker her advice [women, especially grandmothers, often were the first person anxious parents would consult about a sick child] we gave him Barbarie [barberry] barke boyled in beer, with saffron, twice in a day, for two dayes together: and one time saffron alone. Also lice 2 or 3 times, and Tumerick twice."* We hoped that the Jaundise had been cured: because he was sometimes more chearful and had a better appetite, but the last Saterdaie at night he was very unquiet, heavie and could not sleep and upon the Sabbath seemed to look somewhat swart in the face. In the afternoone we gave him about 3 quarters of a grain of your purging powder which we had of Mrs. Haynes which caused him to vomit twice or three and to purge downwards thrice—he slept well the night after and in the

---

* In 1708 Lady Otway[19] gave two recipes for curing jaundice made up mostly of yellow substances. In one she put lemon, turmeric, and saffron; the other consisted of twenty head lice mixed with nutmeg, sugar, and turmeric.

morning was somewhat unquiet again as before, wringing and winding back, his cough seemes to increase, as if he had much fleagme. He seems to be sick at times but without any convulsions or starting fits. When he began to be ill he was costive in his bodie but now is in good temper. He doth not burne often, but a little sometimes. I pray Sir send me word whether he may not take some more of that powder and what quantity. If you thinke it convenient to prescribe anything I pray speake to Mr. Blinman. I know he will procure some Indian to bring your note and I will please him for his journey.

The "purging powder" referred to by the Reverend Mr. Stone was a secret preparation of Winthrop's by the name of *rubila*, which he claimed was a "sovereigne remedy." The belief in panaceas was commonplace in the seventeenth century, as is evident in the letter of John Winthrop, Sr., to his wife Margaret (who was preparing to leave England for America) dated July 23, 1630, advising her that "for physic you will need no other but a pound of Doctor Wrighte's *Electarium lenitium* [Electuarium Lenitivum] and his direction to use it."[20] Wrighte's medicine was a confection of senna and was used as a purgative. Winthrop apparently was unaware that American senna (*Cassia marilandica L.*) was virtually equivalent to European senna.

Oliver Wendell Holmes[26] studied Winthrop's medical cases and from these tried to get an idea of his practice. Holmes found that Winthrop's great remedy was nitre, which he ordered in doses of twenty to thirty grains for adults and three grains to infants. "Measles, colics, headache, sciatica and many other ailments, all found themselves treated" according to Holmes, and "I trust bettered by nitre—a pretty safe medicine in moderate doses and one not likely to keep the good Governor awake at night, thinking whether it might not kill, if it did not cure." Winthrop[1] also liked spermaceti, which he considered "the sovereign'st thing on earth for the treatment of falls and bruises"; he often prescribed it for children's falls and similar injuries. And in one of his letters Winthrop urged his correspondent to "remember that Rubila be taken at the beginning of any illness."

Holmes's curiosity about Winthrop's secret prescription rubila led him to investigate its contents.

I had almost given it up in despair, when I found what appears to be a key to the mystery. In the vast multitude of prescriptions contained in the [Winthrop] manu-scripts, most of them written in symbols, I find one which I thus interpret:—"Four grains of (diaphoretic) antimony, with twenty grains of nitre, with a little salt of tin, making *rubila*." Perhaps something was added to redden the powder, as he [Winthrop] constantly speaks of "rubifying" or "viridating" his prescription; a very common practice of prescribers, when their powders look a little too much like plain salt or sugar.

A principal disadvantage of rubila was the difficulty experienced in keeping it down; its specific advantages even Winthrop failed to define very explicitly.

Governor Winthrop's advice was also sought for pediatric dental problems, as was evident in Danielle Clarke's (1622–1710)[53] letter sent from Windsor, Connecticut, and dated February 11, 1652:

I would intreat a favour from you. My request is this. I have a little one that is now 4 yrs of age that hath bin and is yet much troubled with 4 of his foremost teeth on [the] upper part of his mouth, which began to fade [decay] when he was about three quarters old and soe have continued fadeinge away until this tyme and are now rooted some within his goome [gum] and one close to his goome and in the time of their thus decayinge their hath been a rhume [discharge] that hath followed his goome soe that on the outside of the upper jaw betwixt his lipp and his goome just uppon the foure decaying teeth there would four small pimples arise very redd in colour and after a day or two they would breake and coruption would issue forth and thus they continued for about two yeares space and at last when the teeth were rotted close to the goome the lower end of the tooth that stickt in the jaw bone is come [out] . . . not long Since I perceaved one of the upper teeth a little loose by the end wagging or stirring in the hole that it had made through the goome I went and ript it with a smal silver hooke and gott hold on one side of the tooth with a smal [pair of] pincers and puld it out save one splinter which yet is in and appears at the foresaid hole in the goome and keeps it from healinge. . . . The child is very healthy and growes well and hath bin in a healthy condition for the general only for a certayne space at first when his teeth began to rott he was troubled with the ache in his teeth as my wife and others deemed. My other little one of about a year and quarter old his teeth doe decay even as my little boyes did.

s./ Danielle Clarke

I believe this is the first American description of a recently described devastating dental condition, termed the nursing bottle caries syndrome, in which there is rampant tooth decay associated with prolonged bottle-feeding of sweetened milk to infants beyond a year of age.[39] Typically, the primary maxillary incisors are affected most severely. The primary first molars are second in frequency; the most remarkable finding is that the mandibular incisors are seldom involved. This is thought to be related to the protective effect of the tongue during sucking and to the protective bathing action of saliva from submandibular salivary glands. Mr. Clarke's children would probably not have been given a nursing bottle of sweetened milk as a pacifier, but they may very well have been offered a homemade cloth pacifier soaked with honey or molasses, which would have been even more cariogenic than sweetened milk.

Winthrop's practice, conducted in a most informal manner, experienced a prodigious growth. On March 10, 1656/7, he commenced a regular recording of his prescriptions, a habit continued with only a few interruptions until the summer of 1669. From it, we find that over this period he treated at least seven hundred different patients, an astonishing number when the whole population of New England (which as late as 1675 did not exceed 120,000) is considered.[1]

Obviously seventeenth-century American clerical and lay medicine must have been primitive. It was, as we have seen, a peculiar mixture of religious medicine, folk medicine, and scientific principle. The practitioner invoked the word of God and then let blood or prescribed drugs to the best of his understanding. However, European medicine in this period, even when practiced by physicians, was effective only in exceptional cases. This was the time of Molière's bitter satire about medicine. To Molière the physicians would, of course, speak Latin, but their treatment was essentially limited to *Clysterium donare,/Postea seignare,/Ensuita purgare.**

Colonial Infants Delivered by Midwives

Obstetrics in America had its beginning in the efforts of those midwives who were brought to this country to practice their art.[44] Male physicians considered it beneath their dignity, in both England and America, to compete with midwives.

In colonial times the delivery of the infant was—in

---

* Molière's Latin hodgepodge: Give an enema, then bleed, finally purge.

all the colonies—entirely in the hands of midwives. Midwives did not restrict themselves to obstetrics. They would also serve as nurses and pediatricians, and they often helped lay out the dead. They relied largely on folklore passed down from generation to generation. The quality of their medical care depended almost entirely on the intelligence and common sense of the individual midwife.

Bridget, the third wife of Samuel Fuller, was held in great esteem as a midwife. She was the first to practice midwifery in New England. The records of the town of Rehoboth, Massachusetts, for July 3, 1663, contain this comment: "Voted and agreed that . . . Mrs. Bridget Fuller of Plymouth should be sent for to see if she would be willing to come and dwell among us, to attend on the office of midwife to answer the town's necessity, which at present is great."[24]

Midwives were important to colonial married women because those who survived spent nearly all of their childbearing years either pregnant or nursing an infant.

Midwifery in New York

The midwives of New Amsterdam were no better and no worse than their professional sisters in Holland who aroused the ire of Hendrik van Deventer (1651–1724),[44] the great Dutch obstetrician, who wrote that "they do not understand their business. . . . I cannot sufficiently wonder at the gross ignorance of most midwives." He urged that autopsies of women dying in childbirth be made a matter of law to find out whether the mother and fetus died naturally or "sadly perished by the carelessness and cruel hand of the midwife."

In Virginia, as elsewhere in the colonies, midwives were entirely responsible for the care of mothers and their newborn infants. It was 1753, almost a century and a half after the establishment of Jamestown, before the advent of the man midwife.[3]

A revealing view of the practice of colonial midwifery is found in the well-known and detailed diary of Judge Samuel Sewall (1652–1730).[43]

April 1, 1677—About two of the Clock at night I waked and perceived my wife ill: asked her to call Mother. She said I should goe to prayer, then she would tell me. Then I rose, lighted a Candle at Father's fire, that had been raked up from Saturday night, kindled a Fire in the chamber, and after 5 when our folks up, went and gave Mother warning. She came and bad me call the midwife, Goodwife Weeden, which I did. But my wives pains went away in a great measure after she was up; toward night came on again, and about a quarter of an hour after ten at night, *April 2*, Father and I sitting in the great Hall, heard the child cry, whereas we were afraid twould have been 12 before she would have been brought to Bed. Went home with the Midwife about 2 o'clock, carrying her Stool, whoes parts were included in a bagg.... The first Woman the Child sucked was Bridget Davenport.

Anne Hutchinson and Mary Dyer's Anencephalic Infant

Anne Hutchinson (c. 1591–1643), the first woman to play a leading role in American history, was the most celebrated of the early colonial midwives.[36] She and her husband came from England to Boston in 1634. At that time she was forty-three years of age and was said to be "a woman very helpful in the times of childbirth, and other occasions of bodily infirmities, and well furnished with means for those purposes." However, she was allowed to remain in Boston for only four years because her religious tenets (antinomianism) were not suited to the minds of her neighbors. She held religious meetings in her house at which she would preach and pray. This led to her excommunication and banishment from the Massachusetts Bay Colony. Among Anne's misfortunes was being in attendance when her friend Mary Dyer (d. 1660) was delivered of an anencephalic infant on October 17, 1637, although another midwife, Jane Hawkins, had actually delivered the baby.[36] This is the first report of this congenital malformation in America. The superstitious neighbors were filled with all sorts of questions about the cause of the "monstrous" infant. The civil and religious authorities read it as a sign of God's condemnation of Mary for having been a follower of Anne Hutchinson.[48]

John Winthrop[52] vividly embellished his description of this tragic delivery:

The wife of one William Dyer, a milliner..., a very proper and fair woman ... infected with Mrs. Hutchinson's errors [antinomianism] ... had been delivered of [a] child some few months before, October 17 [1637], and the child buried, (being stillborn,) and viewed of none but Mrs. Hutchinson and the midwife, one Haw-

kins's wife, a rank familist also; and another woman had a glimpse of it, who, not being about to keep counsel, as the other two did, some rumor began to spread, that the child was a monster.... At first she [the midwife] confessed only, that the head was defective and misplaced, but being told that Mrs. Hutchinson had revealed all ... she made this report of it, viz.: It was a woman child, stillborn, about two months before the just time, having life a few hours before; it came hiplings till she turned it, it was of ordinary bigness [newborn infants were not weighed in the seventeenth century]; it had a face, but no head, and the ears stood upon the shoulders and were like an ape's; it had no forehead, but over the eyes four horns, hard and sharp; two of them were above one inch long, the other two shorter; the eyes standing out, and the mouth also; the nose hooked upward; all over the breast and back full of sharp pricks and scales, like a thornback; the navel and all the belly, with the distinction of the sex, were where the back should be, and the back and hips before, where the belly should have been; behind, between the shoulders, it had two mouths, and in each of them a piece of red flesh sticking out; it had arms and legs as other children; but, instead of toes, it had on each foot three claws, like a young fowl, with sharp talons.

It is probably no accident that Winthrop's description was remarkably similar to the pictorial representations of satanic demons dating back well into the middle ages.[27]

Mary Dyer and Anne Hutchinson were banished to Rhode Island, where Anne later gave birth to a grapelike cluster of tissue, probably a hydatidiform mole; the Massachusetts authorities ordered a count of the lumps to see if they equaled the number of heresies for which she had been convicted—twenty-seven. They did, and thus confirmed her status as one displeasing to God.[48] Twenty-one years later Mary Dyer returned to Boston and became the victim of religious persecution. She was executed as a Quaker on Boston Common on June 1, 1660.

Mrs. Hutchinson's tragic end is well known; after leaving Rhode Island she went to Long Island and then to Pelham, New York, where she was killed by Indians.

Birth Defects in Colonial America

Our seventeenth-century ancestors saw the hand of God meting out illness or birth defects as punishment for deviation from His laws. The birth of a child with congenital anomalies was often recorded in colonial diaries whether or not the parents were known to the diarist. Examples are these seventeenth-century entries in Sewall's [43] diary: *Feb. 15 (1681/2)... there is a child born near the north Meeting House, which hath no Tongue at all; or the Tongue grown fast to the roof of the Mouth; one finger too much on one Hand, and one too little on the other. And the Heels right opposite one to another, the Toes standing to the Right and left outward."*

Of historical interest is Sewall's entry for February 13, 1686, because I believe it to be the first recorded case of the sudden infant death syndrome in America: *"Feb. 13 1686. Mr. Eyre's little son dyed, went well to bed; dyed by them in the Bed. It seems there is no Symptom of Over-laying."*

Another important entry is that for June 3, 1689, because it is the earliest description of cretinism I have found in American medical literature.

June 3, 1689. As came home saw one Elisabeth Nash, born at Enfield, about 25 Years old, just about Three foot high, not the breadth of my little finger under or over. Her Hands show Age more than anything else. Has no brests. By reason of her thickness and weight can goe but very sorrily. Can speak and sing but not very conveniently, because her Tongue is bigger than can be well stowed in her mouth. Blessed be God for my Stature, unto which neither, I, nor my Dear Mother, my Nurse, could add one Cubit.

March 28, 1693. Mr. Cotton Mather has a Son born which is his first; it seems was without a Postern for the avoidance of Excrements; died Satterday, [*April 1*]

I believe this latter entry is the earliest American record of an infant born with anal atresia.

Common Accidents and Diseases of Seventeenth-Century Colonial Children

The settlers carried with them the communicable diseases of their native country. In addition, they met with new ones indigenous to America. Smallpox, measles, scarlet fever, and diphtheria, influenza, malaria, yellow fever, dysentery, and also tuberculosis were common diseases of colonial children.[12] An incalculable number also suffered from "convulsive fits," worms, thrush, dental caries, scabies, ringworm of the scalp, and skin infections. It should also be noted that the character of the diseases that prevailed in the seventeenth century in the colonies was on the whole rather indefinite. "Fever" frequently was cited as the only diagnosis. There were many reports of communities having been visited with "epidemical colds, coughs, agues, and fevers."

Accidents

There were frequent reports, especially in colonial diaries, of serious childhood accidents, such as burns from playing with candles or gunpowder, or from falls into open fires.

For example, Cotton Mather's [32] diary contained these entries about two of his children who fell into open fires: *"January 2, 1698.* This day an uncomfortable Thing happened in my Family. My little Daughter Nanny [Hannah (1697–1721)], being in my study with her two Sisters, when I was not there, fell into the *Fire.* The right side of the *Face* especially, and right *Hand* and *Arm*, were sorely burned in this Fall; and we feared a terrible Event." A happier entry was that of *January 30, 1696–1697.* "This Day, my little Daughter, Nibby [Abigail (1694–1721)], fell directly upon the *Fire,* and yett a wonderful Providence of Heaven, was pull'd out without the least scorch upon Hands or Face, to damnify her."

Many children were drowned after falling off wharves or while swimming in treacherous streams. Still more were seriously, if not fatally, scalded from falling into large caldrons of boiling milk or water. For example, Sewall[43] wrote in his diary for January 13, 1687/8: "Mr Moodey hears that Martha, a Grandchild of 4 or 5 years old is scalded to death at Barnstable."

Epidemic Diseases of Colonial Children

SMALLPOX. The terror of smallpox and death from it had been part of English life for centuries before the first settlements were attempted in the New World.[37] The English historian and essayist Thomas Macaulay (1800–1859) wrote in his *History of England* that "the smallpox was ever present, filling the church yards with corpses, tormenting with constant fears all whom it had not yet stricken... turning the babe into a changeling at which the mother shuddered."

The first mention of smallpox affecting the children of settlers in the American English colonies occurred on May 17, 1629, on board the *Talbot* while en route to New England, when the Reverend Francis Higginson (1586–1630)[20] wrote:

This day my two children Samuel and Mary began to be sick of the smallpox and purples [?purpura] together, which was brought into the ship by one mister Browne, who was sick of the same at graves end [Gravesend], whom it pleased God to make the first occasion of bringing that contagious sickness among us [April 25, 1629], where with many were after afflicted.

May 19, 1629. This day towards night my daughter grew sicker, and many blue spots were seen upon her breast [?hemorrhagic smallpox], which affrighted us. At the first we thought they had been the plague tokens, but we found afterwards that it was only an high measure of the infection of the pox, which were struck again into the child, and so it was God's will the child died about six of the clock at night, being the first in our ship that was buried in the bowels of the Great Atlanticke Sea, which as it was a grief to us her parents and a terror to all the rest as being the beginning of a contagious disease and mortality. So in the same judgment it pleased God to remember mercy in that child, in freeing it from a world of misery wherein otherwise she had lived all her days. For being about four years old a year since, we know not by what means [she] swayed in the back so that it was broken and grew crooked, pitiful to see, since which time she hath had a most lamentable pain in her belly and would ofttimes cry out in the day and in her sleep also, "my belly!" which declared some extraordinary distemper, so that in respect of her we had cause to take her death as a blessing from the Lord to shorten her misery.

From the dearth of information in early colonial diaries, journals, and church and town records, it seems that smallpox had been accepted almost perfunctorily as one of the hazards of life along with all the other disasters such as tornadoes, fires, floods, locusts, and Indian raids. Smallpox has been blamed by many for the terrible epidemic of 1617–1618 which devastated the Indians prior to the landing of the *Mayflower*.[17]

The first epidemic of smallpox to be definitely recorded in New England occurred among the Massachusetts Indians in 1633. The English were not spared in this epidemic. Samuel Fuller was one of the victims. Bradford[4] described this epidemic in Plymouth Plantation and the death of Fuller: "It pleased the Lord to visit them this year with an in-fectious fever, of which many fell very sick and upward of 20 persons died, men and women, besides children . . . and in the end, after he had much helped others, Samuel Fuller who was their surgeon and physician and had been a great help and comfort unto them.

Another serious epidemic of smallpox broke out in New England in 1677 and by May of that year hundreds had died.[2] In a single day, September 30, 1677, thirty people died in Boston—the proportional equivalent of more than *sixty thousand* New Yorkers today. This devastating smallpox epidemic, in conjunction with the normal death rate, probably killed one-fifth of Boston's entire population.[51] This epidemic also led to the publication of Thacher's broadside. The broadsheet method of disseminating news of epidemics was a natural one because there was no genuine newspaper in America until *Publick Occurences* was published in Boston in 1690. (However, it offended the authorities, the Governor and Council, and was suppressed after only one issue had appeared.)

MEASLES. Measles received little attention from writers in the eighteenth century. Its relatively low rate of mortality relegated it to a minor role when smallpox would reduce the population by the thousands.

The diary of John Hull (1624–1683),[18] the mintmaster, contained the first record in colonial America of measles, which appeared in Boston during 1657–1658. Hull wrote that "scarce any house escaped; only through the goodness of God, scarce any died of it. The like soon befell most of the towns hereabouts." He also wrote that "about the 2nd of October, it pleased the Lord to send the disease of measles into my family, which took hold of my wife, being great with child; yet it pleased the Lord mercifully to restore her in a week's time to former health. My little cousin Daniel, and my maid, had the same disease, and through favor, found God's restoring mercy."

During the seventeenth century the Atlantic Ocean had been an effective barrier against the epidemics of measles which occurred in England, because the average sailing time was eight to ten weeks and the incubation period of measles less than two weeks; it follows that most shipboard epidemics must have burned out before the ships would reach these shores.

The epidemic described by Hull must have eventually spread to Connecticut, because on September 9, 1658, John Winthrop, Jr.,[11] wrote in a letter to his eldest son, Fitz-John Winthrop (1638–1707): "At Hartford . . . Elizabeth [twenty-two years old] was very sick of the measells, but it pleased the Lord to deliver her from the very dores of death, when we had been little hopes of her recovery. All the rest also had the measells, your cousin Martha also, and your brother in the bay, but it pleased the Lord to recover them all with out much illnesse."

In this first documented epidemic of measles in New England, many of the patients suffered complications; yet, on the whole, the epidemic was not very severe, for out of a large number of cases in Boston "scarce any died of it."

The next epidemic did not stike until 1687–1688, two decades later, and as Ernest Caulfield (1893–1972)[11] noted, "It seems somewhat strange that a disease which appears nowadays [prior to measles immunization] every two, three, or four years and is essentially a childhood disease should disappear from the colonies for a long time, but, as yet, I have not found even any sporadic case [from 1658] until 1687." On December 10, 1687, John Allyn, of Hartford, wrote that "many people in Boston are sick of the measells, but it is not mortall as yet."

The fact that the disease attacked adults as well as children is evident in Sewall's[43] diary:

Jan. 11, 1687–88. Sam [nine years old] falls ill of the Measles . . . *Jan. 13.* Betty Lane [six years old] falls sick of the Measles . . . Betty vomits up a long worm. Satterday, *Jan. 21.* My dear Daughter Hannah [eight years old] is put to bed, or rather kept in Bed, being sick of Measles. Droop'd ever since *Thorsday {Jan. 19}. Monday, Jan. 23.* The Measles come out pretty full on my dear Wife, which I discern before I rise. She was very ill in the night. *Tuesday, Jan. 24th.* About noon, the Physician tells me the Measles are come out in my face, and challenges me for his Patient. *Friday, Jan. 27.* In the afternoon I arise to have my Sweaty Bed made and dri'd. [Friday] *Feb. 3.* Unkle Quinsey visits us, and tells us that one Withrington, a lusty young man of Dorchester, is died of the Measles . . . *Tuesday, Feb. 7.* My Aunt Gerrish died between 7 and 8. *mane:* Had the Measles lately, and now by Flux, vapours and others inconveniencies, expires before I had so much as heard of her being ill, that I know of. This day, my wife, Sam and self purge after the Measles.

At Plymouth, March 7, 1688, was a "Day of Fasting and Prayer, on account of the measles in the winter." Such days of fasting and prayer were common occurrences during epidemics.[18]

DIPHTHERIA. The first recorded epidemic of diphtheria apparently occurred in 1659. According to Cotton Mather, the Reverend Samuel Danforth, of Roxbury, Massachusetts, lost three children within a fortnight during December of that year from an unknown malady (until then) termed "Bladders in the Windpipe," which may well have been diphtheria.[11]

In colonial records diphtheria appears under various other names, such as cynanche trachealis, squinancy, quinsy, bladder, canker, rattles, hives, croup, throat ail, throat distemper, bowel heaves, *suffocatio stridula,* and pleurisy of windpipe. These terms are confusing because some of them were applied to other diseases as well, especially scarlet fever.

Until the nineteenth century, diphtheria for the most part was confused with other, less dangerous forms of sore throat. Worse still, diphtheria was frequently confused with scarlet fever. Practitioners in the seventeenth and eighteenth centuries were unable to make a clear distinction between these two diseases. Thrush and diphtheria were also confused. The modern understanding of diphtheria really begins with Pierre Bretonneau (1778–1862) who in 1821 had the genius to recognize the disease as a specific entity and to separate it from the confused welter of sore throats which were then being described. It was he who named the disease la diphthérite.

During the closing years of the seventeenth century several other outbreaks of what may well have been diphtheria occurred in the colonies, but here the information is scarce. In 1686 there was an epidemic of "throat distemper" in Virginia, according to a letter sent to the editors of *Philosophical Transactions* by John Clayton,[18] a minister in that colony. And, according to John Josselyn (fl.1670–1675),[29] in 1689 "a Distemper of sore throats and ffeaver . . . the Like haveing not been knowne in the Memory of man," brought death to many in New London, Connecticut.

SCARLET FEVER. Sydenham's account of scarlet fever (1676), which was the first English record of it under the name of scarlatina, was not clearly defined, and, strangely enough, Sydenham, usually so precise an observer, made no mention of the sore throat. The name *scarlatina* originally came from Italy and was borrowed by Sydenham. Scarlet fever was often mistaken for measles and diphtheria during our colonial period. It is of interest that it was not until 1703, when seven deaths were attributed to it, that scarlet fever first appeared in the London Bills of Mortality.[18] As will be noted in the next chapter, William Douglass (1691–1752), of Boston, wrote an excellent account of scarlet fever (which he called *angina ulcusculosa*) in New England.

WHOOPING COUGH (Chincough). An extensive epidemic occurred in December, 1659, when John Hull[18] wrote in his diary that "in this same month of December, the young children in this town, and sundry towns here about were much afflicted with a very sore hooping cough; some few died of it." This appears to be the first mention of this disease in colonial records. In reviewing early fragmentary records there is always the possibility of errors in diagnosis, and other diseases in all likelihood passed for whooping cough. Inexperienced observers may well have confused whooping cough with croup or with the "very deep colds among children" described in the occasional colonial records of such epidemics. The younger John Winthrop mentioned cases of "hoping cough" and "great hooping cough" in Hartford. However, Caulfield[12] was unable to locate any other records of whooping cough epidemics until 1738, an interval of nearly eighty years. This cannot be attributed to lack of records entirely, because in neither the Sewall nor the Mather diaries is whooping cough even mentioned.

DYSENTERY. Bloody flux, once called the "most violent and dangerous of all American diseases," should not be confused with the disease termed "common flux" in Massachusetts or "Lax" in Pennsylvania, although in many records it is impossible to separate one from the other. Common flux was in all likelihood a nonspecific diarrhea and was seldom serious except in infants. Though occasionally mentioned in colonial records, it did not receive much attention until described in 1773 as cholera infantum by Benjamin Rush (1745–1813).[12] As towns became larger, summer diarrhea among infants was mentioned

more frequently; but not until the nineteenth century, with its crowded cities and contaminated milk and water supplies, did "cholera infantum" or "summer complaint" reach its peak.

Walter Harris[38] was familiar with what was later termed the "summer complaint": "From the Middle of July to about the Middle of September, the Epidemical Gripes of Children are so rife every Year, that more of them usually die in one Month, than in three or four at any other Time; For the Heat of that Season commonly weakens them at least, if it does not entirely exhause their Strength."

It is equally difficult to differentiate bloody flux from typhoid fever as described in colonial records because these two diseases had the same seasonal distribution, both produced gastrointestinal symptoms, and both occurred in epidemic form. It must also be remembered that accurate diagnoses of the various intestinal infections on the basis of colonial records are often impossible. The same might be said for many of the other childhood infections.

Josselyn[29] wrote in 1674 that "griping of the belly (accompanied with Feavor and Ague) which turns to the bloody flux" was a common disease in New England and that it "together with the smallpox carried away abundance of their children."

As the seventeenth century ended, John Marshall (1664–1732)[12] wrote that "about this time many persons dyed at Boston, especially children, of a bloody flux and feaver and some dyed of it in the country." There is little doubt that bloody flux was one of the most formidable and widespread diseases of the seventeenth century. No age group or area was immune from the contagion and in colonial days it flourished from Massachusetts to Georgia.

Seventeenth-Century Medical Doctrines and Practice

At the beginning of the seventeenth century, medicine was still in the grasp of Greco-Roman and Arabian tradition, and pathology was tied to the humoral theory. It will be remembered that the fundamental theory of Hippocrates was the doctrine of the four humors. Hippocrates (c. 460–c. 375 B.C.) had taught that "the body of man has in itself blood, phlegm, yellow bile and black bile. . . . Now he enjoys the most perfect health when these elements are duly proportioned to one another in respect of compounding power and bulk and when they are perfectly mingled. Pain is felt when one of these elements is in defect or excess, or is isolated in the body without being compounded with all the others." Hippocrates saw health as the proper mixture of the humors, a *crasis* or *eucrasia,* while an improper mixture with one humor, a *dyscrasia,* caused disease. Disease could also be caused by an outside agent, such as the patient's environment. If one of the "qualities"—dryness, cold, heat or dampness—was present in excess in the environment, this tended to produce an excess in the corresponding humor of the body, thus causing a dyscrasia and disease. To restore health, the physician then attempted to counteract this imbalance. There were two ways to accomplish this: first by depletion methods and second by prescribing alteratives. Evacuant or depletion methods were the most widely used; these included sweating and bloodletting by venesection, scarification, cupping, or applying leeches.

In the American colonies bloodletting was practiced by clergymen and other medical amateurs and dabblers to whom the old almanacs pointed out the proper time of the moon for letting blood according to the age of the patient. Bleeding and sweating were thought to free the body of the "poisons" that were making it unhealthy. Alteratives, mostly galenicals, were given by mouth to alter the putative humoral imbalance. Complicated prescriptions including several different herbs were commonly used. This polypharmacy was blessed by antiquity. The irony of all the seventeenth- and eighteenth-century medical theories was that they all rationalized the traditional practices of bleeding, sweating, blistering, inducing vomiting, and purging. Whether the physician thought he was restoring the humoral balance or removing "morbifick" substances, the treatment was the same.

Galen (A.D.130–200), one of the towering figures in medical history, like Hippocrates, held as his fundamental theory of nature that all natural objects were composed of four elements—earth, air, fire, and water—and that all natural objects have four qualities—hot, cold, dry, and moist—and that there were four humors. Blood is hot and moist; phlegm, cold and moist; yellow bile, hot and dry; black bile, cold and dry. The elaborate form in which Galen clothed

the doctrine of humors added importance and attraction to it. For more than fifteen hundred years this doctrine remained the very foundation of all medical thought and the fundamental knowledge each doctor must understand before he could practice medicine intelligently. Without it, diagnoses were impossible and treatment futile. Galen also stressed the Hippocratic doctrine of critical days, a doctrine which, buttressed by his authority, also dominated medical thinking throughout the centuries. Galen's theories were well known to our early preacher-physicians and the Galenic system lasted in America until the beginning of the eighteenth century.

The Doctrine of Signatures

The ancient doctrine of signatures was widely accepted in the colonies.[19] The notion was as old as Hippocrates, but later medical writers amplified, emphasized, complicated, and mystified the doctrine in such a way as to make it seem almost an original discovery of their own time. This doctrine taught that God created plants in a form suggesting the organ upon which they acted. Thus the porosity of the leaves of Saint-John's wort (*Hypericum perforatum*) and the spots which resembled perforations of the leaf indicated the value of this plant in all cases of abrasion, external or internal. The illusory appearance of holes in its leaves meant that it would be of value in the treatment of hallucinations, madness, and assaults of the devil. Reminders of the former acceptance of such beliefs are suggested by plant names such as hepatica, formerly believed to be useful in liver complaints: lungwort, once believed of value for pulmonary infections; and euphrasia, or common eyebright, for diseases of the eyes. The essence of this doctrine was that "like cures like"; thus, yellow plants were good for jaundice; red ones were good for the blood. According to Edward Eggleston (1837–1902),[19] "the world was a cosmic pharmacy; God had placed a signature on each substance to indicate the disease it was good for. What was necessary was to read the label to note the indications of odor, color, form, and other marks."

The influence of the theory of signatures on English medicine in actual transit to the colonies is evident from examining Stafford's letter, quoted earlier in this chapter, to Governor John Winthrop, Jr., of

Connecticut. In his letter Stafford recommended sweet milk with salt for "jaunders." Milk, being white, cleared black humors. This was "contraries cured by contraries," an accepted seventeenth-century principle. Stafford used both methods in one remedy; he added saffron to the milk and salt for jaundice. This was called "curing by the assimilate, a yellow remedy for a yellow disease."

Causes of Disease

Since there was only one strictly medical publication in the colonies before 1700, it is almost impossible to know what the physician thought about the causes of disease. It is largely through the writings of the pastor-physicians that the medical theories of the age are expressed.

In the seventeenth century almost all physicians accepted the importance of the supernatural as a cause of disease as gospel truth.[37] Astrology also had a firm grip and the influence of the moon and stars was widely accepted. Epidemics and many other misfortunes were blamed not only on sinful practices but were also often attributed to meteorologic and planetary influences.

Still births, premature births, and congenital malformations were believed to result from the association of the mother or midwife with demons, witches, and other evil consorts. The belief in witchcraft led to the earliest postmortem in New England of which we have an official record.[25] (Cotton Mather[11] mentions, but gives no details of, an earlier postmortem performed in December, 1659, on one of the three children of the Reverend Samuel Danforth who, as mentioned above, had died in an epidemic, possibly of diphtheria.) It was performed on eight-year-old Elizabeth Kelley of Hartford, Connecticut, who died on March 26, 1662. The autopsy was requested by the General Court of Connecticut because the child's parents had accused a neighbor, Goody Ayers, of practicing witchcraft on their child. Mr. Rossetter, who performed the autopsy on March 31, 1662, for twenty pounds, attributed Elizabeth's death to preternatural causes. What became of Goody Ayers, the putative witch, is not known because she and her husband fled precipitately as soon as they learned of the Court's order.

Child Care and Child Rearing

Although colonial life was woven of many strands, such as English, Scotch-Irish, Dutch, French, and German, all the new groups, whatever their ethnic differences, shared the common belief that the family was, in Benjamin Franklin's (1706–1790) phrase, the "sacred cement of all societies." As Cotton Mather put it in 1693, "Families are the Nurseries of all Societies; and the First Combinations of Mankind. Well-Ordered *Families* naturally produced a *Good Order* in other Societies." Not only was the family thus decreed by custom and by religion as the basis for sound community life, but also in the New World the tradition of family solidarity was made the more urgent by economic need.

Colonial childhood is largely hidden in obscurity. Unfortunately, letters and diaries contain little mention of children except for records of their births, deaths, and illnesses. The day-to-day observations of children at play, at school, or in their joys or griefs, are absent. And we read with sadness that there were no inventories of toys in Pilgrim families.

Childhood as such was barely recognized during the seventeenth century. There was little sense that children might somehow be a special group with their own needs and interests and capacities. Instead, they were viewed largely as miniature adults: the boy was a little model of his father, likewise the girl of her mother. In many seventeenth-century colonial families children of seven or eight years of age were already veteran workers. For example, the Reverend Francis Higginson,[20] in a letter he wrote to friends in England in 1629, claimed that "little children here by setting of corn may earn much more than their own maintenance."

The mortality among colonial infants was appalling. Putrid fevers, epidemic influenzas, bloody fluxes, malignant sore throats, and smallpox carried off, as has been noted, thousands of the children who survived baptism. Perhaps for this reason parents searched for names of deep significance, for names appropriate to conditions, or for those of profound influence—presumably on the child's life. Abigail, meaning father's joy, was frequently given, as was Hannah, meaning grace. Names such as, Comfort, Deliverance, Temperance, Peace, Hope, Patience, Charity, Faith, Love, Submit, Rejoice were not uncommon. Some children of Roger Clap

(1609–1691), were named Experience, Waitsill, Preserved, Hopestill, Wait, Thanks, Desire, Unite, and Supply.

When a baby was safely past the hazards of his first few days of life, he was incorporated into the ongoing routine of his household. The seventeenth-century infant slept in a wicker or wooden cradle (p. 165). Infants were usually baptized within a week of birth irrespective of the weather, as Judge Sewall's[43] first child was baptized seven days after his birth. His diary entry for April 8, 1677, reads: "Sabbath day, rainy and stormy in the morning... Eliz Weedon the midwife, brought the Infant to the Third Church when sermon was about half done in the afternoon Mr. Thacher preaching. After sermon and Prayer, Mr. Thacher prayed for it then I name him John and Mr. Thacher baptized him."

The infant's clothing was probably quite simple. Previous studies of this subject have turned up no seventeenth-century evidence of swaddling or otherwise binding the child so as to restrict his movement. Colonial children were dressed like their parents. Little boys, just as soon as they could walk, wore clothes made exactly like their father's: doublets, which were warm double jackets, leather knee breeches, leather belts, and knit caps; and for girls, chemise bodices, petticoats of linen or dimity, and cotton skirts.[8] Diapers—as we know them—were unknown in this century. In fact, the modern diaper is less than eighty years old.

In the seventeenth century nobody bathed much and infants were probably bathed even less frequently to avoid their taking cold. Soap and towels were scarce.

The baby's nourishment consisted almost entirely of breast milk. The subject is not much discussed in any extant documents, but there are occasional, incidental references to it. (Colonial infant-feeding practices will be considered in Chapter 3.) Especially in Plymouth Plantation, according to John Demos,[16] a baby had a relatively comfortable time for the first year or so. The ebb and flow of domestic life must have been constantly around him: large families in small houses created an inevitable sense of intimacy. These large families, however, were often the product of two, three, or more successive wives.

The relationship of parents to children was often compared with that of God to his children. Life was very real and earnest and the child's first and last duty was to walk obediently in the ways of his elders. Legally, boys reached their majority at sixteen, when they became taxpayers and members of the militia, and at this age some of the girls were already wives and mothers.

Seventeenth-Century Vital Statistics

Unhappily, a high death rate accompanied the high birth rate. Many mothers risked their lives to bring forth infants only for the grave. Inadequate diet, ignorance of hygiene and nutrition, lack of medical care, and poorly heated homes all took their toll. Nor did the more fortunate children always outlast their parents. Of Cotton Mather's fourteen, but one survived him; of Judge Sewall's fourteen, but two; of Thomas Jefferson's six, but one. It is small wonder, therefore, that Mather was in a continual apprehension over the thought that his son Samuel "tho a lusty and hearty infant will die in its Infancy," nor is it cause for surprise to find that Sewall was "much affected" by recurring dreams that his wife or offspring had died. Time and time again such dreams and apprehensions turned out to be prophetic.

Recent demographic studies of colonial New England indicate that childbearing, although a great danger, may have been overestimated as a cause of death.[48] Current evidence suggests that fewer American women died in giving birth than their English contemporaries, probably because the conditions of American life were more healthful. It is estimated that the maternal death rate in American towns was between 66 and 80 percent of the death rate in comparable towns in England and France.[48]

In many communities the American child also had a greater chance of surviving infancy than his English counterpart. For instance, a child in Plymouth had a 75 percent chance of living to the age of twenty-one and in Andover an 83 percent chance, but in London before 1660 one-third of all recorded deaths were those of children younger than age six.[47] Nevertheless, to the colonist death was an ever-present menace that struck the children of the community with a particular vengeance.

One of the problems of mortality figures is their distortion through the almost inevitable underestimation of infant mortality, as demographic analysts freely acknowledge; most infant deaths were unrecorded and their number can only be guessed.[10] Kenneth A. Lockridge[31] made one such guess in his study of Dedham, Massachusetts, in the seventeenth and early eighteenth centuries when he estimated that an upward adjustment of one-ninth of the town's birth rate would likely take account of the unrecorded infant deaths.

Studies of seventeenth- and eighteenth-century Salem indicate a fluctuating infant mortality rate ranging from a low of 105 per 1,000 for eighteenth-century male children to a high of 313 per 1,000 for seventeenth-century female children. "In other words," according to Maris A. Vinovskis,[47] "ten to thirty percent of the children never survived the first year of life." But despite this high infant mortality rate, it has been estimated that youngsters of fifteen years and under made up about half the population as the American Revolution approached.

Philip J. Greven[21] calculated that the average number of children born per family in colonial Andover was 8.8 and of those an average of 5.9 survived to adulthood. He further notes that "approximately three of the close to nine children born to the average family would die before reaching their twenty-first birthday." But the most vulnerable period in life was that "beyond infancy but prior to adolescence—the age group which appears to have been most susceptible, among other things, to the throat distemper prevalent in the mid-1730's." David E. Stannard[41] found that by applying the infant mortality adjustment of one-ninth to Greven's figures, the rate of survival to age ten of all children born between 1640 and 1759 was approximately 74 percent—with a generational high of 83 percent and a low of 63 percent. This latter figure indicates that at one point fewer than two out of three infants lived to see their tenth birthday. During the colonial period as a whole, more than one child in four failed to survive the first decade of life in a community with an average births-per-family rate of 8.8.[21]

Thus a young couple, as they started their married life, did so "with the knowledge and expectation that in all probability *two or three* of the children they might have would die before the age of ten." In certain cases, of course, more than two or three would die. In fact, during severe epidemics, such as the epidemic of diphtheria in 1735–1740, multiple deaths in families were characteristic. There were at least six instances of eight children dying within a

period of a week or ten days.[10] In Boston the death rate for children was much higher, and even the best-cared-for residents of the city were constantly reminded of the fragility of life in childhood.

As the century was approaching its end, American children in all the colonies were already demonstrating a distinctive temperament. Cotton Mather in one of his sermons remarked that "the Youth in this country are verie Sharp and early Ripe in their Capacities." The next century would show how prescient Mather was.

References

1. Black, R. E., III. *The Younger John Winthrop.* New York: Columbia University Press, 1966.
2. Blake, J. B. *Public Health in the Town of Boston, 1630–1822.* Cambridge, Mass.: Harvard University Press, 1959.
3. Blanton, W. B. *Medicine in Virginia in the Seventeenth Century.* Richmond, Va.: W. Byrd Press [1930].
4. Bradford, W. *Of Plymouth Plantation.* S. E. Morison (ed.). New York: Modern Library, 1967.
5. Bremner, R. H. (ed.) *Children and Youth in America,* Vol. 1. Cambridge, Mass.: Harvard University Press, 1970.
6. Bridenbaugh, C. *Vexed and Troubled Englishmen, 1590–1642.* New York: Oxford University Press, 1968.
7. Byrne, J. J. Medicine at Plymouth Plantation. *N. Engl. J. Med.* 259:1012, 1958.
8. Cable, M. *The Little Darlings: A History of Child Rearing in America.* New York: Scribner's, 1975.
9. Caffrey, K. *The Mayflower.* New York: Stein and Day, 1974.
10. Caulfield, E. A history of the terrible epidemic, vulgarly called the throat distemper, as it occurred in His Majesty's New England Colonies between the years 1735 and 1740. *Yale J. Biol. Med.* 11:219, 1939.
11. Caulfield, E. Early measles epidemics in America. *Yale J. Biol. Med.* 14:531, 1942.
12. Caulfield, E. Some common diseases of colonial children. *Trans. Colonial Soc. Mass.* 35:4, 1951.
13. Cone, T. E., Jr. Highlights of two centuries of American pediatrics, 1776–1976. *Am. J. Dis. Child.* 130:762, 1976.
14. Cone, T. E., Jr. *200 Years of Feeding Infants in America.* Columbus, Ohio: Ross Laboratories, 1976.
15. Creighton, C. *A History of Epidemics in Britain,* 2

vols. Cambridge: Cambridge University Press, 1891–1894.

16. Demos, J. *A Little Commonwealth.* New York: Oxford University Press, 1970.

17. Duffy, J. Smallpox and the Indians in the American Colonies. *Bull. Hist. Med.* 25:324, 1951.

18. Duffy, J. *Epidemics in Colonial America.* Baton Rouge: Louisiana State University Press, 1953.

19. Eggleston, E. *The Transit of Civilization from England to America.* New York: Appleton, 1901.

20. Emerson, E. *Letters from New England: The Massachusetts Bay Colony, 1629–1639.* Amherst, Mass.: University of Massachusetts Press, 1976.

21. Greven, P. J. *Four Generations: Population, Land and Family in Colonial Andover* [Mass.]. Ithaca, N.Y.: Cornell University Press, 1970.

22. Guerra, F. *American Medical Bibliography, 1689–1783.* New York: Lathrop C. Harper, 1962.

23. Handlin, O. *The Americans.* Boston: Little, Brown, 1963.

24. Harrington, T. F. Dr. Samuel Fuller, of the Mayflower. *Bull. Johns Hopkins Hosp.* 14:263, 1903.

25. Hoadly, C. J. Some early post-mortem examinations in New England. *Proc. Conn. Med. Soc.,* 1892.

26. Holmes, O. W. *Medical Essays.* Boston: Houghton Mifflin, 1911.

27. Holländer, E. *Wunder, Wundergeburt und Wundergestalt.* Stuttgart: F. Enke, 1922.

28. Jones, G. *The Angel of Bethesda.* Barre, Mass.: American Antiquarian Society, 1972.

29. Josselyn, J. *An Account of Two Voyages to New-England,* Boston: Reprinted in *Coll. Mass. Hist. Soc.* (3rd ser.) vol. 3, 1833.

30. Lampe, K. E., and Fagerström, R. *Plant Toxicity and Dermatitis,* Baltimore: Williams & Wilkins, 1968.

31. Lockridge, K.A. The population of Dedham, Massachusetts, 1636–1736. *Economic Hist. Rev.* (2nd ser.) 19:331, 1966.

32. Mather, C. Diary 1681–1708, 1709–1724. *Coll. Mass. Hist. Soc.* (7th ser.) vols. 7, 8, 1912.

33. Mettler, C. C. *History of Medicine.* Philadelphia: Blakiston, 1947.

34. Morison, S. E. *The European Discovery of America.* New York: Oxford University Press, 1971.

35. Murdock, K. B. (ed.) *Cotton Mather: Magnalia Christi Americana,* Books I and II. Cambridge, Mass. Belknap Press of Harvard University Press, 1977.

36. Packard, F. R. *History of Medicine in the United States* (2nd ed.) New York: Hoeber, 1931.

37. Radbill, S. X. Pediatrics. In A. G. Debus (ed.) *Medicine in Seventeenth Century England.* Berkeley: University of California Press, 1974.

38. Ruhräh, J. Walter Harris, a seventeenth-century pediatrist. *Ann. Med. Hist.* 2:228, 1919.

39. Shelton, P. G., et. al. Nursing bottle caries. *Pediatrics* 59:777, 1977.

40. Stafford, E. Original letter to John Winthrop, Sr., dated May 6, 1643. Countway Medical Library, Boston.

41. Stannard, D. E. *The Puritan Way of Death.* New York: Oxford University Press, 1977.

42. Steiner, W. R. Governor John Winthrop, Jr., of Connecticut, as a physician. *Bull. Johns Hopkins Hosp.* 14:294, 1903; 17:357, 1906.

43. Thomas, M. H. (ed.). *The Diary of Samuel Sewall, 1674–1729* (2 vols.). New York: Farrar, Straus and Giroux, 1973.

44. Thoms, H. The beginnings of obstetrics in America. *Yale J. Biol. Med.* 4:665, 1932.

45. Viets, H. R. *A Brief History of Medicine in Massachusetts.* Boston: Houghton Mifflin, 1930.

46. Viets, H. R. Thomas Thacher and his influence on American medicine. *Va. Med. Mon.* 76:384, 1949.

47. Vinovskis, M. A. Mortality rates and trends in Massachusetts before 1860. *J. Economic Hist.* 32:200, 1972.

48. Wertz, R. W., and Wertz, D. C. *Lying-In: A History of Childbirth in America.* New York: Free Press, 1977.

49. White, J. Journal of His Voyage to Virginia in 1587. In S. Lorant (ed.), *The New World.* New York: Duell, Sloan and Pearce, 1965.

50. Willison, G. E. *Saints and Strangers.* New York: Time, Inc. 1964.

51. Winslow, O.E. *A Destroying Angel: The Conquest of Smallpox in Colonial Boston.* Boston: Houghton Mifflin, 1974.

52. Winthrop, J. *Journal.* New York: Scribner's 1908.

53. Winthrop, J. Letters. Countway Library of Medicine.

Children Discovered

It is clear enough that children were "discovered" in America also during the later eighteenth century. Life had been hard for them in the 1600's; and in New England at least their elders' teachings had made it even grimmer—if that was possible. Books written for children carried such titles as War with the Devil *or* Spiritual Milk for Boston Babes. *But parental attitudes apparently began to relax by the 1740's and the devil was at least partly replaced in juvenile literature by our old friend Mother Goose. Rising standards of living and growing secularism doubtless encouraged this trend.*

Richard H. Shryock (1960)

By the dawn of the eighteenth century only a fringe of our land nowhere more than forty or fifty miles from the seacoast or a navigable river had been brought under cultivation or settlement. As the century began our population was slightly more than two hundred thousand and at its end this figure would rise to about four million, a twentyfold increase.

In the continental area, our population, small as it was, had set the main pattern of government and society for the future United States. In less than a century English culture had been transferred to America. The colonies now had two colleges, Harvard and William and Mary, and in 1701 Yale would be added. For almost all white boys primary education was available in most of the colonies north of Maryland. Boston's printing presses had a greater output than any English city except London, and Philadelphia would soon be actively competing with Boston.

Crossing the Atlantic was even tougher for young and old than in the seventeenth century. Gottlieb Mittelberger,[40] who came to Philadelphia in 1750, described the misery during his voyage: bad drinking water, rotten salt meat, unbearable heat, overcrowding, and lice so thick that they could be scraped off the body; passengers dying of dysentery, scurvy, typhus, canker, and mouth-rot. Children under seven, he said, rarely survived the voyage, and in his own ship no fewer than thirty-two died, all of whom were finally thrown into the ocean, and their parents grieved all the more "since their children do not find repose in the earth, but are devoured by the predatory fish of the ocean." The children who had not had either measles or smallpox often got them on board ship and for the most part perished as a result.

Medical Training and Practice

Medicine was beginning to shake off the shackles of antiquity and for the first time since Hippocrates clinical observation was viewed as a fertile field of study. Experimental science developed rapidly during the seventeenth century and came into its own in the eighteenth. The period of clerical medicine was nearing its end as the apprentice method of learning medicine became increasingly important.

Young men planning a career in medicine who did not attend a European medical school were all trained under the apprentice method, which may not have been without its advantages. The apprenticed student might lack the theoretical knowledge to be gained at a European medical school, but he learned "practical" medicine by daily bedside contact with patients. At European medical schools students would more likely accept the unproved assertions of their learned teachers, which justified their heroic therapeutic regimens of bleeding, purging, blistering, vomiting, and sweating on theoretical rather than empirical grounds. The American historian Daniel Boorstin[6] believes the colonial American patient had an advantage over his European counterpart because the less educated American practitioners were not bogged down "with so much learned error" as were the British confreres. For this reason, the less educated American physician may have been less of a threat to his patient's life.

Of the ten practitioners in Boston in 1721, only William Douglass had a *bona fide* doctor's degree.[54] At the outbreak of the Revolution there were about thirty-five hundred practitioners in the colonies, and of these it is estimated that no more than four hundred had attended medical school on either side of the Atlantic.[4]

At the beginning of the eighteenth century some progress had been made in pediatrics in that certain diseases such as rickets (1645), chorea (1686), scarlet fever (1641 and 1676), whooping cough (1640 and 1675), and measles (1676) were now recognized as diseases *sui generis.* But medical progress in general was sluggish, not because of any lack of writers on the subject but because, as Francis Bacon (1561–1626) had noted in his *Advancement of Learning* (1605), medicine was "more laboured than advanced; the labour having been . . . rather in circle than in progression. For I find much iteration but small addition."[49]

In the eighteenth century the concept of child health hardly existed. Children when sick were treated like their elders. Physicians treated both young and old patients with emetics, purges, bleeding, sweating, and blistering. Drug therapy consisted largely in the use of calomel, tartar emetic, jalap, the bark (quinine), and opium. Inasmuch as little or nothing was known about the pharmacologic action of these drugs, they were used indiscriminately and often without therapeutic effect. This led to a vigorous quest for and a willingness to accept the existence of panaceas such as theriac, the "unicorn horn," bezoars, and tar water.

Sanitation was extremely primitive. Flies and mosquitoes were described merely as simple nuisances and no one thought of them as highly dangerous carriers of disease. Lice, fleas, and "the itch" mite were plentiful. Frequent admonitions were made about the need for a vigorous attack on the vermin carried by new servants in a household, often to the extent of boiling their clothes.

Many remedies were kept at home and used very freely. This practice probably saved the lives of numerous sick children because it spared them the heroic and drastic therapy prescribed by most physicians. For example, Douglass[20] complained:

The physical practice in our Colonies is so perniciously bad that excepting in surgery and some acute cases it is better to let nature take her course than to trust to the honesty and sagacity of the practitioner. Our American practitioners are so rash and officious that the saying in the Apocrypha may with propriety be applied to him: "He that sinneth before his maker let him fall into the hands of the physician." Their general method of treatment . . . was uniformly bleeding, blistering, purging, anodynes, etc. If the illness continued, there was *repetendi* and finally *murderandi.*

There was no American medical literature to

speak of until well after the Revolution. The first periodical with medicine as its central theme was the *Medical Repository*, founded in New York City in 1797, and the first medical transactions published by a medical society in the United States, *The Cases and Observations of the Medical Society of New-Haven County*, appeared nine years earlier (1788). The Massachusetts Medical Society published a number of papers in 1790; and the *Transactions* of the Philadelphia College of Physicians began in 1790. The only medical publication during the entire seventeenth century was Thacher's broadside about smallpox (p. 12).

In 1708 Nicholas Culpeper's (1616–1654)[16] *The English Physician* became the first real medical book to be published in America. This small book (approximately 3 by 5 inches) of only 94 pages, meant for the lay reader, contained some of the author's "choicest Secrets in the Art of Physick" (Fig. 2–1). Culpeper included about ten "secrets" to cure "Children's Infirmities."

One wonders how effective his treatment of worms would have been, since the medications prescribed would not be taken by mouth but rather would be applied to the patient's navel: "Take Myrrh and Aloes of each alike, finely powdered and with a few drops of Chymical Oyl, or Savin, with a little Turpentine, mix them, and make them up for a Plaister for the Childs Navel."

Culpeper's books, especially *The English Physician* and *A Directory for Midwives*, were popular in colonial America because they were easy to read and offered practical medical advice.[14]

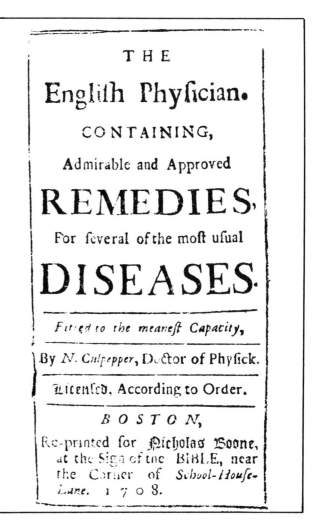

Figure 2–1. *Title page of Nicholas Culpeper's* The English Physician *(1708). This page has a variant spelling of Culpeper's name. (Courtesy of the Countway Library of Medicine.)*

Epidemic Diseases

The tragic role played by sickness and disease in the history of the American colonies was more dramatically revealed and reported in the eighteenth century than during the seventeenth. Frequent epidemics of smallpox, diphtheria, scarlet fever, yellow fever, and measles, some of extraordinary severity, would often carry away several children in a family within a few days. Ernest Caulfield[10] considered the epidemic of diphtheria during the years 1735–1740 "the most frightful epidemic of any childhood disease in American history."

Rather than giving a detailed account of all the epidemic diseases in colonial America, only those in which colonial Americans made a major contribution to the history of these diseases and thus to pediatrics will be cited. Interestingly, Cotton Mather and Benjamin Franklin, the two eighteenth-century Americans who made the most original contributions to medicine, were not physicians.

It was in the field of epidemiology that colonial America made the greatest contributions. A strong case could be made that the major problems of contagious diseases and epidemics were solved on this continent. The large number of publications on diphtheria, scarlet fever, and measles rank second only to the abundant literature on the subject of smallpox, the latter represented by the important works of Zabdiel Boylston, (1679–1766), William Douglass, and Cotton Mather.

Smallpox

No disease was regarded with greater terror than was smallpox, and it is in connection with this disease that the first significant advance of American medicine occurred, namely the introduction of inoculation (variolation) against smallpox in 1721 by Zabdiel Boylston at Cotton Mather's suggestion.

On May 26, 1721, Mather[35] wrote in his diary, "The grievous Calamity of *Small-Pox* has now entered the Town." The next day the *Boston News-Letter* reported that there were eight cases of smallpox in town. As the last epidemic of smallpox had occurred in 1702, nineteen years earlier, this meant that no child born during those nineteen years had a chance of protection from acquired immunity to this disease. It also meant that a large proportion of the total adult population had little familiarity with the necessary precautions and responsibilities which a major epidemic imposed upon young and old.

Smallpox epidemics occurred almost simultaneously in both London and Boston in 1721. In the former city, at the urging of Lady Mary Wortley Montagu (1689–1762), twenty persons were inoculated in the hope that they would suffer mild cases of smallpox and be protected thereafter against infection. Lady Montagu had learned about inoculation soon after her arrival in Constantinople, where her husband had been appointed Ambassador Extraordinary to the Court of Constantinople in 1718. This well-known episode is usually said to mark the beginning of inoculation in the Western world. What actually happened, however, was that one or two deaths occurred following these inoculations; hence there was much opposition and no extensive experimentation with the practice occurred in England that year.

In Boston, meantime, Mather[35] wrote further in his diary on May 26, 1721: "The Practice of conveying and suffering the *Small-Pox* by *Inoculation,* has never been used in *America,* nor indeed in our Nation, but how many Lives might be saved by it, if it were practiced? I will procure a Council of our Physicians, and lay the Matter before them."

And on June 24, 1721, Mather[57] wrote to Boylston, the only one of Boston's ten physicians who did not condemn inoculation as both dangerous and irreligious:

You are many ways, Sir, endeared unto me, but in nothing more than in the very much good which a gratious God employs you and honours you in a miserable world.

I design it, as a testimony and esteem that I now lay before you, the most that I know (and all that was ever published in the world) concerning a matter, which I have the occasion of its being much talked about. If upon mature deliberation, you should think it admissable to be proceeded in, it may save many lives that we set a great store on. But if it be not approved of, you will have the pleasure of knowing what is done in other places. . . .

But now think, Judge, do as the Lord our healer shall direct you, and pardon the freedom of

Sir, Your hearty friend and Servant, co. Mather

Boylston wrote of this letter: "Upon reading of which I was very pleas'd, and resolved in my Mind to try the Experiment." He did so two days later, June 26, 1721, when he inoculated his six-year-old son Thomas for smallpox, the first person to be inoculated in the New World (Fig. 2–2). During a period of five months Boylston inoculated 247 persons. This was to be the first experiment with active immunization ever carried out in the Western World.

Boylston's method of inoculation was to use infected matter from the pustules of a person with a mild case of smallpox (inoculated or natural) who was otherwise healthy. Taken on the ninth to fourteenth day after eruption, the infected matter was stored in a closely sealed vial. Unlike the Turks, who made scratches on the skin, Boylston made two incisions through the "true skin" with a lancet either on the outside of the arm or on the inside of the leg. Pus was inserted into the incisions, which were then covered with a simple dressing, usually a cabbage leaf, which he found to be better than the Turkish method of covering the incision with half a nutshell.

Even as the epidemic of smallpox had begun to weaken, Boston's war of words over inoculation, which had begun on June 26, 1721, with Boylston's first use of it, continued to be waged for almost a year in the Boston newspapers. The anger and bad feeling toward Mather was so intense that he comon reading of which I was very well pleas'd, and resolv'd in my Mind to try the Experiment ; well remembring the Deftruction the Small-Pox made 19 Years before, when laft in *Bofton* ; and how narrowly I then efcap'd with my Life. Now, when my Wife and many others were gone out of Town to avoid the Diftemper, and all Hope given up of preventing the further fpreading of it, and the Guards were firft removed from the Doors of infected Houfes, I began the Experiment ; and not being able to make it upon myfelf, (fuch was my Faith in the Safety and Succefs of this Method) I chofe to make it (for Example fake) upon my own dear Child, and two of my Servants.

JUNE the 26th, 1721, I inoculated my Son *Thomas*, of about fix, my Negro Man, *Jack*, thirty fix, and *Jackey*, two and an half Years old. They all complain'd on the 6th Day ; upon the 7th, the two Children were a little hot, dull, and fleepy, *Thomas* (only) had twitchings and ftarted in his fleep. The 28th, the Children's Fevers continued, *Tommy's* twitchings and ftartings in fleep increafed ; and tho' the Fever was gentle and his Senfes bright, yet as the Practice was new, and the Clamour, or rather Rage of

Figure 2–2. The inoculation of Zabdiel Boylston's son and servants on June 26, 1721. (From Zabdiel Boylston, An Historical Account of the Small-Pox Inoculated in New England. *Courtesy of the Countway Library of Medicine.)*

plained in his diary[35] of "the monstrous and crying wickedness of this Town, and the vile abuse which I . . . suffer, for nothing but my instructing our base Physicians, how to save many precious Lives." The Mather-Boylston achievement, according to Richard Shryock (1893–1972),[47] the medical historian, "may be viewed as the chief American contribution to medicine prior to the mid-nineteenth century."

Mather,[35] however, recorded the anguish he suffered for his having his son Sammy inoculated against smallpox:

[May] 26 [1721]. The grievous Calamity of the *Small-Pox* has now entered the Town. The Practice of conveying and suffering the *Small-Pox* by *Inoculation*, has never been used in *America*, nor indeed in our Nation. But how many Lives might be saved by it, if it were practised? . . .

[June] 13. What shall I do? what shall I do, with regard unto *Sammy?* He comes home, when the *Small-Pox* begins to spread in the Neighbourhood; and he is lothe to return unto *Cambridge*. I must earnestly look up to Heaven for Direction. . . .

[July] 16. At this Time, I enjoy an unspeakable Consolation. I have instructed our Physicians in the new Method used by the *Africans* and *Asiaticks*, to prevent and abate the Dangers of the *Small-Pox*, and infallibly to save the Lives of those that have it wisely managed upon them. The Destroyer, being enraged at the Proposal of any Thing, that may rescue the Lives of our poor People from him, has taken a strange Possession of the People on this Occasion. They rave, they rail, they blaspheme; they talk not only like Ideots but also like *Fanaticks*, and not only the Physician who began the Experiment, but I also am an Object of their Fury. . . .

[August] 1. Full of Distress about *Sammy;* He begs to have his Life saved, by receiving the *Small-Pox*, in the way of *Inoculation*, whereof our Neighbourhood has had no less than ten remarkable Experiments: and if he should after all dy by receiving it in the common Way, how can I answer it? On the other Side, our People, who have Satan remarkably filling their Hearts and their Tongues, will go on with infinite Prejudices against me and my Ministry, if I suffer this Operation upon the Child. . . .

15. My dear *Sammy*, is now under the Operation of receiving the *Small-Pox* in the way of *Transplantation*. The Success of the Experiment among my Neighbours, as well as abroad in the World . . . [has] made me think, that I could not answer it unto God, if I neglected it. . . .

25 d. VI m. Friday. It is a very critical Time with me, a Time of unspeakable Trouble and Anguish. My dear *Sammy*, has this Week had a dangerous and threatening Fever come upon him, which is beyond what the Inoculation for the *Small-Pox* has hitherto brought upon my Subjects of it. In this Distress, I have cried unto the Lord; and He has answered with a Measure of Restraint upon the Fever. The Eruption proceeds, and he proves pretty full, and has not the best Sort, and some Degree of his Fever holds him. His Condition is very hazardous. . . .

[September] 5. *Sammy* recovering Strength, I must now earnestly putt him on considering, what he shall render to the Lord!

[November] 19. Certainly it becomes me and concerns me, to do something very considerable, in a way of Gratitude unto GOD MY SAVIOUR, for the astonishing Deliverance, which He did the last Week bestow upon me, and upon what belong'd unto me.

Cotton Mather was born in Boston on February 12, 1663, the eldest son of Increase (1639–1723) and grandson of John Cotton (1584–1652), for whom he was named. He graduated from Harvard in 1678 and, sharing his father's interest in science, studied

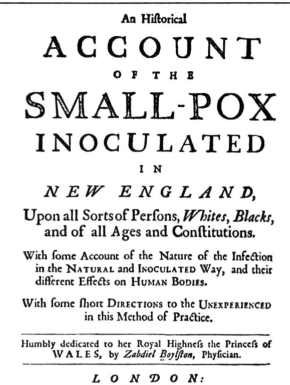

An Hiftorical
ACCOUNT
OF THE
SMALL-POX
INOCULATED
IN
NEW ENGLAND,
Upon all Sorts of Perfons, *Whites, Blacks,*
and of all Ages and Conftitutions.

With fome Account of the Nature of the Infection
in the NATURAL and INOCULATED Way, and their
different Effects on HUMAN BODIES.

With fome fhort DIRECTIONS to the UNEXPERIENCED
in this Method of Practice.

Humbly dedicated to her Royal Highnefs the Princefs of
W A L E S, by *Zabdiel Boylfton,* Phyfician.

L O N D O N:
Printed for S. CHANDLER, *at the* Crofs-Keys *in the* Poultry.
M. DCC. XXVI.

Figure 2–3. Title page of Zabdiel Boylston's An Historical Account of the Small-Pox Inoculated in New England. *(Courtesy of the Countway Library of Medicine.)*

medicine for a time. He turned to the ministry, however, and in 1685 joined his father in the pulpit of Boston's Second Church, where he remained for the rest of his life. He took great interest in the proper training of children, organized a school for the education of blacks, and concerned himself with ministering personally to his parishioners. In 1713 he was elected to the Royal Society, one of the first native-born Americans to be so honored.[47]

Boylston's account of his own experience with inoculation in Boston during the 1721 outbreak of smallpox, written as a first-person story, was entitled *An Historical Account of the Small-Pox Inoculated in New England;* it was originally printed in London in 1726 and was reprinted in Boston in the same year (Fig. 2–3). His book recorded the 280 cases of inoculation he performed in 1721 with careful observation and emphasis on the success or failure of the operation for each case; the very abbreviated case histories bring alive much of the atmosphere of

this time of crisis in beleaguered Boston. The book contained the first clinical investigation, outlined in tabular form, in American medical literature (Fig. 2–4). This was also the advent in America of a strictly "preventive" medicine. By using a simple calculus of probability, in itself a pioneer use of quantification in medicine, Boylston demonstrated that smallpox case mortality dropped from 15 percent "in the natural way" to 1 to 2 percent after inoculation.

Boylston's severest critic, William Douglass, the leader of the opposition to inoculation during the epidemic of 1721, finally accepted inoculation during the 1730 outbreak in Boston but never offered an apology to Boylston for the abuse he had heaped upon him. During the 1721 epidemic Douglass bitterly criticized Boylston for mischievously "Propogating the Infection" and he was vigorously opposed to "this novel and dubious practice" because he deemed it "a sin against Society to propogate infection by this Means." Surprisingly, the ministers, including Mather's father, Increase, supported

Figure 2–4. Boylston's tabular summary of his inoculation experiment.

Their Ages.	Perfons inoculated.	Had the Small-Pox by Inoculation.	Had an Imperfect fmall Pox.	Had no Effect.	Sufpected to have died of Inoculation.
From 9 months to 2 years old.	06	06	00	00	00
2 to 5	14	14	00	00	00
5 to 10	16	16	00	00	00
10 to 15	29	29	00	00	00
15 to 20	51	51	00	00	01
20 to 30	62	60	00	02	01
30 to 40	44	42	00	02	01
40 to 50	08	07	00	01	00
50 to 60	07	06	00	01	02
60 to 67	07	07	00	00	01
Total	244	238	00	06	06
Inoculated by Drs. Roby and Thompfon in Roxbury and Cambridge.	36	36	00	00	00
Total	280	274	00	00	06

It appears by the foregoing Table, that Inoculation upon fix Perfons did not produce the Small-Pox, by Reafon they had had it before. And that out of **274**, fix died, though they had not all the Small Pox only by Inoculation, as we have Reafon to believe, but were fome of them infected in the natural Way, **before**

Several REASONS

Proving that Inoculating or Tranſplanting the *Small Pox*, is a Lawful Practice, and that it has been Bleſſed by GOD for the Saving of many a Life.

By *Increaſe Mather*, D. D.

Exod. XX. 13. *Thou ſhalt not kill.*
Gal. I. 10. *Do I ſeek to pleaſe Men? if I pleaſe Men, I ſhould not be a Servant of* CHRIST.

It has been Queſtioned, Whether *Inoculating* the *Small Pox* be a Lawful Practice. I incline to the Affirmative, for theſe Reaſons.

I. BEcauſe I have read, that in *Smyrna*, *Conſtantinople*, and other Places, Thouſands of Lives have been ſaved by Inoculation, and not one of Thouſands has miſcarried by it. This is related by Wiſe & Learned Men who would not have impoſed on the World a falſe Narrative. Which alſo has been publiſhed by the *Royal Society*; therefore a great Regard is due to it.

II. WE hear that ſeveral *Phyſicians* have Recommended the Practice hereof to His *Majeſty*, as a Means to preſerve the Lives of his Subjects, and that His Wiſe and Excellent *Majeſty* King GEORGE, as alſo his *Royal Highneſs* the *Prince* have approved hereof, and that it is now coming into practice in the Nation. In one of the Publick Prints are theſe Words, "*Inoculating the Small Pox is a ſafe and* "*univerſally Uſeful Experiment.* Several Worthy Perſons lately arrived from *England* inform us, that it is a ſucceſsful Practice there: If Wiſe & Learned Men in *England*, declare their Approbation of this *Practice*, for us to declare our Diſapprobation will not be for our Honour.

III. GOD has graciouſly owned the *Practice of Inoculation*, among us in *Boſton*, where ſome Scores, yea above an hundred have been *Inoculated*, & not one miſcarried; but they Bleſs GOD, for His diſcovering this Experiment to them. It has been objected, that one that was Inoculated, died, viz. Mrs. *D——ll*: but ſhe had the *Small Pox*, in the common way before, & her Friends and neareſt Relations declare that ſhe received no hurt by *Inoculation*, but was by a fright put into Fits that cauſed her Death. It is then a wonderful Providence of GOD, that all that were *Inoculated* ſhould have their Lives preſerved; ſo that the Safety and Uſefulneſs of this Experiment is confirmed to us by Ocular Demonſtration: I confeſs I am afraid, that the Diſcouraging of this Practice, may cauſe many a Life to be loſt, which for my own part, I ſhould be loth to have any hand in, *becauſe of the Sixth Commandment*.

IV. IT cannot be denied but that ſome Wiſe and Judicious Perſons among us, approve of Inoculation, both *Magiſtrates* and *Miniſters*; Among Miniſters I am One, who have been a poor Preacher of the Goſpel in *Boſton* above Threeſcore Years, and am the moſt Aged, Weak and unworthy Miniſter now in *New-England*. My Sentiments, and my Son's alſo, about this *Matter* are well known. Alſo we hear that the Reverend and Learned Mr. *Solomon Stoddard* of *Northampton* concurs with us; ſo doth the Reverend Mr. *Wiſe* of *Ipſwich*, and many other younger Divines, not only in *Boſton*, but in the Country, joyn with their Fathers. Furthermore, I have made ſome Enquiry, Whether there are many Perſons of a Prophane Life and Converſation, that do Approve and Defend *Inoculation*, and I have been anſwered, that they know but of very few ſuch. This is to me a weighty Conſideration. But on the other hand, tho' there are ſome Worthy Perſons, that are not clear about it; nevertheleſs, it cannot be denied, but that the known Children of the Wicked one, are generally fierce Enemies to Inoculation. It is a grave ſaying of Old *Seneca*, *Peſſimi Argumentum Turba eſt.* For my part I ſhould be aſhamed to joyn with ſuch Perſons; *O my Soul come not thou into their Secret, unto their Aſſembly be not thou United.* I am far from reflecting upon all that are againſt *Inoculation*. I know there are very worthy Perſons (with whom I deſire to Live and Die) that are not clear in their Judgments for it, and they are greatly to be commended and honoured in that they will not act againſt a doubting Conſcience; yet it may be ſome of them might change their minds, if they would adviſe with thoſe who are beſt able to afford them Scripture Light in this as well as in other Caſes of Conſcience.

Novemb. 20. 1721.

That the Cauſe may have Two Witneſſes, here are ſubjoyned the Sentiments of another, well known in our Churches, of which I declare my hearty Approbation.

Sentiments on the Small Pox Inoculated.

A moſt Succeſsful, and Allowable Method of preventing Death, *and many other grievous Miſeries, by the* Small Pox, *is not only* Lawful *but a* Duty, *to be uſed by thoſe who apprehend their Lives immediately endanger'd by the terrible Diſtemper.*

But the Method of managing and governing the Small Pox *in the way of* Inoculation, *is a moſt ſucceſsful and allowable Method of preventing* Death, *and many other grievous Miſeries by this dreadful Diſtemper. Therefore, 'tis not only* Lawful, *but alſo*

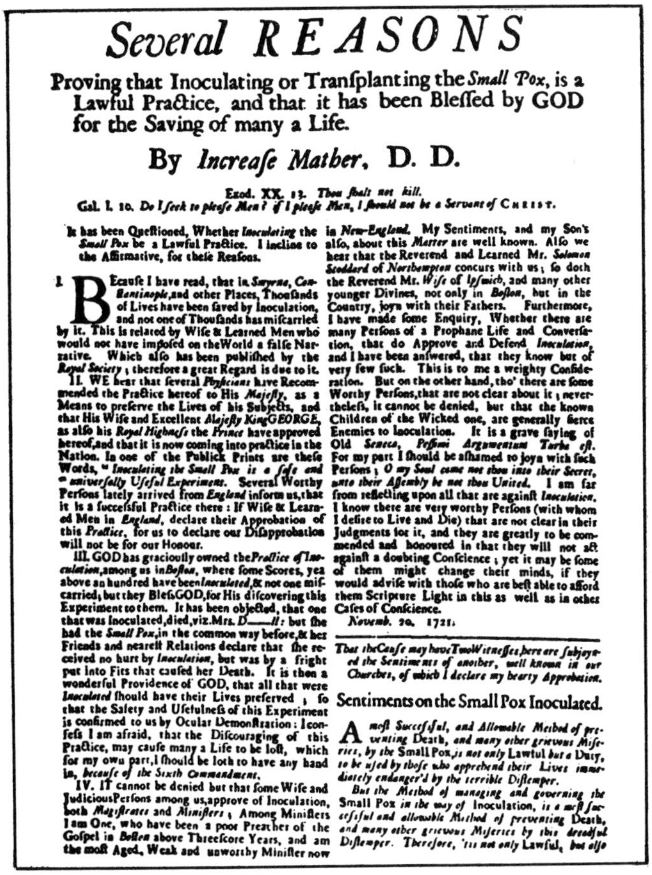

Figure 2–5. Increase Mather's support of inoculation (1721).

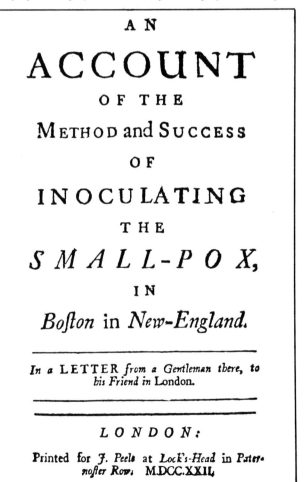

inoculation while most of the doctors opposed it (Fig. 2–5).

Douglass's attitude was that taken by most of the profession in the colonies, with the sole exception of Boylston. It was not until 1754 that the College of Physicians of London ventured to urge a general use of inoculation. However, general adoption of inoculation was never reached and its real value was always a matter of heated controversy.

Mather's position in American medicine becomes clearer when one considers both the number and scope of his medical writings. From the date of the first medical imprint in America in 1677 to 1724, the year Mather completed his *The Angel of Bethesda*, all the published medical works by Americans were limited to a few pamphlets. Save for Thacher's *Brief Rule* (1677), the only other American publication of a primarily medical nature prior to 1721 was Mather's own pamphlet of 1713 on measles. During 1721 and 1722, Mather published in Boston and London seven items dealing with smallpox inoculation. His *An Account of the Method and Success of Inoculating the Small-Pox*[37] was published in London in 1722 (Fig. 2–6). In 1724 he completed *The Angel of Bethesda*,[38] the first general treatise on medicine to be prepared in the English Colonies. In these terms, there was no parallel figure among American contemporaries.[28]

Even more significant than Mather's role in introducing smallpox inoculation in America was the reason he did so. He, alone among his fellow colonists, knew of and espoused the animalcular theory first postulated by Athanasius Kircher (1602–1680) in his *Scrutinium Physico-Medicum Contagiosae Luis, quae Pestis Dicitur* (1658), namely that the tiny "worms" seen in the blood under the microscope were the cause of infectious diseases. It remained for Louis Pasteur (1822–1895) to demonstrate the soundness

Figure 2–6. Title page of Cotton Mather's An Account of the Method and Success of Inoculating the Small-Pox *(1722). (Courtesy of the Countway Library of Medicine.)*

AN

ACCOUNT

OF THE

METHOD and SUCCESS

OF

INOCULATING

THE

SMALL-POX,

IN

Boſton in *New-England*.

In a LETTER *from a Gentleman there, to his Friend in* London.

LONDON:

Printed for *J. Peele* at *Lock's-Head* in *Pater-noſter Row*. MDCCXXII.

of this theory more than two centuries later. Mather[38] in *The Angel of Bethesda* suggested that these minute animals could corrupt the body and cause disease.

While New England suffered only periodically from smallpox, New York, New Jersey, and Pennsylvania were rarely free from this disease during any five-year period. The southern colonies were not affected quite so much during this period; this may be attributed to their scattered population and comparative isolation from the other sections of the country. The death of a ten-month-old infant girl named Mary Roche in Charleston, South Carolina, following inoculation performed on June 28, 1738, might be claimed, according to Joseph I. Waring (1897–1977),[53] as "the first infant of the country to achieve the distinction of recorded pediatric interest." James Killpatrick (c. 1700–1770),[34] an active advocate of inoculation who performed the operation, described the circumstances:

Miss Roche was about ten months old, a very hale plump child, and a hoarse pipe for an infant. I was consulted about her inoculation, and advised deferring it till the fall. . . . The Parents doubting this, and being urged by my colleague, Thomas Dale, M.D., to inoculate her at all events, it was performed the 28th of June [1738]. She sickened the 6th of July following, in a violent manner, took a little puke, which operated four times, and, a glyster which produced one free stool, after 48 hours costiveness. She was very tense and hot all night; it was impossible to open a vein: She took a drachm and half of Diacodium [an opiate], and had it repeated in better than an hour, which abated her fever and tension a little; but next morning everything was exasperated, and she expired suddenly in convulsions.

The controversy between Killpatrick and Dale was not on the propriety of inoculation but on the necessary preparation for the procedure. In his later work on inoculation, published in England, Killpatrick (by now calling himself Kirkpatrick) devoted seven pages to a discussion of the use of this measure in children.

Boston would have four more smallpox epidemics during the eighteenth century, each approaching major proportions: in 1729–1730, 1751–1752, 1764, and 1775–1776. An increasing number of residents would flee the city each time an epidemic struck, and of those who remained more were inoculated. This led to a decrease in the mortality from smallpox, but the danger of death from inoculation and its cost continued to deter many adults from taking the risk themselves or having their children inoculated.

One of the strongest advocates of inoculation was Benjamin Franklin, who had lost his four-year-old son in 1736 to smallpox; rumor had it that the boy's death had resulted from inoculation. Franklin, on hearing the rumor, immediately published an article in his newspaper, the *Pennsylvania Gazette*, denying it and reasserting his confidence in the practice of variolation (inoculation).

By 1780, however, it became evident that inoculation was not adequately controlling the incidence of smallpox, for the number of epidemics was actually increasing. There was need for a completely new and more effective method of control. The new method happened to be vaccination, established and popularized in 1798 by Edward Jenner (1749–1823).

Inoculation just was not good enough, and it could not be denied that wherever inoculation was used, and no matter how carefully, smallpox contagion would spread, and neither strict quarantine nor inoculation hospitals could avail. Another serious drawback was the increasingly elaborate preparation, with fees to match, and the longer recovery period that was required. The cost had risen until only a few could afford inoculation in either price or time. The poor and ignorant were almost entirely excluded.

With Jenner's[33] publication in 1798 of *An Inquiry into the Causes and Effects of Variolae Vaccinae*, describing twenty-three successful vaccinations, inoculation as a preventive measure against smallpox disappeared almost overnight. Since inoculation had a specific meaning, it was used to describe the technique utilizing smallpox virus, while vaccination was the descriptive term when cowpox was used.

Diphtheria

In May, 1735, at Kingston, New Hampshire, a strange throat distemper developed which was different from any disease with which the townspeople were familiar. They knew that measles and smallpox could spread among children, but this disease attacked here and there, "not according to the effects of contagion or qualities of the soil," and so was beyond their understanding. This vicious epidemic has long been accepted by medical historians as the beginning of unquestionable diphtheria in America.[10]

The epidemic raged most violently during the summer and fall of 1735. Twenty families buried all their children. Within one year the town of Hampton Falls, New Hampshire, was more than decimated by the epidemic of this "new disease" (210 died out of a population of about 1,200, and 95 percent of the victims were less than twenty years of age).

The same disease spread to Haverhill, Massachusetts, fifteen miles south of Kingston, in November, 1735. Haverhill, with a population of about 1,200 people, recorded 116 deaths in 1736 and 130 deaths in 1737 from this disease, 98 percent in children and youths under twenty years of age. The previous records of Haverhill showed about 10 deaths a year, so that the "throat distemper" caused a mortality of about 90 per 1,000 population. It was said that "more than half of the Haverhill children died."[10] At least sixty families lost two or more children; some of them lost four or five apiece. Twenty-three families were left childless.

The epidemic's horrible mortality led to bewilderment and fright. To colonial minds the sudden epidemic of what was considered a "new" disease that killed so many of their children seemed mysteriously disruptive of the natural process wherein the eldest die first.[48] The fierceness with which diphtheria struck led to bafflement and perturbation.

This epidemic of "throat distemper," unlike many other contagious diseases which usually subsided after having reached epidemic proportions, continued to break out sporadically in New England between 1735 and 1740, and out of a population of about two hundred thousand people, there were at least five thousand deaths. Except in an occasional town, one finds no evidence of any great confusion or the loss of self-control that people usually exhibit during great epidemics. Perhaps this apparent outward calm did not completely show the inner feelings of the people, but there is good reason to think that it did, because with complete faith in God—as is evident in many contemporary sermons and pamphlets—they did not question the meaning or justice of their misfortunes.

In retrospect, it appears that their emotions may have been only temporarily suppressed, for almost immediately following these five years of sickness and death, indeed so near in time that the causal connection might be suspected, there occurred a period of intense excitement—the great psychological and religious upheaval better known as the Great Awakening. At this period people still gave a religious interpretation to every event of their daily lives and still considered each adversity as a just punishment for sin. One finds surprisingly little evidence of bitterness or despair in their writings.[48]

Two minister-physicians played a significant role during the great "throat-distemper" epidemic. The first was the Reverend Jabez Fitch (1672–1746),[23] minister of the North Church in Portsmouth, New Hampshire. His pamphlet entitled *An Account of the Numbers That Have Died of the Distemper in the Throat, Within the Province of New Hampshire* (1736) was a commendable piece of scientific research and is of great epidemiological value, for not only does it give the total numbers that died in the various towns but also the deaths are grouped according to age. According to his estimate, nearly a thousand persons succumbed to the infection, and more than 80 percent were children under ten years of age. Fitch was particularly interested in the theological interpretation of his figures and when he found that the disease vented its fury upon the children he attributed it to "The Woful Effects of Original Sin."

The second minister-physician to make an important contribution to the history of diphtheria was the Reverend Jonathan Dickinson (1688–1747),[17] the first president of the College of New Jersey (now Princeton). Dickinson's *Observations on That Terrible Disease Vulgarly Called the Throat-Distemper* (1740), the second medical publication by a Yale graduate, is one of the few outstanding contributions to early American pediatrics. He clearly differentiated "a variety of types" of "throat-distemper"; he distinguished scarlet fever from diphtheria and was aware that the mortality from the latter was much greater than from the former disease. However, he, like William Douglass,[19] insisted that the various types of "throat-distemper" were different manifestations of one disease, which was naturally accompanied by a rash, and his intention was "to bring out the Eruption as soon as possible." Dickinson saw patients who had both diseases (scarlet fever and diphtheria) at different times and he thought they were second attacks of the same disease, although he added: "I have never seen any upon whom the Eruption could be brought out more than once."

The important facts as told by Dickinson were that an epidemic appeared in New Jersey in February, 1735/6; it was chiefly an epidemic of diphtheria. This epidemic was also complicated by the presence of scarlet fever; and, like the scarlet fever in New England, it was comparatively mild.

During the eighteenth century scarlet fever and diphtheria were almost always regarded as different manifestations of the same disease. Diphtheria came to be known as "canker" and scarlet fever as "canker rash," but during epidemics many cases of laryngeal diphtheria were seen and then the condition was often described as "canker quinsey."

Physicians explained the difference in the mortality of these two diseases in a clever way. Their theory was that the "distemper" was caused by some "morbifick matter" in the blood and that all one had to do was prescribe remedies that would allow the poisons to reach the skin surface, evaporate through the pores, and thus produce a rash ("canker rash"). If the rash was not "brought out," the mortality from the distemper ("canker") was noted to be greatly increased. In certain ways, this "morbifick matter" theory influenced kitchen medicine for generations and in isolated areas persists down to this day. Many of our grandmothers believed that some diseases were more serious "when the rash strikes inward" and this belief was the basis for that well-known treatment for measles which consisted of trying to "bring out a good rash" by warm baths and thereby rid the body of its "poisons."

The most important and complete description of the epidemic of "throat distemper" first appeared in the *Boston Gazette* and was copied by the publisher of the *New-York Gazette* (Feb. 17–24, 1735/6).[10] Although it was originally published in Boston, the unknown writer said that his description also applied to the New Hampshire epidemic:

No Disease has never raved [sic] in *New-England* (except the Small-Pox) which has struck such a universal Terror into People, as that which has lately visited *Kingston, Exeter, Hampton* and other Parts of the Province of *New-Hampshire*, and tho' something has been divers Times said of it in the publick News Papers, it yet wants a Name. It has been among young People and Children, pretty universal and very mortal; but what surprizes me most is, that the Physicians in those Parts (altho' their bad Success evidently shews that they have no manner of Notion of the Nature of the Disease or Method of Cure)

yet persist in one invariable Method to kill very successfully, *secundem Artem*. This Disease invades generally such as are very young, but they feel at the first somewhat listless and heavy for a Day or two, and then begin to complain of a Soreness in the Throat, and if you look into the Motion you'l discover upon the Uvula and Parts adjacent the Cuticula raised in Spots of different Sizes, sometimes to a quarter of an Inch Diameter, and fill'd with a laudable coloured Pus. This is the pathognomonick Sign of the Disease. In a Day or two more, they have the same Cough as in the common humorous Quinzey; the next Day a Fever rises, and the Cough is often between whiles very loose; the Patient now begins to breath hard, and almost loses his Voice, being able only to whisper; and a Day more makes (with Coughing) only a whistling kind of Noise, and the next Day pays his Debt to Nature. These are the different Stages of the Disease, which, as the Disease is more or less fierce, are longer or shorter. . . .

This article, which appeared at about the same time as Douglass's[19] account of the Boston epidemic (which was scarlet fever and not diphtheria), not only established the diagnosis of the New Hampshire epidemic, but also was the first printed description of unquestionable diphtheria to appear in America.[10]

It was said in traditional colonial folktales that during the Kingston epidemic, "Children while sitting up at play would fall and expire with their playthings in their hands."[10] This is an accurate, concise textbook description of a late complication of diphtheria that could still be found in some American textbooks of pediatrics published in the 1920's or 1930's. For example, the 1921 edition of Holt and Howland's[29] textbook *Diseases of Infancy and Childhood* contained this comment: "Sudden heart failure may be seen late in diphtheria. . . . It may occur with few or no premonitory symptoms; as when a child falls dead after walking across a room, or suddenly sitting up in bed, or from some other muscular effort, or possibly as a consequence of passion or excitement. We knew of one little girl who was considered well enough to go coasting and who died suddenly after the effort."

In 1771 Samuel Bard (1742–1821)[2] published his *Angina Suffocativa* as a result of his studies of a virulent epidemic of diphtheria in New York City in the early 1770's (Fig. 2–7). Osler[45] considered this book "an American medical classic of the first rank." Abraham Jacobi (1830–1919)[32] considered Bard's

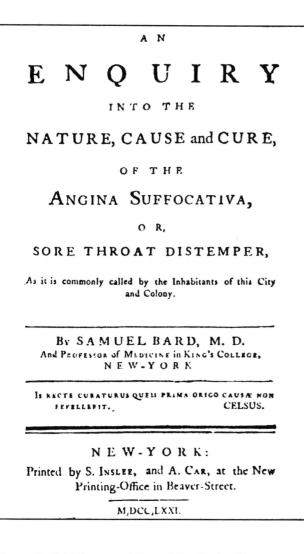

A N

E N Q U I R Y

IN TO THE

NATURE, CAUSE and CURE,

OF THE

ANGINA SUFFOCATIVA,

O R,

SORE THROAT DISTEMPER,

As it is commonly called by the Inhabitants of this City and Colony.

By SAMUEL BARD, M. D.
And Professor of Medicine in King's College,
NEW-YORK

Is recte curaturus quem prima origo causæ non fefellerit. CELSUS.

NEW-YORK:
Printed by S. Inslee, and A. Car, at the New Printing-Office in Beaver-Street.

M,DCC,LXXI.

Figure 2–7. Title page of Samuel Bard's An Enquiry into the Nature, Cause and Cure, of the Angina Suffocativa, or Sore Throat Distemper *(1771).*

little book to be among the calmest, wisest, and most accurate ever written on diphtheria, both before and during his time. Bard clearly described the various forms of pharyngeal diphtheria; his observations on cutaneous diphtheria are accurate, and his historical review of diphtheria is sound.

Bard had the foresight to believe that diseases described by others under different names were in fact the same diseases, i.e. *angina suffocativa*, or diphtheria:*

Upon the whole, I am led to conclude that the *morbus*

* In the eighteenth century diphtheria was also known as garrotillo, phlegmone anginosa, and aphthae malignae, especially in Europe. The term diphtheria (diphthérite) was first suggested by Bretonneau in 1826 (p. 22).

strangulatorius of the Italians, the croup of Dr. Home, the malignant ulcerous sore-throat of Huxham and Fothergill, and the disease I have described . . . however they may differ in symptoms, do all bear an essential affinity and relation to each other; or are apt to run into each other, and, in fact, arise from the same lever. The disease I have described appeared evidently to be of an infectious nature, and being drawn in by the breath of a healthy child, irritated the glands of the throat and wind-pipe. The infection did not seem to depend so much on any prevailing disposition of the air, as upon effluvia received from the breath of infected persons. This will account why the disorder sometimes went through a whole family, and yet did not affect the next-door neighbors. Here we learn a useful lesson, viz.: to remove young children as soon as any one of them is taken with the disease, by which many lives have been saved and may again be preserved. . . .

Bard's[2] description of diphtheria reveals the clarity and modernity of his style:

In general, this disease was confined to children under ten years old. . . . Most of those who had it were observed to droop for several days before they were confined. . . . At the same time, or very soon after, such as could speak, complained of an uneasy sensation in the throat, but without any great soreness or pain. Upon examining the tonsils or *almonds*, appeared swelled and slightly inflamed, with a few white specks upon them, which, in some, increased as to cover them all over with a general slough, and in a few the swelling was so great, as almost to close up the passage of the throat. . . .

These symptoms, with a slight fever at night, occurred in some for five or six days, without affecting their friends; in others a difficulty of breathing came on within twenty-four hours, especially in the time of sleep, and was often suddenly increased to so great a degree as to threaten immediate suffocation. In general, however, it came on later, increased more gradually, and was not constant; but the patient would now and then enjoy an interval of an hour or two, in which he breathed with ease, and then again a laborious breathing would ensue, during which he seemed incapable of filling his lungs, as if the air was drawn through a too narrow passage.

This stage of the disease was attended with a very great and sudden prostration of strength; a very remarkable dry cough; and a peculiar change in the tone of the voice; not easily described, but so singular, that a person who had once heard it, could almost certainly know the disease again by hearing the patient cough or speak. . . . A constant fever attended this disease, but it was much more remarkable in the night than in the day time; and in some there was a remarkable remission towards morning. . . .

Lionel Chalmers (1715–1777),[13] a Scotsman who had emigrated to South Carolina, wrote in his *An Account of the Weather and Diseases of South-Carolina* (1776) that "an *angina* resembling that which is called putrid, appears now and then amongst us, but never *epidemically* that I have observed." He had noticed that it usually affected children under ten or twelve years of age. Despite his statement, he described an epidemic occurring in the fall of 1770 as having all the characteristics of the "throat disease." Most of the patients described by Chalmers had an inflammation of the throat and tonsils, which gradually became ulcerated; the voice would become hoarse, and when the infection spread down to the glottis the patient almost always died. Chalmer's description of epidemics of diphtheria in South Carolina were almost identical with those emanating from New England.

One of the primary concerns of Chalmer's *Account*[13] was with the weather as a cause of disease, but his two-volume work covered a wide variety of medical conditions, among them a large number relating to children. For this reason he deserves a prominent place in eighteenth-century American pediatrics. Waring[53] believed that Chalmer's "book gave more direct attention to pediatric problems than any other American work of the 18th century."

Chalmer's text was based entirely on his own personal experience. He considered acidity to be the root of all evil in childhood and directed his treatments to "correct" this condition. He was less enthusiastic about bloodletting than was Rush, reserving it for a few conditions such as "suffocative or catarrhal peripneumony." Purging, vomiting, and blistering were his chief remedies.

Scarlet Fever

Brief references to an epidemic of scarlet fever in Boston between September and December, 1702, can be found in the diaries of John Marshall and Cotton Mather; this epidemic occurred concurrently with the Boston smallpox outbreak of 1702.

Cotton Mather[35] in a letter to Samuel Penhallow wrote: "My Daughter Katy [1689–1716] is yesterday taken Dangerously and Violently sick of the Scarlet Feavour and were with much Care and Fear waiting the Event of the Sickness. My next Daughter, was taken ill of the same Distemper, at the same Time, and, my only son [Increase (1699–1724)], who has been longer down is yett very ill of it."

The next major epidemic of scarlet fever occurred in 1735, but it was then described as a "new disease" by the doctors in New England, largely because they confused it with the virulent epidemic of diphtheria which occurred at the same time. Douglass[19] in his *The Practical History of a New Epidemical Eruptive Miliary Fever, with an Angina Ulcusculosa* (1736), described a disease which he claimed was a new one, yet his decription of a "new epidemical eruptive fever" was, according to Weaver, "the first adequate clinical description of scarlet fever in English and probably in any language; . . . it stands as the first real important work on the disease."[54] Douglass's account was published twelve years before John Fothergill (1712–1780),[24] the English physician, issued his classic account of both diphtheria and scarlatinal angina, although Fothergill failed to differentiate between the two conditions.

Douglass[19] wrote:

The first attack is somewhat of a *chill* or shivering; soon after follows *Head ake* or some other versatile *spasmodick pains*, as pain in the back, joints, side etc; a vomiting or nausea, or in some constitutions, which are not easily provoked to vomit, only a certain uneasiness or sickness at Stomach; at the same time the *Uvula*, but chiefly the Tonsils, were tumified, inflamed and painful, with some white specks, then follows a flush in the Face and some *miliary eruptions* therewith a benign *mild fever*, the same efflorescence soon after appears on the neck, chest and extremities; the 3rd or 4th Day, Eruption is at the hight and well defined with fair intervals; the flushing goes off gradually with a general *itching*; and in a Day or two more the *cuticle* scales or peels off, especially in the extremities: At the same time the cream coloured sloughs or specks in the *Fauces* become loose and [are] cast off. . . . The tongue from the beginning is furr'd as in a *Mercurial Ptyalism*, urine high coloured . . . in the whole course of the Distemper [there is] a very *great prostration* of strength and faintness . . . [and a] loss of *en bon point*. As in the Measles there is a peculiar smell, so in our Distemper the *effluvia* from the Patient have a proper smell; in children as if troubled with *Worms*, in grown Persons the rancid smell of foul Bed Linnen.

This is a Real History of the distemper as *it appeared in Boston New-England*, taken clinically from the life and not copied. There is no stroak or cause but which I can vouch by real not imaginary cases. It is founded only upon observations, . . . that is upon the Symptoms that appeared in the course of this Epidemical disease, it must therefore be of permanent truth.

Douglass[19] was certain that the two epidemics, the one in New Hampshire, and the other in Boston, were caused by the same "new" disease. Medical historians agree that the Boston epidemic was a single disease, but they differ in the diagnosis. Caulfield[10] and Charles Creighton (1847–1927)[15] considered this to be the first great epidemic of scarlet fever in this country. Others, such as Abraham Jacobi[32] and Francis R. Packard (1870–1950),[43] thought it was diphtheria.

Between 1735 and 1770 there were few records of even isolated cases of scarlet fever, but during the last quarter of the century the disease became increasingly common; during these years there were records of numerous epidemics as well as a few excellent clinical descriptions. Among the latter was Chalmers's[13] account of an epidemic in Georgia and South Carolina in 1770. He described what seemed to him to be an alarming disease with chills, fever, vomiting, delirium, sore throat, and a scarlet rash followed by desquamation and painful, swollen extremities [?joints]. Most of the patients recovered.

Benjamin Rush[46a] described a widespread epidemic of scarlet fever, which he termed *scarlatina anginosa*, that occurred in Philadelphia in the years 1783 and 1784:

The month of September [1783] was cool and dry, and the scarlatina anginosa became epidemic among adults as well as young people. In most of the patients who were affected by it, it came on with a chilliness and a sickness at the stomach, or a vomiting; which last was so invariably present, that it was with me a pathognomonic sign of the disease. The matter discharged from the stomach was always bile. The swelling of the throat was, in some instances so great, as to produce a difficulty of speaking, swallowing, and breathing. In a few instances, the speech was accompanied by a squeaking voice, resembling that which attends the cynanche trachealis [diphtheria]. The ulcers on the tonsils were deep, and covered with white, and in some instances, with black sloughs. In several cases there was a discharge of thick mucus from the nose, from the beginning, but it oftener occurred in the decline of the disease, which most frequently happened on the fifth day. Sometimes the subsiding of the swelling of the throat was followed by a swelling behind the ears.

An eruption of the skin generally attended the symp-

toms. . . . This symptom appeared with considerable variety. In some people it preceded, and in other followed the ulcers and swelling of the throat. . . .

The disease frequently went off with a swelling of the hands and feet . . . during the decline of the disease.

Rush's treatment of this disease was characteristic of the period. He began "the cure with a vomit joined with calomel." The "vomit was either tartar emetic or ipecacuanha" and the throat was "kept clean by detergent gargles." Rush also advised that "in cases of great difficulty of swallowing, the patients found relief from receiving the steams of warm water mixed with a little vinegar, through a funnel into the throat." He also noted that "a perspiration kept up by gentle doses of antimonials and diluting drinks impregnated with wine, always gave relief." But if the patient was not better in three days, "I applied a blister behind each ear or one to the neck, and I think, always with good effects."

In an additional report on *scarlatina anginosa* Rush claimed that "camphor suspended in a bag from the neck, as a preservative against this disease . . . possesses little or no efficacy for this purpose. . . . I have had reason to entertain a more favorable opinion of the benefit of washing the hands and face with vinegar and of rinsing the mouth and throat with vinegar and water every morning, as a means of preventing this disorder."

Measles

A widespread and severe epidemic of measles occurred in the colonies during the years 1713–1716; this was the first big epidemic since that of 1687–1688. All other descriptions of the epidemic, which struck Boston in October, 1713, are overshadowed by Cotton Mather's[35] melancholy account of the distress in his own household: *"October 18, 1713. The Measles coming into the Town, it is likely to be a Time of Sickness and much Trouble in the Families of the Neighbourhood."* Every member of the household caught the disease except Mather himself, who probably had come down with measles during the 1687–1688 epidemic, the last one to strike Boston prior to the 1713–1716 epidemic. Of the seven adult cases mentioned in the Mather and Sewall diaries, four were fatal.

A summary of the entries in Mather's[35] diary between *October 18, 1713,* and *November 21, 1713,* makes one aware of the virulence of measles in the colonial period:

October 17, 1713. Increase Mather, fourteen years old, began to have symptoms of measles but recovered after being moderately sick.

October 27. Nibby, the nineteen-year-old daughter, very ill with measles.

October 30. Mrs. Mather gave birth to twins. Katy, the twenty-four-year-old daughter, became sick but recovered after a very severe illness lasting thirteen days.

November 4. Mrs. Mather down with measles: Nanny, a sixteen-year-old daughter, sick; Lizzy, a nine-year-old daughter, very sick; daughter Jerusha, two and a half years old, became ill.

November 5. A son, Samuel, seven years old, taken with a case of average severity. The maid was very sick with measles.

November 7. "Not only are my children, with a servant, lying sick, but also my consort is in dangerous condition and can get no rest. Either Death, or Distraction is much feared for her."

November 9. Mrs. Mather, "My dear, dear, dear Friend expired." She died "between 3 and 4 in the afternoon."

November 14. The maid died with "malignant Feavor." "'Tis a Satisfaction to me, that tho' she had been a wild, vain, airy Girl, yett since her coming into my Family, she became disposed unto serious Religion."

November 17. "Little Eleazer," one of the twins, died "about midnight"—eighteen days old.

November 20. "Little Martha," the other twin, died "about ten o'clock A.M."—twenty-one days old.

November 21. "My lovely Jerusha died on her 17th day of illness, between 9 h. and 10 h. at Night."

In spite of all his domestic tragedies, Mather, at the height of the epidemic, not only preached a number of sermons but on December 23, 1713, gave to the printer a short manuscript entitled *A Letter about the Right Management of the Sick under the Distemper of the Measles.* Mather[36] said of this *Letter:* "I purpose to scatter it into all parts, and propose with the Blessing of Heaven, to save many Lives. Tho' doubtless my action may dispose me to some Invectives."

Mather modeled his *Letter* after Thacher's *Brief Rule,* and in it he outlined the symptoms, complications, and treatment of the disease. Although written for the lay person, it happens to be one of the classics of American pediatrics and compares favorably with any eighteenth-century European description of measles.[11]

The *Measles* are a Distemper which in *Europe* ordinarily proves a light Malady: but in these parts of *America* it proves a very heavy Calamity; a Malady *Grievous* to most, *Mortal* to many, and leaving pernicious Relicks behind it in All. Because the Sickness is now spreading in all Parts; and its *Malignity* increases, as the *Winter* advances, and *Good Physicians* are not every where at Hand, for the Relief of the Sick, and a very *nice Management* of the Case is very requisite: You are now addressed with a short Letter of Advice concerning it. . . .

The Unusual Symptoms of an *Arrest* from the *Measles* are, an *Head-ake;* or Troubles in the *Eyes;* a Dry *Cough;* an Oppression on the *Breast* or *Stomach;* or a pain there, and in the *Back* and *Limbs;* and sometimes a *Faintness,* with *Sickness,* perhaps *Vomiting,* or *Griping* and *Purging;* A *Thirst,* with a constant Fever, which is mild at first, but grows high enough before it has done. . . .

If a *Cough* continue, then fly to the usual Remedies. To take a Spoonful of shavings of *Castile Soap* in a Glass of Wine or Beer, for a few Nights following, has been very successful for the cure of that Inconvenience. If a *Flux* follow, whether a *common,* or a *Bloody,* a *Tea* made of *Rhubarb,* and sweetened with a Syrup of *Marshmallows,* given daily, so much as to cause one or two Stools, is a way to carry it safely off. The same *Tea* will also carry off the *Worms,* that so often follow the *Measles;* especially in *Children.*

A Purge would be necessary for all that would not have Venome of the *Measles* remaining in them, and follow'd with many Evil Consequences.

A *Fever,* (perhaps that which they call, *The Pleuretick*) too often follows the *Measles.* But for this, I do not now offer any Directions. A skillful *Physician* must be consulted withal. . . .

Colonial epidemics of measles had a few characteristics not often seen today. Although no statistics revealing the age of the patient or the incidence of the disease have been located, it is certain that many adult cases occurred. In most of the epidemics it was not unusual to find fathers and mothers having the disease along with their children.

Whooping Cough (Chincough)

In the seventeenth century, and also in the eighteenth, whooping cough was commonly called chincough. Save for the reference to an extensive epidemic of it in 1659 in John Hull's diary (p. 23), no mention of it on such a scale occurred until 1738, when an epidemic broke out in South Carolina. Three epidemics of whooping cough took place in that colony, and in each outbreak all age groups were affected.

Chalmers[13] gave an excellent description of these epidemics of whooping cough in his *An Account of the Weather and Diseases of South-Carolina* (1776). Although Guillaume de Baillou (1538–1616) described an epidemic of whooping cough that occurred in 1578, as did Thomas Willis (1621–1675) in 1675, neither of their descriptions was as succinct as Chalmers's:

Though the *hooping-cough* be not *epidemick* of this climate, but is brought hither from other parts, its approach having always been heard of before it appeared amongst us, I have given it a place in this essay, as perhaps, somewhat new may be said of that dangerous and obstinate complaint. In the space of twenty-six years this disease was *epidemick* here at three different times; twenty-one years elapsing between its first [1738] and second appearance [1759] . . . and a little more than five years between the second and third; when like most contagious disorders, it did not spare any one who had not passed through it before. . . . [This may have been the first major epidemic of whooping cough in the colonies.]

This disease, commonly begins with a frequent but dry cough; nor have the patients *that running* at the nose, *snuffling* or hoarseness, which often ensues from catching cold. The *coughing* by degrees holds longer, and becomes so severe in a few days, that the sick scarcely have time to breathe during the fits. For so *spasmodically* affected are the lungs and their appendages, that one interrupted act of *violent expiration* continues, till the patient, being ready to be stifled, is obliged to fetch breath with all his might, in spite of the convulsed condition of these organs. . . .

The cough however does not cease with one or two such vehement efforts to breathe. For, as the fit may continue for the space of a minute or longer, the patient will be obliged to exert several such forcible inspirations, before the coughing ceases; nor will *this* be, till more or less of *viscid* phlegm is brought up; and only so far does a vomiting contribute to the paroxysm, by assisting in the expulsion of the *mucus.* When the fit is over, the person pants and is almost lifeless for a while, as being in a manner spent with the violent exercise he had undergone.

From the shrill or hollow sort of noise, that is made by the rushing of the air into the aperture of the windpipe, which is now convulsively constricted, the disease hath the name of *hooping-cough.* . . .

Chalmers wrote that the use of *"balsamics* and *pectorals"* were "without any advantage; oily and other relaxants rather did harm, and *opiates* alone were of but little use. For though I indiscreetly stupified some patients, *they* nevertheless coughed as often and severely when overwhelmed with sleep as if nothing at all had been given." Despite their lack of significant therapeutic value, he advised that "for an infant three or four months old, one *drachm* of spirit of *hartshorn,* as much *tincture* of *cantharides,* five or six drops of *laudanum,* and about twenty drops of *essence* of *antimony* should be mixt together, of which five or more drops may be given every second hour or oftener with a little warm tea."

Mumps

Epidemics of mumps were rarely mentioned prior to the mid-eighteenth century, although the disease was known in this country at least as early as May, 1699, when John Marshall[22] of Braintree wrote in his diary: "I did not hear of any great matter which happened: only we had severall sick with an unusual distemper called the mumps of which some were bad. But none dyed that I heard of."

According to Chalmers,[13] there were epidemics of "serious Quinsey," or mumps, in South Carolina in 1744 and 1768. Rush[46] mentioned epidemics of "cynanche parotidea" in Philadelphia during the winter of 1786–1787. Save for his erroneous inclusion of swollen axillary and inguinal nodes as common manifestations of mumps, Chalmers's otherwise excellent account described the involvement of the testicles and the permanent immunity resulting from the initial attack of mumps. His was the only clinical account of this disease in English prior to 1790, when Robert Hamilton's (1721–1793)[27] account of the occurrence of an epidemic of mumps was published in Scotland.

Chalmers[13] wrote:

It commonly attacks with more or less fever, and presently a swelling will be perceived under the chin, which continues to increase for a few days, so as to extend itself sometimes from the temples quite to the clavicles, and all around the neck; but the greatest swelling happens mostly, across the throat from one ear to the other, projecting outwards, in a manner that much deforms the patient. The danger, however, is not great; for I never heard of one person dying of this complaint. In general, *degluti-*

tion is but little obstructed; for the *uvula* and *tonsils* are seldom so much enlarged as the other glands, that lie within the mouth, or in the forepart of the neck; but the patient hath some pain in opening his jaws. Yet, large as this tumour may be, the colour of the skin is rarely changed; nor is there any extraordinary heat or acute pain in the part when it is touched, as happens when the sanguiferous vessels are obstructed . . . it also appears that those who have once passed through it, escape it for the future. . . .

He recommended that

some blood must be taken away, if the patient be strong and the fever high; and there may even be necessity for repeating this operation when the *testicles* are inflamed. . . . The mouth and throat should often be gargled with mustard whey, to which a few drops of spirits of hartshorn or of *sal ammoniacum* ought to be added when it is used, in order to promote a discharge from the *salivary* gland; and other *apophlegmatizers* may also be tried at times. Every six hours, the swellings must be fomented with a decoction either of *camomile flowers, fennel, wormwood,* or some other moderately warm plant made with water; to each quart of which two ounces of brandy, and one hundred drops of the spirit of *sal ammoniacum* ought to be added, when it is used. Covering the parts afterwards with a poultice made with same liquor and *oatmeal* or *crumb* of *bread.*

Benjamin Rush and Pediatrics

To the three thousand doctors he trained, Benjamin Rush remained an inspiring example, and he was generally considered the ablest American clinician of his time; he probably had more influence on American medicine than any other single man.[44] He was a close friend of Benjamin Franklin and was one of the five physicians who signed the Declaration of Independence (the other four were Josiah Bartlett (1729–1795) and Matthew Thornton (1714–1803) of New Hampshire; Oliver Wolcott (1726–1797) of Connecticut; and Lyman Hall (1724–1790) of Georgia).

Of Rush's many contributions to pediatrics, John Ruhräh (1872–1935),[45] among others, considered his paper *An Inquiry into the Causes and Cure of Cholera Infantum* (1777) the most important, because he was the first writer to give anything like a systematic account of this serious disease and to connect its appearance with that of hot weather in various locations. Summers in Philadelphia were often unbear-

ably hot, so much so that it led the French statesman and diplomat Talleyrand to remark, "At each inhaling of air, one worries about the next." In Philadelphia during Rush's time, the disease was called "the vomiting and purging of children," and from the regularity of its appearance in the summer months it was also known as the "disease of the season."[44] It is indeed curious that the diarrheal diseases of children received so little attention until the mid-nineteenth century, for the mortality in children from the "fluxes" and "summer complaints" was enormous during the entire colonial period. Those who did write about diarrhea in children ascribed its cause to various things; an "acid condition" was one of the favorites.

As Rush[46] described cholera infantum:

It prevails in most of the large towns of the United States. It is distinguished in Charlestown, in South Carolina, by the name of "the April and May disorder," from making its first appearance in those two months. It seldom appears in Philadelphia till the middle of June, or the beginning of July, and generally continues till near the middle of September. Its frequency and danger are always in proportion to the heat of the weather. It affects children from the first or second week after their birth, till they are two years old. It sometimes begins with a diarrhoea, which continues for several days without any other symptom of indisposition; but it more frequently comes on with a violent vomiting and purging, and a high fever. The matter discharged from the stomach and bowels is generally yellow or green, but the stools are sometimes slimy and bloody, without any tincture of bile. In some instances they are nearly as limpid as water.

Rush's[46] treatment of cholera infantum was learned and practiced by medical students and physicians even as late as the beginning of this century. It consisted of first evacuating "the bile from the stomach and bowels . . . by gentle doses of ipecacuanha, or tartar emetic. The bowels should be opened by means of manna, castor oil, or magnesia." But "in those cases, where there is reason to believe that the offending contents of the *primae viae* have been discharged by nature, (which is often the case) the emetics and purges should by no means be given; but, instead of them, recourse must be had to opiates. A few drops of liquid laudanum combined in a testaceous julip, with pepper-mint or cinnamon-water would soothe the stomach and bowels." He further advised the use of "demulcent and diluting drinks" because they "have an agreeable effect in this disease. Mint and mallow teas, or a tea made of blackberry roots infused in cold water, together with a decoction of the shavings of hartshorn and gum arabic with cinnamon, should all be given in their turns for this purpose."

To alleviate the tenesmus and abdominal pain associated with cholera infantum he recommended "glysters made of flaxseed tea, or of mutton broth, or of starch dissolved in water, with a few drops of liquid laudanum in them" because they "give ease, and produce other useful effects." And he also had found that "plasters of Venice treacle applied to the region of the stomach, and flannels dipped in infusions of bitter and aromatic herbs in warm spirits, or madeira wine, and applied to the region of the abdomen" would often "afford considerable relief."

Of interest to the modern pediatrician, keenly aware of the fluid and electrolyte losses in diarrheal disease in infants, would be this comment by Rush: "I have seen my children recover from being gratified in an inclination to eat salted fish, or the different kinds of salted meats" (to correct hyponatremia?).

Rush[46] did not believe—as did most of his contemporaries—that dentition, worms, or summer fruits caused cholera infantum, nor was he impressed with the value of the remedies prescribed for this condition:

After all that has been said in favor of the remedies that have been mentioned, I am sorry to add, that I have very often seen them all administered without effect. My principal dependence, therefore, for many years, has been placed upon Country air. . . . Where the convenience of the constant benefit of country air cannot be obtained, I have seen evident advantages from taking children out of the city once or twice a day. It is extremely agreeable to see the little sufferers revive, as soon as they escape from the city air, and inspire the pure air of the country.

Sources of Pediatric Information for Colonial Parents

Almanacs

The scarcity of colonial medical practitioners led to the widespread popularity of almanacs containing medical material. Almost seventeen hundred almanacs are known to have been printed before 1783; o these over five hundred contained medical informa tion, much of it of pediatric interest.[25] These alma nacs had tremendous influence because they founc their way into the remotest homes and supplied a reading public which could not be reached by eithei medical or general literature, or even by the newspapers.[50] Since there was no continuous American newspaper before 1704 (the Boston News-Letter) and no American magazine before 1741 (the American Magazine), the colonial almanac served a dual literary purpose: topical items were blended with informative and entertaining essays, stories, and verse. The almanac was the earliest consecutive colonial publication, preceding the newspaper by almost seventy years, and its influence completely overshadowed that of any other publication of this period.[26]

For all but a few American colonists, the almanac was the only secular source of useful information about many things, including medicine. Cotton Mather avowed that "such an anniversary compiler comes into almost as many hands as the best of books" (the Bible). In Massachusetts, for example, eighty almanacs made up four-fifths of the secular literature published there before 1700. In sheer quantity, almanac publications during the seventeenth and eighteenth centuries actually outnumbered all other books combined, including religious ones.[25]

In these almanacs parents would often find a host of suggested cures for the common infectious diseases which plagued the colonial child. For example, there were many essays on smallpox, on inoculation for it, and on premedication techniques for inoculation. One of the best presentations on pediatrics appeared in Poor Richard's Almanack for 1763, in which space was given to several excerpts from Theophilus Lobb's (1678–1763) Directions for the Management of Children in Health; and with an Account of the Distempers Common to Them. These excerpts also appeared in Hutchins's Almanack for 1778.[26] Articles on infant nursing were popular almanac items; especially popular were long excerpts from William Cadogan's (1711–1797) An Essay upon Nursing (1748).[9]

Books on Domestic Medicine

In addition to almanacs as a source of medical information, books on domestic medicine, or do-it-your-

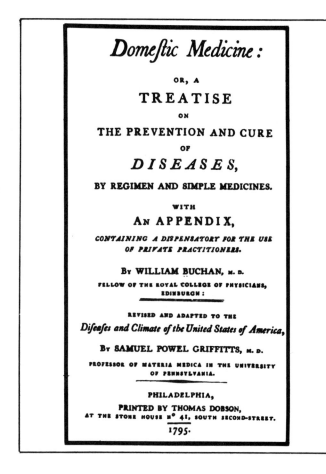

Figure 2–8. Title page of William Buchan's Domestic Medicine, *first American edition (1795).*

self handbooks, were extremely popular in an America desperately short of professionals. One of the favorites was William Buchan's (1729–1805)[8] *Domestic Medicine: or, The Family Physician,* a comprehensive book on health care that was first published in Edinburgh in 1769 (Fig. 2–8). Buchan qualified in medicine in Edinburgh and became director of the Foundling Hospital at Ackworth, Yorkshire, in 1759, which accounts for his emphasis upon pediatric care. His book went through over twenty British editions and there were at least fourteen American editions running well into the nineteenth century.

In the eighteenth century people doctored one another much more extensively than they do today. For many, Buchan's *Domestic Medicine* was their textbook. His therapy was moderate for the time and he stressed that the role of medicine was to "gradually assist nature in removing the cause of the disease." He gave practical advice on the twelve pediatric problems which he believed would be most frequently encountered: thrush, acidities, galling and excoriation, stoppage of the nose, vomiting, looseness, eruptions, croup or hives, teething, rickets, convulsions, and water in the head.

Another do-it-yourself medical book, also with a wide American audience, was the Reverend John Wesley's (1703–1791)[55] *Primitive Physick,* which went through thirty-two English and seven American editions between 1747 and 1829. Wesley was the founder of Methodism and had spent two years as a missionary in Georgia between 1735 and 1737. Although he included a few of the esoteric eighteenth-century remedies, Wesley advised his readers against excessive bloodletting and powerful drugs, a caution that probably helped the sale of his book. Another reason, perhaps, for the book's widespread distribution was that it enabled the patient to save medical fees. Wesley was not enamored of the medical profession and strongly advised his followers to "consult only godly doctors if they could be found."

Wesley offered a number of reasons for writing the book; the two chief ones were to rescue mankind (including children) "from the jaws of destruction" and to prevent them "from pining away in sickness and pain either through the ignorance or dishonor of physicians." He claimed that his book was the only one available which "contains only safe, and cheap, and easy medicines." Wesley was intensely opposed to the "compounding and recompounding [of] too many ingredients in the same prescription." He believed that "experience shows that one thing will cure most disorders at least as well as twenty put together. Then why do you need nineteen? Only to swell the apothecary's bill. Nay, possibly on purpose, to prolong the distemper, that the doctor and he may divide the spoil."

One wonders how effective were some of Wesley's pediatric prescriptions. For example, to treat childhood convulsions he advised parents to "scrape piony roots, fresh digged. Apply what you have scraped off to the soles of the feet." And for jaundice he recommended that parents "take half an ounce of fine rhubarb, powdered, mix with it thoroughly, by long beating, two handfuls of good well cleansed currants. Of this give a tea-spoonful every morning."

From the year 1704, when publication of the *Boston News-Letter* began, to the end of the century, more than two hundred titles of newspapers appeared—most of them printed in English, though a small number were printed in German and even a smaller number in French.[25] With few exceptions colonial newspapers published items of medical interest. Some included essays on the prevention and treatment of disease. Other items frequently published were reports of epidemics with detailed information on the number and location of cases and measures calculated to prevent their spread; such coverage was especially comprehensive in the case of smallpox, the scourge so dreaded by colonial Americans. By reading these newspapers it is possible to date the establishment of medical societies, trace the beginnings of medical education by private practitioners, pinpoint the exact dates for the inception of medical teaching in Philadelphia, New York, and other cities, follow the spread of epidemics, and identify the patent medicines available for sale.

Drug advertisements were surprisingly frequent and appeared in the vast majority of these early newspapers.[25] For example, the *Boston News-Letter* for October 4, 1708, contained an advertisement for "DAFFY'S" Elixir Salutis, "very good, at four shillings and six pence *per* half pint bottle." Daffy's Elixir, one of the scores of British-made patent medicines with which our colonial ancestors dosed themselves and their children, was a compound senna tincture that had been concocted about 1650 by a British clergyman. Patent medicines containing opium, meant to be given to children, were also widely advertised. Through newspaper advertisements one even learns that wet-nursing was not uncommon in colonial America (p. 56).

Newspapers were also the prime source of information, even more so than almanacs, of the signs, symptoms, complications, and treatment of childhood illnesses. Of course, much of the therapy recommended was wrong, such as the use of calomel and rhubarb for rickets, advocated in the *Royal American Magazine* (Boston) in 1774. But many of the descriptions of the signs and symptoms of the common diseases of colonial children were just as accurate as those found in the standard medical texts of the period.

Accidents and Common Diseases of Eighteenth Century American Children

Accidents

Descriptions of childhood accidents occurred frequently in colonial diaries. For example, Mather's diary[35] contained many descriptions of accidents that happened to his children. One of them was the following: *"August 30, 1713.* Two of my Children, Cresy and Lizzie, have newly been scorched with Gunpowder, wherein tho's they have received a non-merciful Deliverance, especially of their Eyes, yett they undergo a Smart that is considerable."

Elizabeth Sandwith Drinker (1734–1807)[21] wrote in her diary that her fifth child, Henry (b. 1770), "fell into the river this afternoon [August 30, 1780] and after a quarter of an hour remaining in wet clothes, came home very cold and coughing. We stript him, and after rubbing him well with a coarse towel, put on warm dry clothes, gave him some rum and water to drink and made him jump a rope till he sweated."

And Eliza, her young granddaughter, "put a piece of a nut shell up her nose." Dr. Adam Kuhn (1741–1817), professor of theory and practice of medicine at the University of Pennsylvania, attempted to remove it with an instrument but without success; "the child's eyes were bound and she was held down, but she cried so hard that nothing could be done." Dr. Kuhn then ordered "her nose syringed with warm water and swabbed with oil." Two days later, Dr. William Shippen, Jr. (1736–1808), whom Kuhn called in, "tried with an instrument to take the shell out of the poor child's nose, but could not effect it." She later fought off Dr. Kuhn's second attempt to remove it. Failing, he concluded that "perhaps it might rot away by itself," but it did not and Eliza's nose gave off a most offensive odor. Eliza's father finally pulled the shell out with a hooked instrument, but only while three people held her down as she howled.[21]

Another granddaughter, on October 29, 1799, swallowed a pin (the safety pin was not patented until 1849). Mrs. Drinker made her "take a raw egg white and yolk" and told the father to give his child another "in an hour's time—it is what frequently happens to Children, and it is admirable that so few bad consequences follow it as it slips down the common sewer, with other things, and kind Nature often eludes calamity."[21]

Colonial newspapers often printed reports of childhood poisonings; for example, in the *Boston Gazette* for September 25–October 2, 1738, there appeared a clinical description of the poisoning of two children who ate thorn-apple seeds *(Datura stramonium L.)*.[25]

Common Diseases of Colonial Children

TINEA CAPITIS Tinea capitis, also called scald-head, scabbed head, or *porrigo scutulata,* must have been extremely common in colonial children, judging from the frequency with which cures for it were published in almanacs, newspapers, and books on domestic medicine. Lionel Chalmers[13] gave a novel and, he claimed, effective method of treating this complaint that a countrywoman had taught him.

Having recollected that a woman had cured several *tineas,* which were said to have baffled all the methods that were tried by others, I enquired how she treated them. . . . Two or three purges must be given, at the distance of three days from each; and the hair being closely cut off, she applied some *colewort* [cabbage] leaves one above another over the head, every morning and evening. . . . Having done so for a week, a plaster should be prepared by boiling two ounces of rosin and a proper quantity of wheat flour with a quart of malt liquor called *porter,* 'till the whole acquire the consistence of a stiff paste . . . spread on soft leather . . . laid over the whole head. . . . This paste is so adhesive, that much of the hair comes away with it . . . so that, after some time, the head is quite bald. The bulk of a hazelnut of *Roman vitriol* [copper sulfate] ought then to be dissolved in a pint and a half of rum, with which the part must be washed every morning and evening daily, and afterward covered with a plaster, made with *bees-wax* and mutton suet, till the hair begins to grow thick.

Buchan[8] considered *tinea capitis* "the most obstinate of all the eruptions incident to children . . . often exceedingly difficult to cure, and sometimes indeed the cure proves worse than the disease." He warned that he had frequently known children who died soon after their scabbed heads had been healed by the applications of drying medicines. After washing the scalp and cutting off the hair, Buchan recommended shaving the head once a week and then anointing the scalp with a "liniment made of train oil eight ounces, [and] red [mercury] precipitate, in fine powder, one drachm." Buchan, like others of his day, feared that "stoppage of the discharge" from the scalp would retain "peccant humors." To prevent this, he advised, "especially in children of a gross habit," making "an issue* in the neck or arm, which may be kept open till the patient becomes strong."

Wesley's treatment for all cutaneous inflammations, including pimples and scabs, was the simplest of all: bathing in cold water. This was in keeping with his plan to make his treatments as simple and direct as possible.

WORMS Worm infestations must also have been extremely prevalent. Worms were thought responsible for paleness and at other times for flushing of the face, picking the nose, grinding of the teeth at night, swelling of the upper lip, a sour or "stinking breath," great thirst, frothy urine, colicky pains, a dry cough, unequal pulses, palpitations of the heart, cold sweats, palsy, epileptic fits, and—according to Buchan[8]—"many other unaccountable nervous symptoms, which were formerly attributed to witchcraft, or the influence of evil spirits."

To treat a four- or five-year-old child, Buchan[8] recommended "six grains of rhubarb, five of jalup, and two of calomel." These "may be mixed in a spoonful of syrup of honey and given in the morning." The dose "may be repeated twice a week for three or four weeks." And on "the intermediate days," Buchan recommended that the child "may take a scruple of powdered tin and ten grains of aethiops mineral† in a spoonful of treacle twice a day. . . . To prevent the recurrence of worms, half a drachm of [Peruvian] bark‡ in powder may be taken in a glass of red port wine, three or four times a day."

Wesley,[55] like Culpeper[16] (p. 31), advised treating worms by external means rather than by oral medications. "Boil a handful of rue and wormwood in water; foment the belly with a decoction, and apply the boiled herbs as a poultice; repeat the application night and morning."

* "Issue" was an induced suppurating sore. The discharge from it was promoted by dressing it with a mild blistering ointment.
† Aethiops mineral contained equal parts of flowers of sulfur and clean crude mercury, ground together in an iron mortar until they turned into a black powder.
‡ Peruvian bark contained quinine and other alkaloids.

An unusual and unfastidious remedy to kill worms was included in a widely read mid-eighteenth-century American almanac, *Poor Tom's Almanac,* in 1750:[50] "There is not a faster or surer Remedy to kill worms in children than to take 6, 8, or 10 red Earth-Worms, and let them purge in Bay Salt, then slit them open and wash them in fair Water, then dry them in an Earthen Dish and beat them to a powder, and give them to the Child in the morning fasting, for 3 or 4 Mornings, but let them eat nothing for an hour after."

Chalmers[13] wrote extensively about the treatment of worms, finding that "of all the vermifuges, *lonicera* [honeysuckle] hath the best effect." He also recommended "the use of common salt" because "it is both ancient and universal." Salt had been recommended by Celsus eighteen centuries before. Rush had also used it effectively in treating many cases of worm infestation. Another effective vermifuge, according to Chalmers, was Carolina pinkroot (*Spigelia marilandica* L.). But because "instances of death have been associated with its use," he advised the use of "less certain, but more safe medicines for destroying worms."

Colonial grandparents, like Elizabeth Drinker,[21] were certainly more curious about the internal anatomy of worms than are modern-day grandparents—at least those I know. In her diary on June 11, 1799, she wrote: "Elizabeth Skyrin [a granddaughter] voided a worm 9 ½ inches long, I cut it open with my Sicers and found several young ones in it—she has taken medicine this evening on [that] account."

THRUSH OR APHTHAE. Thrush, which is not looked upon as a particularly serious problem today, was viewed quite differently in the eighteenth century. Michael Underwood (1737–1820)[52] wrote that "it is a vulgar error" to consider thrush as "a very harmless complaint," although he acknowledged that it is "a much milder disorder in this island [Britain], than in most parts of the Continent, particularly in France, where it reigns as a malignant epidemic, especially in the Hôtel Dieu, and Foundling Hospitals, and where it is known by the names of Muguet and Millet."

In colonial America thrush was believed to be a common cause of diarrheal disease. Most American writers concurred with Chalmers's *caveat* of not trying to rub off the aphthae with a piece of gauze or with the gloved finger. If this "barbarous custom of rubbing of the aphthae" went unchecked, he wrote, "convulsions would be the immediate consequence of this cruel treatment." Chalmers[13] treated thrush in infants by first taking "the most expeditious methods to clear the stomach and intestines of... sharp humours, with *rhubarb, magnesia* or crabs' eyes:* the patient must... be confined to a diet of broth made with lean meat... till the stools are of a proper colour," after which he advised that a mixture be prepared by "boiling one fig together with a little *liquorice* and barley in water to two ounces; to which ten or twelve grains of *borax* [was] added, a tea-spoonful of it should be given frequently warm to moisten and relax the affected parts, during their present inflamed state."

Of Wesley's[55] three remedies for thrush, the most curious was his recommendation to "burn scarlet cloth to ashes and blow them into the mouth. This seldom fails." Why the cloth had to be scarlet is not revealed.

Buchan[8] advised the "nurse to rub the child's mouth frequently with a little borax and honey, or with... fine honey an ounce, borax a drach, burnt alum half a drachm, rose water two drachms."

TEETHING. Buchan[8] quoted John Arbuthnot's (1667–1735) comment that "about a tenth part of [British] infants die in teething from the irritation of the tender nervous parts of the jaws, occasioning inflammations, fevers, convulsions, gangrenes, etc." Buchan also mentioned the belief, generally accepted since the time of Hippocrates, that teething was often accompanied by many serious symptoms, especially convulsions.

Treatment usually consisted of purging, vomiting, or sweating and if "inflammation appears... a leech should be applied under each ear." Contrary to most of his contemporaries, Buchan was not impressed with the benefit of cutting the infant's gums with a blade to allow the tooth to erupt.

CONVULSIONS AND FITS. Many deaths of colonial infants and children were attributed to convulsions; these included the terminal convulsions of any disease, especially when the exact diagnosis was in doubt. Unrecognized tetany was in all likelihood considered under the term "convulsions."

* Crabs' eyes are concretions found in the stomach of the European crayfish at the time the animal is about to change its shell.

Comment about childhood convulsions or fits are frequently found in colonial diaries, letters, and newspapers. For example, in Mather's diary[35] there are several poignant descriptions of convulsions:

Feb. 15, 1700. On Friday this week, my only and lovely Son [Increase (1699–1724)], a Son given to me in Answer to many Prayers among the People of God, was taken with *Convulsion-Fits. March 6.* Another Thing, which brought me, on my Knees this Day before the Lord, is that my lovely and only Son, is again the last Night arrested with Convulsions, and the Life of the Infant is exceedingly in Danger.

Feb. 7 {1701}. The Evil that I feared is come upon me. On Tuesday night . . . my little Son Samuel, was taken with very sad Convulsions. They continued all *Wednesday* incurable, and we were all the Day in continual Expectation of his Expiration. But he lived all Thursday, too, and outlived more than an hundred very terrible Fitts.

Despite all of Mather's personal tragedies, his belief in the rightness of God's decrees, however inscrutable, never wavered.

Tetanus of the newborn, or "nine-day fits," was also a cause of death. As late as 1782, especially in Dublin, tetanus caused the death of 17 percent of all infants delivered at the Lying-In Hospital, while in London this disease was responsible for the deaths of 4 percent of the newborn.[49]

Eighteenth-Century American Pediatric Publications

One of the last American medical publications of the eighteenth century and the first pediatric monograph published in the United States was an inaugural dissertation of sixty-nine pages by Charles Caldwell (1772–1853) for the degree of doctor of medicine from the University of Pennsylvania. It was titled *An Attempt to Establish the Original Sameness of Three Phenomena of Fever (Principally Confined to Infants and Children) Described by Medical Writers under the Several Names of Hydrocephalus Internus, Cynanche Trachealis and Diarrhoea Infantum* (1796). The inaugural dissertation had been an established requisite for European medical graduates long prior to the eighteenth century and was first required in America at the Medical Department of the University of Pennsylvania in 1771. After 1800 there were an increasing number of American pediatric publications of this type, most which were of only transitory value. Caldwell's theory and practice were greatly influenced by the tension theory of medicine developed by two Scottish physicians, William Cullen (1710–1790) and John Brown (1735–1788). Caldwell considered the three entirely unrelated diseases in the title of his dissertation as "the genuine and destructive offspring of *arterial action* [increased excitability], morbid in its *nature*, excessive in its *violence,* and by causes of particular tendency determined by the *encephalon,* the *trachea,* or the *intestines.*" Thus, the treatment for all three diseases —supposedly of common origin—considered of rest, cool temperature, mild diet, acidulated beverages, bleeding, purgatives, diaphoretics, diuretics, and sialagogues.

The tortuous and illogical arguments adduced by Caldwell to support his hypothesis were (1) that the three diseases were of a general and not a local nature; (2) that the topical affections were preceded by general fever; (3) that the diseases were confined to infants and children of similar age and constitution who were considerably alike in all their general habits; (4) that they exhibited a reciprocal alternation with each other; and (5) that the same remedies were effective in all three diseases.

A few pediatric case reports appeared in the first volume of transactions ever published by a medical society in the United States, that of the New Haven County Medical Society, in 1788.[5] Two were of particular interest. The first was Leverett Hubbard's[31] (1722–1794) report of a fetal "monstrosity" with a large sacral teratoma, described in considerable detail by the author and accompanied by a very presentable wood engraving, the only illustration in the volume (Fig. 2–9). The second was Hezekiah Beardsley's (1748–1790)[3] report of a case of scirrhus in the pylorus of an infant. This has become one of the classics of American pediatrics since 1903, when it was discovered by Sir William Osler[42] (1849–1919) and reprinted in the *Archives of Pediatrics.* Beardsley described not only the symptoms but also the pathology of the lesion, which consisted of "scirrhosity of the pylorus which completely obstructed the passage into the duodenum [so] as to admit with the greatest difficulty the finest fluid." Beardsley's case report is noteworthy both for its superiority to George Armstrong's[42] (1719–1789) account written

the feet and legs, but to my great furprife the body ftopt. Then with my left hand extended the
thighs of the fœtus as far afunder as I could, and
flipt the two fore fingers of my right hand, in
order to obtain the extremity of the inteftinum
rectum. But to my aftonifhment, I found there
was no inteftinum rectum, but the fame feeling
below the thighs as there was in the firft touch,
as I mentioned before, which proved to be the
pendulous body which prefented to the birth, as
delineated in the plate.

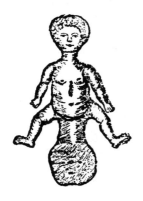

Finding I could do nothing that way, I then
returned the legs into their former pofition, and
by repeated trials, turned the child fo as to feel
one of the hands, after that the fhoulder, and
then the head which I caufed to prefent, and
foon after that obtained a delivery in the natural way.
    I fhould not have troubled you with this cafe,
if the formation of the fœtus had not been very
                                                fingular.

Figure 2–9. Leverett Hubbard's case of a fetal "monstrosity" with a large sacral tumor (1788). (Reprinted from Cases and Observations Medical Society of New-Haven County.)

during the previous decade (1777), and for being one of the very first American contributions to nosography.

The first volume of the *Medical Repository*, the pioneer American medical journal, contained the earliest formal paper on a pediatric subject published in this country. This paper about "cholera or bilious diarrhea" of infants by Edward Miller[39] included the first reference to the value of the cold bath in the treatment of fever. Miller advised that "several times a day the patient should be washed with vinegar and water, salt and water, or water alone, by means of a sponge, as he lies in bed, with as little motion, disturbance, or fatigue, as possible." Fur-

ther, it was necessary to "discharge the stomach and intestines of their acrid and often offensive contents." When this had been accomplished, he advised the use of a "pill" containing ⅙ grain of opium and ⅓ grain of calomel for a child of two years, to be repeated every two to six hours or "sometimes oftener according to the urgency of symptoms." (In almost all eighteenth-century papers dosage recommendations were given rather loosely.)

In the same volume of the *Medical Repository*, Edward Augustus Holyoke (1728–1829)[30] of Salem, recommended the use of calomel in the treatment of "throat distemper." This was nothing new; calomel was recommended for almost any childhood illness and, like bloodletting, it became a panacea for all ills. Many physicians believed that the omission of calomel in desperate cases was tantamount to abandoning the patient without a final saving effort.

American contributions to pediatrics during the eighteenth century, while not many, numbered a few that became widely acclaimed abroad. The most important of these were Bard's study of angina suffocativa, or diphtheria, in 1771; Chalmers's clinical description of the same disease in 1766, and Rush's description of cholera infantum, which for the first time also contained a systematic account of this devastating pediatric disease.

Colonial America also made significant contributions to epidemiology, especially in regard to smallpox. The contributions of Boylston and Mather toward the amelioration of smallpox are universally recognized as classics in the history of medicine.

References

1. Armstrong, G. *An Account of the Diseases Most Incident to Children, from Their Birth till the Age of Puberty*. London: T. Cadell, 1777.
2. Bard, S. *An Enquiry into the Nature, Cause and Cure, of the Angina Suffocativia, or Sore Throat Distemper*. New York: S. Inslee & A. Car, 1771.
3. Beardsley, H. Case of a scirrhus in the pylorus of an infant: *Cases Obs. Med. Soc. New-Haven Co.* 1:81, 1788.
4. Bell, W. J. *The Colonial Physician and Other Essays*. New York: Science History Publications, 1977.

5. Blumer, G. The first medical transactions in America. *Yale J. Biol. Med.* 6:299, 1934.

6. Boorstin, D. *The Americans: The Colonial Experience.* New York: Random House, 1958.

7. Boylston, Z. *An Historical Account of the Small-Pox Inoculated in New England.* London: S. Chandler, 1726. Reprinted, Boston, 1730.

8. Buchan, W. *Domestic Medicine; or, A Treatise on the Prevention and Cure of Diseases, by Regimen and Simple Medicines.* Philadelphia: Thomas Dobson, 1795.

9. Cadogan, W. *An Essay upon Nursing and the Management of Children, from Their Birth to Three Years of Age.* London: J. Roberts, 1748.

10. Caulfield, E. A history of the terrible epidemic, vulgarly called the throat distemper, as it occurred in His Majesty's New England colonies between 1735 and 1740. *Yale J. Biol. Med.* 11:219–277, 1939.

11. Caulfield, E. Early measles epidemics in America. *Yale J. Biol. Med.* 15:531, 1942–1943.

12. Caulfield, E. Infant feeding in colonial America. *J. Pediatr.* 41:673, 1952.

13. Chalmers, L. *An Account of the Weather and Diseases of South-Carolina.* London: E. & S. Dilly, 1776.

14. Cowen, D. L. The Boston editions of Nicholas Culpeper. *J. Hist. Med.* 11:156, 1956.

15. Creighton, C. *A History of Epidemics in Britain.* Cambridge: Cambridge University Press, 1891–1894.

16. Culpeper, N. *The English Physician.* Boston: Nicholas Boone, 1708.

17. Dickinson, J. *Observations on That Terrible Disease, Vulgarly Called the Throat-Distemper.* Boston: S. Knelland and T. Green, 1740.

18. Dittrick, H. The nursing can: An early American infant feeding device. *Bull. Hist. Med.* 7:696, 1939.

19. Douglass, W. *The Practical History of a New Epidemical Eruptive Miliary Fever, with an Angina Ulcusculosa, Which Prevailed in Boston New-England in the Years 1735 and 1736.* Boston: T. Fleet, 1736.

20. Douglass, W. *A Summary, Historical and Political, of the First Planting, Progressive Improvements, and Present State of the British Settlements in North America.* Boston: Rogers and Foyle, 1747–1752.

21. Drinker, C. K. *Not So Long Ago: A Chronicle of Medicine and Doctors in Colonial Philadelphia.* New York: Oxford University Press, 1937.

22. Duffy, J. *Epidemics in Colonial America.* Baton Rouge: Louisiana State University Press, 1953.

23. Fitch, J. *An Account of the Numbers that Have Died of the Distemper in the Throat within the Province of New-Hampshire, with Some Reflections Thereon.* Boston: Eleazer Russel, 1736.

24. Fothergill, J. *An Account of the Sore Throat Attended with Ulcers.* London: C. Davis, 1748.

25. Guerra, F. Medical almanacs of the American Colonial period. *J. Hist. Med.* 16:234, 1961.

26. Guerra, F. *American Medical Bibliography, 1639–1783.* New York: Lathrop C. Harper, 1962.

27. Hamilton, R. An account of a distemper, by the common people in England vulgarly called the mumps. *Trans. R. Soc. Edinb.* 2:59, 1790.

28. Holmes, T. J. *Cotton Mather: A Bibliography.* Cambridge, Mass.: Harvard University Press, 1940.

29. Holt, L. E., and Howland J. *Diseases of Infancy and Childhood* (7th ed.). New York: Appleton, 1922.

30. Holyoke, E. A. A letter to Dr.——— in answer to his queries respecting the introduction of mercurial practice in the vicinity of Boston, Mass. *Med. Repository* 1:490, 1800.

31. Hubbard, L. Case of a deformed foetus. *Cases Obs. Med. Soc. New-Haven Co.* 1:38, 1788.

32. Jacobi, A. History of American pediatrics before 1800. *Janus* 7:460, 518, 590, 626, 1902.

33. Jenner, E. *An Inquiry into the Causes and Effects of the Variolae Vaccinae.* London: S. Low, 1798.

34. Killpatrick, J. *A Full and Clear Reply to Doct. Thomas Dale.* Charles Town, S.C.: P. Timothy, 1739.

35. Mather, C. Diary, 1681–1708, 1709–1724. *Coll. Mass. Hist. Soc.* (7th ser.) vols. 7, 8, 1912.

36. Mather, C. *A Letter about a Good Management under the Distemper of the Measles.* Boston: John Allen, 1713.

37. Mather, C. *An Account of the Method and Success of Inoculating the Small Pox in Boston in New England.* London: J. Peels, 1722.

38. Mather, C. *The Angel of Bethesda: An Essay upon the Common Maladies of Mankind* (1724). G. W. Jones (ed.). Barre, Mass.: American Antiquarian Society and Barre Publishers, 1972.

39. Miller, E. Remarks on the Cholera or bilious diarrhoea of infants. *Med. Repository* 1:85, 1798.

40. Mittelberger, G. *Journey to Pennsylvania.* O. Handlin and J. Clive (eds.). Cambridge, Mass.: Harvard University Press, 1960 (first published in 1754).

41. Nelson, J. *An Essay on the Government of Children.* London: R. and J. Dodsley, 1753.

42. Osler, W. Congenital hypertrophic stenosis of the pylorus. *Arch. Pediatr.* 20:355, 1903.

43. Packard, F. R. *History of Medicine in the United States* (2nd ed.) 2 vols. New York: P. B. Hoeber, 1931.

44. Radbill, S. X. The pediatrics of Benjamin Rush. *Trans. Coll. Physicians Phila.* (4th ser.) 40:168, 1973.

45. Ruhräh, J. *Pediatrics of the Past: An Anthology.* New York: Hoeber, 1925.

46. Rush, B. An inquiry into the cause of the cholera infantum. In his *Medical Inquiries and Observations* (2 vols.) vol. 1, p. 112. Philadelphia: Prichard & Hall, 1789.

46a. Rush, B. Scarlatina anginosa. In his *Medical Inquiries and Observations* (2 vols.), vol. 1, p. 101. Philadelphia: Prichard & Hall, 1789.

47. Shryock, R. H. *Medicine in America*. Baltimore: Johns Hopkins Press, 1966.

48. Shute, M. N. A little great awakening, an episode in the American enlightenment. *J. Hist. Ideas* 37:589, 1976.

49. Still, G. F. *The History of Paediatrics*. London: Oxford University Press, 1931.

50. Stowell, M. B. *Early American Almanacs: The Colonial Weekday Bible*. New York: Burt Franklin, 1977.

51. Thacher, T. *A Brief Rule to Guide the Common-People of New-England How to Order Themselves and Theirs in the Small Pocks, or Measels*. Boston: J. Foster, 1677 (1678).

52. Underwood, M. *A Treatise on the Diseases of Children*. London: J. Mathews, 1784.

53. Waring, J. I. Early interest in pediatrics in South Carolina. *Pediatrics* 8:413, 1951.

54. Weaver, G. H. Life and writings of William Douglass, M.D. (1691–1752). *Bull. Soc. Med. Hist. Chicago* 2:229, 1921.

55. Wesley, J. *Primitive Physick, or an Easy and Natural Method of Curing Most Diseases*. Philadelphia: Joseph Crukshank, 1770.

56. Winslow, C.-E. A. The colonial era. In F. H. Top (ed.), *The History of American Epidemiology*. St. Louis: Mosby, 1952.

57. Winslow, O. E. *A Destroying Angel: The Conquest of Smallpox in Colonial Boston*. Boston: Houghton Mifflin, 1974.

The {colonial} baby's nourishment consisted, it appears, entirely of breast milk. The subject is not much discussed in any documents extant today.

John Demos (1970)

Breast-Feeding

The prohibitive mortality that usually accompanied artificial feeding of infants in seventeenth- and eighteenth-century England made breast-feeding essential to the survival of the race, yet the technique of such an important custom was seldom mentioned by the early American colonists. There is ample evidence that nearly all infants were breast-fed, but little was written about this either in printed or manuscript material. Even the diligent diarist Ebenezer Parkman (1703–1782), father of seventeen breast-fed children, never mentioned how often they were fed, whether they were fed when they cried or according to a schedule, or any other details of what to him must have been a commonplace procedure.[10] According to John Demos,[10] the most knowledgeable historian of this period, there are occasional incidental references to breast-feeding in the records of the Plymouth colony. For example, Lidia Standish, testifying in connection with a trial for fornication, spoke of herself as "a mother of many children my selfe and have Nursed many."

There is also the indirect evidence that derives from the study of birth intervals at the Plymouth colony, where in the average family children were spaced roughly two years apart (or a bit longer near the end of the wife's child-bearing span). This pattern is consistent with a practice of breast-feeding a child for about one year, since lactation may present a biological impediment to conception. Demos[10] claims that "the exceptions can nearly always be explained in the same terms," because "when one finds an interval of only twelve or fifteen months between two particular deliveries, one also finds that the older child died at or soon after birth." Here there would be either a very short period of breast-feeding or none at all, and hence nothing to delay the start of another pregnancy. Demos suggests an alternative explanation for the spacing of the birth intervals: it may have been that the settlers in Plymouth maintained a taboo against sexual relations between husband and wife whenever the latter was nursing a child. There is evidence for such a practice, but this is not the kind of information that would tend to be documented in written comment from the Plymouth colony.

In Samuel Sewall's[19] diary, in which he set down a full record of how life was lived in his time, there were only a few details about the feeding of his first child, who was born on April 2, 1677, and who died fifteen months later of an unknown cause. "*April 7, 1677* . . . first laboured to cause the child [John (1677–1678)] suck his mother, which he scarcely did at all. In the afternoon my Wife set up, and he sucked the right Breast bravely, that had the best nipple. *April 9.* The Child sucked his Mothers left Brest [sic] well as she laid in the Bed, notwithstanding the shortness of the Nipple."*

In the six-day period between her child's birth and Mrs. Sewall's first attempt to breast-feed him, the Sewalls undoubtedly made use of a wet nurse, a common practice during the first week or two of an infant's life while the mother recovered from her "groaning" or lying-in period.

Wet-Nursing

Although wet-nursing was a well-accepted seventeenth-century practice in Europe, it is difficult to

*Sewall's remarks about his wife's nipples were omitted from the 1878–1882 edition of his *Diary* published by the Massachusetts Historical Society. The editors deemed such remarks unsuitable for publication, probably because of Victorian reticence about such matters.[19]

find definite evidence of its widespread use in seventeeth-century America, but by the eighteenth century there were many references to the availability of wet nurses in colonial newspapers.[15]

Examples[15] are:

A certain person wants a Wet Nurse to Suckle a child in the House: Inquiries at the Post-Office in Boston.

—*Boston News-Letter*
July 23–30, 1711

Wanted a wet nurse to go into a family.

—*Essex Journal* (New Hampshire)
December 5, 1776

A wet nurse, who has a good breast of milk only five weeks old, would be willing to suckle a child on reasonable terms. Inquire at the Printers.

—*Royal Pennsylvania Gazette*
March 27, 1778

A wet nurse with a good breast of milk, would take a Gentleman's child to suckle. Inquire of the Printer.

—*Continental Journal,* (Boston)
November 11, 1779

A woman with a good breast of milk will take in a Nurse Child, about six miles from Boston.

—*Morning Chronicle* (Boston)
April 6, 1780

A good wet Nurse that lives in that part of Milton [Massachusetts] call'd the Blue Hills, and under the same Roof with a well known skilful Woman for weakly Children, would take a Child to Nurse. Inquire of the Printer.

—*New England Weekly Journal*
April 26, 1737

This last advertisement, according to Caulfield,[6] "reveals America's first baby specialist": He also located this fascinating observation about Marblehead, Massachusetts, in Captain Francis Goelet's journal for 1750: "This Place is Noted for children and Noureches the most of any Place for its Bigness in North America, it's Said the Chief Cause is attributed to their feeding on Cod Heads, etc. which is their Principall Diet."

Newspapers were also extremely important in bringing to the attention of colonial parents the pediatric writings of English authors such as Cadogan[4] and James Nelson (1710–1794).[16a] Excerpts from Cadogan's *Essay upon Nursing* and from Nelson's *An Essay on the Government of Children* (1753) were widely and frequently printed. Extensive excerpts from Cadogan's *Essay* appeared first in the *South Carolina Gazette* of March 6, 1749, less than a year after its first publication in London. In *Ames' Almanack* for 1762, readers would have found this paragraph, which contains many of Cadogan's ideas as well as a few of Stephen Hales (1677–1761):[6]

It is an Error in Judgment on the Part of the Mother, who, only for Preservation of her Beauty, and fine Shape of Body, would put her Infant to Nurse; since suddenly to dry up a full Breast of new Milk in a healthy Woman does such Violence to Nature, as greatly exposes the mother to such diseases as many marr [sic] her Beauty and Shape both . . . for the Infant to be deprived of the Aliment that was congenital to its Nature, and put to the Breast of a Nurse, who differs in Constitution from the Child's, as much as one Species differs from another— happy! thrice happy for many a poor Infant, in such Cases, if its Nurse had been a Goat and not a Woman! The former feeds on the tender Browse, and drinks only at the cool Fountain, but the Latter sometimes feeds foul, and drinks deeply of the Liquor, which can and often does kill the Infant at second Hand, from the Breast of the Nurse; . . . when so delicate a Machine as the Body of an Infant is (whose very Bones were lately a fluid Mass) I say, when such a delicate Thing from the Lap and Care of Nature, comes to be jounced on the hard Knees, or handled with the rough Fingers of a cruel Nurse, or ignorant Mother: it is a Wonder that there are not more crooked Limbs, dislocated Joints, and Cripples from Infancy, than there are.

The old belief still survived and was widely held that undesirable moral characteristics might be imbibed with the nurse's milk unless she had been chosen with the greatest care.

There were, as there had been in all previous centuries, elaborate rules for selecting a wet nurse but probably only the wealthy could observe them. For example, Alexander Hamilton (1739–1802),[16] of Edinburgh, whose influence on our medical practice must have been strong because his books were widely published in the colonies, offered these hints in choosing a wet nurse:

The appearance of health, an unexceptionable moral character, plenty of wholesome milk, and breasts well formed in every respect, with prominent nipples, are always expected in a NURSE. But these are not the only circumstances which ought to be ascertained. Her child should be healthy and thriving; and no woman who bears a dead child can in general be chosen; for, unless the death happened in consequence of some particular accident during delivery, there is always, in such cases, some reason to suspect a fault in the constitution.

Women addicted to the use of tobacco in any form, and those who have never had the Smallpox, or are very much marked by them, make improper Nurses.

It is not sufficient to avoid Nurses who are suspected of having some *disease* which may be communicated to the child; for some blemishes may also be attended with the same bad effects such as immoderate Squinting. . . . No woman should be hired as a nurse who has not already given proofs, by nursing her own child, that she is well qualified for the task.

With all its faults, nursing was thought to be so far superior to "dry-nursing," or artificial feeding, that in court cases in America involving foundlings, orphans, or illegitimate infants, wet nurses were supplied to the county, town, or parish. This was sound policy, because in the late eighteenth century the infant mortality in the Paris Foundling Hospital, where artificial feeding was practiced, was 85 percent of the 32,000 infants received, while in Dublin of 10,000 infants admitted to the hospital during the years 1775 to 1796, only 45 survived—in other words, 99.6 percent died.[5] This frightful mortality makes it plain why artificial feeding was regarded with such suspicion and why it made so little headway in the eighteenth century.

Sending Boston infants to wet nurses in the country was a common practice, because it was generally acknowledged that infants thrived better in the country air. The farming-out of babies to be nursed had become a well-established custom in seventeenth century England; and, as Ernest Caulfield[6] noted, this practice received some scientific support in the eighteenth century when Jonas Hanway (1712–1786), an English philanthropist, after comparing the infant survival rate of London parishes with that of country parishes, attributed the differences to the salubriousness of country air. In this country Benjamin Rush had found that moving infants with cholera infantum to the country was the best of all treatments known to him. Bad air became the accepted explanation for the spread of diseases from person to person. Colonial cities grew at the expense of public health.

Popular practice in infant feeding in our colonial period did not keep pace with the latest medical advances as it does today. The colonist followed the common practices of the home countries, especially England. The writings of English physicians about infant care have a particular historical interest for American readers, for England was our mother in medicine as she was in language, literature, manners, and political institutions. And although cases might differ somewhat in the two countries, American colonial medicine was in principle essentially a replica of medicine in the old country. Except in isolated frontier areas, infants were fed much as they were over there. But on this point, as on many others, the English record is better documented than ours and is thus a good deal easier to follow.[13, 14]

In view of the paucity of original American instructions for feeding infants "by hand" it may be assumed that most mothers followed English folk customs or popular English medical books such as those by Nicholas Culpeper[9] and Cadogan[4] (Fig. 3–1). These English authors, notably Cadogan, with an ingrained prejudice against boiled cow's milk, strongly advocated feeding nothing but breast milk until the child was three to six months old. After that, but only in case of necessity, one could give "thin light broths with a little bread or rice boiled in them" alternating with "toasted bread and water boiled almost dry and then mixed with fresh milk, not boiled."

Cadogan, physician to the Foundling Hospital in London, in his popular *Essay upon Nursing* (1748), issued in the form of a letter to a governor of the hospital, warned mothers of the great perils of wet-nursing. In his *Essay*, Cadogan[4] laid down rules on the nursing, feeding, and clothing of infants. This filled a great need at a time when infant welfare was much neglected because of ignorance and lack of interest. As has been mentioned, extracts from Cadogan's book often appeared on the first pages of colonial newspapers or in almanacs (p. 46). His book was reprinted in Boston in 1772 and a year later in Philadelphia; he was still being quoted in American textbooks nearly a hundred years after his *Essay* first appeared in print.

It is not surprising that Cadogan's work made an impression; what is surprising is that the governors of the London Foundling Hospital should have been so sympathetic to his ideas, which must have appeared revolutionary to them. At a time when infants were heavily swaddled to keep them from chills and to straighten their limbs and when respected authorities such as Jacques Ballexserd (1726–1774),[2] of Geneva, advised that they be kept from direct sunlight lest "the light damage their eyes," Cadogan insisted that they were not "hot-bed plants" and that "the lighter and looser their clothing the better they would be."

Artificial Feeding

David Forsyth (1877–1941),[14] in his scholarly history of infant feeding from Elizabethan times, noted that no mention was ever made of artificial feeding being substituted for the breast before the late

Figure 3–1. William Cadogan, M.D. (1711–1797), pioneer in infant hygiene.

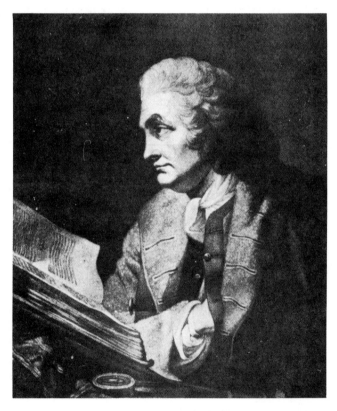

seventeeth and early eighteenth centuries; hand feeding, or artificial feeding, as a reasonably reliable means of infant feeding existed only from the middle of the nineteenth century. It is impossible to say whether this was a consequency of industrialization, or whether it meant that wet nurses were more difficult to find or were regarded with more suspicion. One, and perhaps the best, reason for the paucity of information about infant feeding practices in the seventeenth and eighteenth centuries, both in England and in colonial America, was that fathers, and even mothers, in either their diaries or correspondence, seldom mentioned their children except in formal terms. They seem not to have allowed themselves to show great interest in the daily management of their children's lives, although occasionally parental reserve melts away, especially in the diaries kept by men like Mather and Sewall.

Artificial feeding was hampered by many practical difficulties, such as the lack of an efficient feeding bottle, and by an almost complete ignorance of the most rudimentary principles on which successful artificial feeding is founded. Although the dangers associated with this mode of feeding were realized in this country, there must have been instances of infants successfully raised without the breast. Indirect evidence that infants were brought up on the bottle may be noted in occasional colonial records of nursing bottles; such bottles were imported into Boston in 1690, if not long before, and were sold by various retail merchants.[6] Very little information has been found concerning the kind of fluid mixture used in feeding utensils before the Revolution.

Each generation accepted the tradition handed down by the one preceding. Until the last part of the eighteenth century, as we have seen, breast-feeding was practically the only means of nourishing an infant. The infant was given no choice but the breast, either of its mother or a wet nurse. But as that century was ending, it was finally considered safe to give water-pap as soon as the first tooth had erupted. The breast was not withdrawn altogether until the child had passed its first birthday. Water-pap made of bread and baked flour proved so successful that other foods were introduced; weak broth was offered with the first tooth, and with the second, the minced wing of a chicken. And for the first time sugar was added, being given with bread boiled in water.[8]

Michael Underwood,[20] who many believe laid the foundation of modern pediatrics, was probably the first English author who seriously attempted to find some substitute for breast-feeding. When the breast was not available he considered milk the most proper food for infants. In his *A Treatise on the Diseases of Children* (1784), a book superior to anything that had previously appeared, he wrote that he was puzzled by the nature of the mixtures given in the past (Fig. 3–2): "It has indeed been a wonder to me how the custom of stuffing newborn babies with bread [pap] 'and such like could become so universal, or the idea first enter the mind of a parent that such heavy food could be fit for the babies' nourishment at the age of 6 or 7 months."

Recognizing the importance of choosing a milk as

Figure 3–2. Title-page of the first edition of Michael Underwood's treatise on diseases of children (1784).

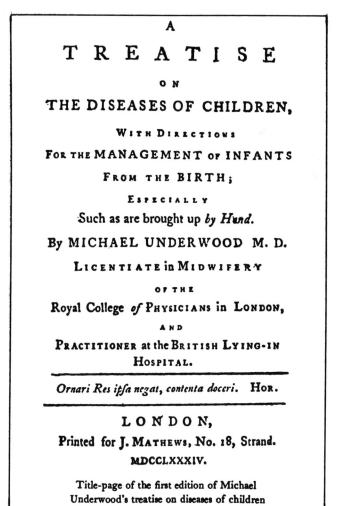

A

TREATISE

ON

THE DISEASES OF CHILDREN,

WITH DIRECTIONS

FOR THE MANAGEMENT OF INFANTS

FROM THE BIRTH;

ESPECIALLY

Such as are brought up *by Hand.*

By MICHAEL UNDERWOOD M. D.

LICENTIATE in MIDWIFERY

OF THE

Royal College *of* PHYSICIANS in LONDON,

AND

PRACTITIONER at the BRITISH LYING-IN HOSPITAL.

Ornari Res ipsa negat, contenta doceri. HOR.

LONDON,

Printed for J. MATHEWS, No. 18, Strand.

MDCCLXXXIV.

Title-page of the first edition of Michael Underwood's treatise on diseases of children

near as possible to mother's milk, Underwood included comparative analyses of the milk of women, cows, goats, asses, sheep, and mares. Such analyses had never been previously published. He concluded that cow's milk was best suited for the ordinary case, but for the very young, or in bad cases of diarrhea, ass's milk was to be used, as "it is thinner and has far less curds than other milks." To this milk the addition of barley water as a diluent was suggested. This, the beginning of milk dilution, marked a decided step in advance. Some years later than this (after 1800) other diluents besides barley water were mentioned by other writers, the preferred one being a small quantity of light jelly made from hartshorn shavings, boiled in water to the consistency that veal broth acquires when cold.

Alexander Hamilton on Infant Feeding

Alexander Hamilton[16] gave clear, concise direction about infant feeding in his *Treatise on the Management of Female Complaints and of Children in Early Infancy* (1792); this popular book went into a seventh edition and was published in at least four colonial cities by the beginning of the nineteenth century.

He suggested that "the child should be put to the breast as soon after birth as the situation of the woman will allow; by which the black viscid substance contained in the intestines will be better evacuated than by any means which art can furnish." He added that "the pernicious practice of giving children purging medicines as soon as [they were] born, cannot be too much reprobated."

Hamilton took issue with "many authors [who] have recommended the practice of allowing the child to suck only at stated periods" because "experience has proved the difficulty which attends such an attempt, and the bad effects which often follow it when carried into execution." And at this point Hamilton's recommendations for feeding "on demand" seem quite modern: "Although those children are most healthy and thriving who are least restricted, and who are permitted to take the breast at pleasure; yet every woman should avoid becoming the slave of her child, as many unguardedly do. The infant ought therefore never to be allowed to sleep at the breast, nor accustomed constantly to overload the stomach by sucking till vomiting ensues."

His views on offering supplemental feedings after nursing on the breast were in line with the belief of most medical writers of the eighteenth century:

Although Nature seldom renders any other food than milk during early infancy necessary, yet, with the view of introducing a change of diet by degrees, the practice of early beginning to give the child daily a little pap or panada, appears to be rational; for when it is neglected till the time of weaning approaches, the habit is with difficulty established; and there is great hazard that the infant may suffer from the sudden change. . . .

Although the panada or pap be now almost universally used for the first food of childen, as a substitute for the mother's milk; yet some more suitable meal may perhaps be given with more advantage, such as cow-milk, mixed with a little water and sugar, to which a small proportion of rusk biscuit may be added; or weak beef-tea may be substituted for the milk and water and sugar.

Hamilton was opposed to the use of cradles, but his was not the conventional view in colonial America. One recalls, for example, that Peregrine White, born on the *Mayflower*, was soon placed in

Figure 3–3. Peregrine White's cradle. Pilgrim Hall, Plymouth, Massachusetts. (Courtesy of the Pilgrim Society, Plymouth, Massachusetts.)

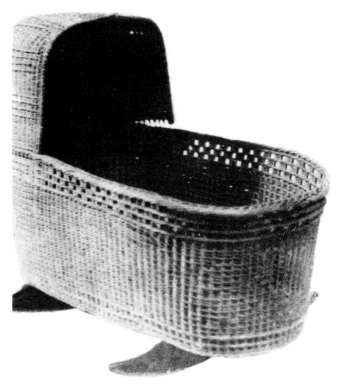

the wicker cradle which her parents had brought with them from Leyden (Fig. 3–3). Sewall[19] recorded a swinging wicker cradle he bought on January 9, 1701/2, for his thirteenth child at a cost of sixteen shillings.

Hugh Smith on Infant Feeding

A book that attained great popular appeal in both England and America during the last three decades of the eighteenth century was *Letters to Married Women on Nursing and the Management of Children* (1772), by the English physician Hugh Smith (?1736–1789).[17] His book, first published in 1772, passed through many editions and was well known on this side of the Atlantic, where it was also printed. In the book's introduction Smith wrote that during the period from 1762 to 1771, about two-thirds of the children born in London died before the age of five years, and about 75 percent of these deaths occurred under the age of two years. As there are not comparable figures for America, one wonders if our child mortality rates were as bad. Smith also claimed that "disease and death are the usual consequences of the present erroneous method of bringing children up by hand. Scarcely one in four of these little innocents live to get over the cutting of their teeth; and the vitiated blood of those that escape, occasioned by improper nourishment generally renders them infirm or short lived."

Sir George F. Still (1868–1941)[18] believed that Smith should have the credit for being the first writer in England to teach the sufficiency of breast milk alone for the feeding of infants up to the age of six or seven months. Before him, most writers had permitted—and even recommended—the addition of pap or panada at the age of three months, and at times it was given much earlier. Smith was strongly in favor of maternal nursing, but if a surrogate was necessary, he preferred feeding with cow's milk to wet-nursing. As his book was popular in our country, it was likely that his teachings helped to shape public opinion about the use of cows' milk for infant feeding in America:

The milk of cows appears, I think, to be the properest substitute we can make for the use of the breast, and will answer best, after the first month or two, without boiling,

unless it purges the child; in which case, boiling it will generally prevent the inconvenience, proceeding in all likelihood from its oily particles. I have no objections to a small quantity of Lisbon sugar being mixed with it, particularly if the child be costive; and indeed this may very frequently be of use, to prevent its too great tendency to become acid, from which disorders of the bowel sometimes arise.

Smith was the first author to mention the actual quantities of undiluted cow's milk to be given to infants of various ages. During the first month of life one pint a day was to be offered equally divided into four feedings; this was to be increased gradually to two pints a day in five feedings by the age of three months, and then further increased to three pints if the infant was still hungry.

Smith was the inventor of a milk or "bubby-pot," the object of which was to imitate nature in making the infant labor for its food (Fig. 3–4). His invention was an important stage in the evolution of the modern nursing bottle. He described his milk pot as follows:

There is nothing therefore wanting, I hope, to complete our system [for hand feeding] but a contrivance to supply the place of the nipple, that the child may still labour to obtain its support; which alone will greatly prevent the error in quantity.... I have contrived a milk-pot for my own nursery ... it appears to my family, and to many of my patients, preferable to those now in use, and may probably be still further improved.... This pot is somewhat in form like an urn, it contains a little more than a

Figure 3–4. Bubby-pot baby feeder, as described by Hugh Smith in 1777. (Courtesy of the Wellcome Historical Medical Library.)

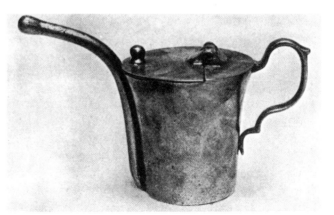

quarter of a pint; its handle, and neck or spout, are not unlike those of a coffee-pot, except that the neck of this arises from the very bottom of the pot, and is very small; in short, it is upon the same principle as those gravy-pots which separate the gravy from the oily fat. The end of the spout is a little raised, and forms a roundish knob, somewhat in appearance like a small heart; this is perforated by three or four small holes: a piece of fine rag is tied loosely over it, which serves the child to play with instead of a nipple, and through which, by the infant's sucking, the milk is constantly strained. The child is equally satisfied as it would be with the breast; it never wets him in the least; he is obliged to labour for every drop he receives, in the same manner as when at the breast; and, greatly in recommendation of this contrivance, the nurses confess it is more convenient than a boat, and that it saves a great deal of trouble in the feeding of an infant; which is the greatest security to parents, that their servants will use it, when they themselves are not present.

Howard Dittrick (1877–1954)[11] described an early American infant feeding device, made out of tin and similar in shape to Hugh Smith's "bubby-pot," that was used by Pennsylvania German parents as early as the 1790's. They called these cans *mammele*, the pronunciation being invariable but the spelling uncertain. The suffix, Dittrick believed, "may be a corruption of the German diminutive ending *lein,* as in kinderlein." In southern Germany, according to Dittrick, "this diminutive lein is contracted to *le . . . Mammele . . .* means 'little breast' or 'little mother.' The nursing device may be appropriately considered as a 'little breast.' "

The early American nursing cans matched Smith's "bubby-pot" quite closely. Dittrick described one specimen thus:

Ten cm in height, 6 cm in diameter at the base, tepering toward the top. A flat handle is soldered to the can. A convex cap is fitted over the top, overlapping to a depth of 1.5 cm. The cover is so well fitted that there is a spout extending from the side of the can opposite the handle, ending in a rounded knob with a small perforation. Inside the can a vertical cyclindrical tube, also of tin, extends to within 1 cm of the bottom of the can. . . . The capacity of the can is 170 cc [Fig. 3–5].

Another specimen is similar to the first except that the inner end of the spout is soldered to the top of the inner cylindrical tube, making, according to Dittrick, "an entirely closed channel from the bot-

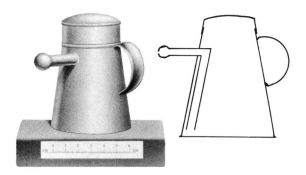

Figure 3–5. *Pennsylvania German tin nursing can, with schematic. (Courtesy of the Cleveland Medical Library Museum.)*

tom part of the can to the perforation in the spout." These cans, Dittrick believed, were copied by Pennsylvania Germans during "their sojourn in England . . . perhaps [from] the design of Hugh Smith's bubby-pot."

Lionel Chalmers on Infant Feeding

Of all the colonial authors on infant feeding, none was more informative than Lionel Chalmers,[7] of South Carolina. His closing comments on "preposterous" methods of infant feeding offer the fullest account of infant feeding practices in the colonies:

It is of the utmost consequence to their welfare, that infants should early be taught to feed, lest they suffer when it become necessary to keep the breast from them, which happens more frequently than most people are aware. And as before weaning they seldom are troubled with any other sort of acrimony than an acid one, the best diet for them is broth of different strength, according to the age and condition of the child. *This* may be made with any kind of lean meat, excepting pork, in which a few tops of parsley, and some grains of black pepper should be boiled, more especially for those who are troubled with flatulency: but it were better not to thicken it at all, though a little salt may be added. On *this* they would willingly feed from the first, if their tastes had not been vitiated by the sugar which is commonly put in whatever is given them. But these sweetened slops, the flour with which their food is usually made, together with the breast milk, are the causes whence they suffer in a greater degree from acidity, than they would do were broth substituted in the place of every other nourishment, excepting the milk they suck. I do not however confine them altogether to the broth of flesh meats; but, by way of change, they are allowed the liquor of stewed *whitings*, or of any other fish that is not oily: of which young children are generally fond. And when they are eight or ten months old, their broth may be a little thickened with the crumb of bread; and the latter may likewise be mixed with either the clear gravy of roasted lean meat, finely minced, chicken or veal once in a day. Neither should a sip of sweet wine (such as that of *Malaga* or *Canary*) or even of some distilled spirit well diluted with water, be denied them once or twice daily, more especially if they be weakly or much depressed by the heat of the weather....

The preposterous manner of feeding infants with *pap*, and other such indigestible food nauseously sweetened, is highly censurable at all times....

During the *summer* and *autumn*, sucking infants ought to be daily allowed a little spirituous drink oftener than once in this country.

And experience proves, that no children thrive so well here as those who every day, sip either a small quantity of *Canary* or other sweet wine, mixt with an equal proportion of water; or a little *rum* well diluted, at all seasons, when nothing forbids; and they might be accustomed to this from the time they are four or five months old.

Chalmers's comments about the use of wine for infants had the sanction of many of the ancient writers on infant feeding. For example, Hippocrates[18] in his *On the Regimen of Health* wrote: "Children and infants for a long time should be washed in warm water, and for a drink should be given wine diluted with water and not quite cold; this should be given because it does not distend the belly and cause wind. These things are done to lessen the liability to convulsions and make the child grow bigger and stronger."

Pap and Panada

If the infant was still hungry after having been offered milk, pap or panada were the most commonly used supplementary food. Pap consisted of flour or bread cooked in water with or without the addition of milk. Panada was the term used for preparations of various flours, cereals, or bread with butter or milk, which were usually cooked in broth. Some authors used the two terms synonymously. The use of pap and panada is of great antiquity. In 1565, Simon de Vallembert (fl. 1565), who wrote the first work on pediatrics in French, stated that panada was one of the most ancient prescriptions known for infant feeding. He quoted Galen as having recommended that "the infant could be fed bread soaked in the broth of flesh or legumes."[12]

In this country mothers were advised that as a supplemental feeding to breast milk the crumbs of a fresh-baked roll or bread boiled in water to the consistency of pap were usually well tolerated by the infant. This pap should be sweetened with sugar but should not be made sweeter than new milk. Egg yolk or whole egg was occasionally added and sometimes beer or wine was used in making pap, or the broth could be made from meat or table vegetables. These "spoon meats," as they were called, were frequently seasoned with anise seed.[3]

One recipe for panada called for steeping bread in water for six hours, pressing it through a cloth, and boiling it with sufficient water for eight hours. It was to be stirred from time to time and diluted with warm water. For seasoning, 59 grains of anise and an ounce of sugar for each pound of bread were used. And finally, the whole thing was passed through a hair sieve. The user was cautioned to "take care to reheat each time only the necessary quantity."[3]

The following recipes for panada were included in an early American cookbook:[3]

PANADA: MADE IN FIVE MINUTES
Set a little water on the fire with a glass of white wine, some sugar, and a scrape of nutmeg and lemonpeel; meanwhile grate some crumbs of bread. The moment the mixture boils up, keeping it still on the fire, put the crumbs in and let it boil as fast as it can. When of proper thickness just to drink, take it off.

CHICKEN PANADA
Boil it till three parts ready in a quart of water, take off the skin, cut the white meat off when cold, and put into a marble mortar; pound it to a paste with a little of the water it was boiled in, season with a little salt, a grate of nutmeg, and the least bit of lemonpeel. Boil gently for a few minutes to the consistency you like; it should be such as you can drink, though tolerably thick. This conveys great nourishment in small compass.

Paps and panadas were fed from a spoon or boat. A pap boat was a vessel, usually made from pewter, silver, or pottery, with a long spout, that was used for feeding liquids and soft foods to infants and chil-

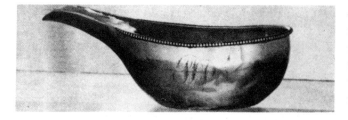

Figure 3–6. Papboat. (Yale University Art Gallery, The Mabel Brady Garvan Collection.)

dren and perhaps to invalids. It was usually about four and one-half inches in length, excluding the handle (Fig. 3–6). A pap spoon (Fig. 3–7) was filled and the lid closed, and the speed of feeding was controlled by the pressure of the finger on the end of the hollow handle.[12]

Seventeenth- and Eighteenth-Century Views on Weaning

Weaning was considered an important episode in an infant's life because it could not be foretold whether or not a serious illness would occur during the process. Cotton Mather, when his daughter Elizabeth was being weaned, used the occasion to preach a sermon entitled "A Soul as a Weaned Child." Other diarists recorded the weaning of their children as seriously as they wrote about births and deaths.[6]

An inordinate prolongation of breast-feeding had been customary up to the early part of the eighteenth century. In the English version (1746) of Jean Astruc's (1684–1766)[1] Treatise, parents were advised not to wean their children "until they are eighteen months, or two years old." Underwood[20] wrote that "a child ought to be in good health, especially in regard to its bowels; and ought first to have cut, at least four of its teeth" before weaning should begin. As this seldom "takes place till the child is near a twelve month old," Underwood's advice was not to consider weaning until the end of the first year of life.

Cadogan[4] had this to say about weaning: "About a TWELVEMONTH, when, and not before, they may be weaned; not all at once, but by insensible degrees; that they may neither feel, not fret at the want of the breast. This might be very easily managed, if they were suffered to suck only at certain times."

Demos,[10] in his study of family life in the Plym-outh Colony, writes that "the second year of life was for many children bounded at either end by experiences of profound loss. Somewhere near its beginning, we have surmised, the child was likely to be weaned; and near its end the arrival of a new baby might be expected."

The season for weaning was extremely important, and seldom was a healthy child weaned in the colonies during July, August, or September. Though there are not many records of children suffering as the results of weaning, most parents appeared pleasantly surprised when all went well, as though they had anticipated some serious illness or at least a spell of boisterous commotion. The technique of weaning must have been handed down from mother to daughter by word of mouth. The earliest printed information on weaning in America will be found in Culpeper's[9] English Physician, published in Boston in 1708:

Wean it not till the Teeth are bred, lest when the eye-teeth come forth, it causeth-Feavers, and ach of Gums, and other symptoms.

The strong children must be sooner weaned than the weak, some in the twelfth, some in the fifteenth month. It is good to wean them at a year and half, or two years old; but give it not suddenly strong food, but bring it by degrees while it sucks.

It is best to wean in the Spring or Fall, in the increase of the moon, and give but very little wine.

Lionel Chalmers,[7] writing in 1776, shared some of Culpeper's views on weaning:

It seems a prevailing mistake, that children ought to be weaned when they are nine or ten months old, whether they be strong or weakly. For having most of their teeth still to cut, and being oftentimes, much disordered thereby, it then becomes necessary to administer

Figure 3–7. Pap spoon. (Courtesy of Mrs. T. G. H. Drake.)

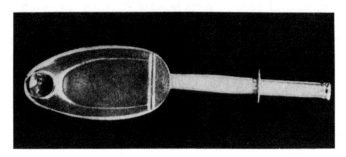

medicines which are not always agreeable to the taste; so that from *this* time, some of them are so suspicious of whatever is attempted to be given, that they will not suffer a cup or spoon to touch their lips. And thus I have know many of them to be lost, when the disease could not be soon removed; for they could not be made to suck again, though their lives might have been saved by it.

It is therefore safest, not to wean infants before they have all or most of their teeth, that they may have somewhat to trust to in case of sickness; for they will take the nipple when all other nourishment is refused. The above rules have been followed in my own family, and they were also recommended to others with success, who, as well as myself, had lost several children by too early weaning and adhering to the usual way of dieting them. And even were they ever so strong and healthy, they should never be weaned till the month of October, when the weather begins to be cool and bracing; for during the relaxing heat of the summer, they are very generally liable to disease in this climate.

No real progress was made in the care and feeding of infants during our colonial period. But at the very end of the eighteenth century (1799) there appeared, in the fourth edition of Michael Underwood's treatise on the diseases of children, the first mention of the chemistry of milk. This marked the beginning of the scientific approach to infant feeding by the clinician. G. F. Still claimed that with Underwood "paediatrics . . . had crossed the Rubicon: the modern study of disease in childhood had begun." However, scientific progress in infant feeding did not take place until the end of the nineteenth century.

References

1. Astruc, J. *A General and Compleat Treatise on All the Diseases of Children.* London: Printed for J. Nourse, 1746.
2. Ballexserd, J. *Dissertation sur l'Education Physique des Enfants.* Paris: Vallat-la-Chapelle, 1762.
3. Bracken, F. J. Infant Feeding in the American Colonies. In *Lydia J. Roberts Award Essays.* Chicago: American Dietetic Association, 1968.
4. Cadogan, W. *An Essay upon Nursing and the Management of Children, from Their Birth to Three Years.* London: J. Roberts, 1748.
5. Caulfield, E. *The Infant Welfare Movement in the Eighteenth Century.* New York: Hoeber, 1931.
6. Caulfield, E. Infant feeding in colonial America. *J. Pediatr.* 41:673, 1952.
7. Chalmers, L. *An Account of the Weather and Diseases of South Carolina.* London: E. & S. Dilly, 1776.
8. Cone, T.E., Jr. *200 Years of Feeding Infants in America.* Columbus, Ohio: Ross Laboratories, 1976.
9. Culpeper, N. *The English Physician.* Boston: Nicholas Boone, 1708.
10. Demos, J. *A Little Commonwealth.* New York: Oxford University Press, 1970.
11. Dittrick, H. The nursing can, an early American infant feeding device. *Bull. Hist. Med.* 7:696, 1939.
12. Drake, T. G. H. Pap and panada. *Ann. Med. Hist.* (n.s.) 3:289, 1931.
13. Drummond, J. C., and Wilbraham, A. *The Englishman's Food: A History of Five Centuries of English Diet.* London: Jonathan Cape, 1939.
14. Forsyth, D. The history of infant feeding from Elizabethan times. *Proc. R. Soc. Med.* 4:110, 1911.
15. Guerra, F. *American Medical Bibliography, 1639–1783.* New York: Lathrop C. Harper, 1962.
16. Hamilton, A. *A Treatise on the Management of Female Complaints, and of Children in Early Infancy.* Worcester, Mass.: Isaiah Thomas, 1793.
16a. Nelson, J. *An Essay on the Government of Children.* London: R. and J. Dodsley, 1753.
17. Smith, H. *Letters to Married Women on Nursing and the Management of Children.* London: C. and G. Kearsley, 1772.
18. Still, G. F. *The History of Paediatrics.* London: Oxford University Press, 1931.
19. Thomas, M. H. (ed.) *The Diary of Samuel Sewall* (2 vols.). New York: Farrar, Strauss and Giroux, 1973.
20. Underwood, M. *A Treatise on the Diseases of Children.* London: J. Mathews, 1784.

The Nineteenth Century

"Perplexing Obscurity and Embarrassing Uncertainty"   *4*

The belief that the disease of children almost constantly present nothing but perplexing obscurity or embarrassing uncertainty, has much retarded the progress of inquiry, by engendering doubts of their susceptibility of successful investigation, lucid explanation, or useful arrangement, and, of course, that every prescribed remedy has but an uncertain aim, and consequently, a contingent or doubtful effect.

William P. Dewees (1829)

As the nineteenth century began, our population was only 5 million and by mid-century it had increased more than fourfold to reach just over 23 million. It was a period of great expansion and unrest. The Industrial Revolution was beginning and with it the movement from the farm to the cities. Children when ill were still cared for almost exclusively by parents, grandparents, and neighbors. Physicians were rarely consulted, nor, save for a few, did they make any effort to seek out infants and children as patients. Young people were numerous despite the high infant mortality rate because our birth rate in 1800 was about 56 per 1,000 population and about 42 per 1,000 population in 1850; this is in contrast to the birth rate of only 14.8 per 1,000 in 1975, the lowest ever recorded in the United States. We have no accurate measure of infant mortality because there were not always exact records of birth, but some idea of the terrible infant mortality can be imagined from the ratio of infant deaths to total deaths. This ratio was approximately 17 percent in 1850 as compared with only 4 percent in 1970.

There was no permanent pediatric hospital in North America until November 23, 1855, when the Children's Hospital of Philadelphia was opened for the reception of children suffering from acute diseases and accidents. This was more than half a century after the Hôpital des Enfants Malades in Paris with three hundred beds for sick children from two to fifteen years of age, the first hospital exclusively for the care of children, had been opened in 1802.[2] In England, the Children's Hospital in Great Ormond Street, London, was founded in 1852, as was a similar institution at Edinburgh in 1860. The Boston Children's Hospital, the second North American children's hospital, was established in 1869.

The germ theory of infectious disease was not firmly established until the 1870's through studies such as those by Robert Koch (1843–1910) and Louis Pasteur (1822–1895) which indisputedly linked a specific organism with a specific disease.

The word *pediatrician* was not coined until near the end of the century. Beginning about 1875, physicians caring for children usually were known as *pediatrists* rather than pediatricians; in fact, the former term persisted until the early decades of the twentieth century. The specialty itself was known as *pediatry* or *pedology*; the word *pediatrics* replaced these terms toward the end of the century, probably to prevent confusion with the term *podiatry*.

There was no discipline of pediatrics, strictly speaking, in American medical schools until the latter years of the nineteenth century; the problems of infancy and childhood were dealt with by the departments of medicine or of obstetrics and diseases of women. But fortunately in the early years of the nineteenth century a changing light had begun to illuminate medicine with what may be termed the scientific outlook, whereby observation, experiment, and inference were as mental processes rated more highly than untrammeled speculation. This outlook eventually led to the realization, but not until the second half of the century, that the young child was not just a diminutive adult and that the physiologic and biochemical differences between infants, children, and adults were sufficiently different to warrant establishing pediatrics as a specific discipline, separate from internal medicine.

Despite improvements in medical theory and practice during the first half of the century, it was obvious that American mortality rates were rising.[70] The first part of the century was characterized by a series of great epidemics. These really began in 1793 in Philadelphia with an outbreak of yellow fever which caused the death of nearly one-eighth of the population. Benjamin Rush[67] attributed the epidemic to a pile of rotting coffee on Ball's Wharf. Terrible epidemics of yellow fever occurred in port cities during this period and alarming epidemics of cholera were frequent occurrences. It was these two diseases, whose nature were best calculated to arouse terror, which inspired public health measures to a greater degree than the more devastating tuberculosis. But during the period of great epidemics between 1800 and 1870 the principal causes of death were not cholera, smallpox, and yellow fever, but rather pulmonary tuberculosis, diarrheal diseases of infancy, bacillary dysentery, typhoid fever, and the infectious diseases of childhood, particularly scarlet fever, diphtheria, and lobar pneumonia.[72]

Medical Education

Until the second quarter of the nineteenth century most medical students obtained their education by serving for a period of time as an apprentice to a physician, called a preceptor. As apprenticeship became institutionalized, medical societies began to adopt rules to govern the relationship between the preceptor and apprentice. The average apprenticeship program was three years at a yearly fee, usually one hundred dollars. This fee might be modified according to the preceptor's fame. The preceptor provided all the books and equipment and provided the apprentice with an appropriate certificate when the term of instruction was completed.[66]

Medical schools gradually replaced the apprenticeship method as the dominant mode of medical education beginning about 1830. William Rothstein,[66] a present-day sociologist, claims that because "medical schools were operated as commercial enterprises, physicians tended to open new ones whenever they found it possible to do so, which increased the number of schools considerably." On the whole the quality of American physicians declined after 1830, owing to small, inefficient private schools of medicine that gradually supplanted the old apprentice system of training and to a lack of medical regulation despite the efforts of the American Medical Association.

The American Medical Association, founded in 1847, established a committee in 1848 to assess the state of medical education in this country. The committee's first report[63] found that our system, in general, was defective and lagged behind the great European centers. "In the United States alone," the committee warned, "is continued an obsolete system of teaching demonstrative sciences by description, of teaching the manipulations of surgery, and the art of recognizing and healing diseases without exhibiting the practice of either, and of explaining the movements and changes of living bodies to those who are ignorant of the laws which govern inert matter." Although apprenticeship was much discussed and questioned in the early years of the nineteenth century, it was, according to Brieger,[13] "an effective means of transmitting practical knowledge in the days before hospitals were widely used for teaching and when medicine was less theoretical and scientific than it is today." As one preceptor saw his role: "We are the janitors at the temple gates of our Profession, and upon our vigilance and discrimination depend the character and usefulness of those who enter its honored portals."[13]

The Influence of French Medicine

An increasing number of American students during the second quarter of the nineteenth century sought postgraduate medical training abroad, especially in Paris, which at that time was the unquestioned center of medical progress and discovery, the *Civitas Hippocratica*. French medicine exerted great influence on American medicine during this period, largely as a result of the great increase in the number of French articles published in American medical journals and because of the many American students who had studied in Paris.[2] French medical articles tended to be detailed clinical studies, seriously concerned with pathology, whereas almost all of the early American medical papers were anecdotal, devoted to individual cases and cures. As a result of the French teachings, diagnosis became the main objective and therapeutics gradually tended toward less regard for drugs and more respect for the natural processes of healing. The work of the "Paris School" initiated the era of strictly modern medicine, and the Parisian hospitals between 1794 and 1848 provided the first environment in which a present-day doctor would have felt in some degree at home.[2]

Modern pediatrics, like internal medicine, had its inception in the medical renaissance in France at the close of the eighteenth and the beginning of the nineteeth century. However, the French school exerted relatively little influence on pediatrics until Charles Michel Billard (1800–1832) developed the long-neglected details of pediatric pathology.

It was first necessary to establish reliable normal criteria for the weight, size, and shape of the growing child and his organs and then to classify and delineate infantile diseases. Billard[10] did much of the preliminary work himself and included it in his *Traité des Maladies des Enfans Nouveau-nés et à la Mamelle* (1828), which was infinitely superior to anything previously published in the field of infants' diseases. Many old superstitions like "dentition diseases" among infants, were discarded. However, it was not until 1875 that problems of physical growth of American children first received really adequate treatment from the very careful statistical study of Henry P. Bowditch (1840–1911).[21] (Fig. 4–1).

Because the French school of 1800–1850 identified diseases by symptoms as well as by lesions detected at autopsy, it developed methods for improving clinical observation, for example, the stethoscope and clinical statistics. By the use of the

Figure 4–1. Henry P. Bowditch (1840–1911). (Courtesy of the Countway Library of Medicine.)

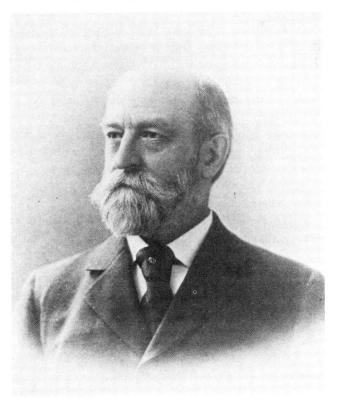

latter, Pierre C. A. Louis (1787–1872),[49] in particular, showed the ineffectiveness of bleeding in the treatment of pneumonia. But these attitudes made slow progress across the Atlantic and even in mid-century the average American practitioner still was ready to physic, bleed, and sweat his patients. Public suspicion of such drastic treatment and the reactionary teachings of the Thomsonians, the hydropaths, and the homeopaths allowed these sectarian practitioners to make great inroads in countering the therapeutic horrors of violent allopathic therapy. To escape the drastic therapy of the latter, many parents turned toward the irregular or sectarian practitioners for help when their children were ill.

Medical Practice

Because of their ignorance of the pharmacologic effect of the drugs they prescribed, most early nineteenth-century physicians plodded through their professional lives with a dreary, inflexible, and often fatal routine of drastic therapeutic regimens. No wonder the sectarians, such as Samuel Thomson (1769–1843) with botanical remedies; Samuel Hahnemann (1755–1843) with homeopathy, based in large part upon the healing power of nature; Vincenz Priessnitz (1799–1851) with hydrotherapy, or cold water therapy; and Sylvester Graham (1794–1851) with his popular health movement, had such an easy time winning converts to their medical systems.[55] An increasing number of the laity found many aspects of regular, or allopathic, practice repugnant. Then, too, physicians in the early part of the century, with little knowledge of the structural changes produced by disease and even less of the chemical and functional alterations caused by illness, were unable to visualize what was happening. This was the greatest handicap of medicine in the eighteenth century, and it would require most of the nineteenth century before the laborious and lengthy process of correlating clinical signs and symptoms with the evidence found at the autopsy table would be accomplished. A great leap forward was made in the understanding of disease when the study of pathology was directed toward structural as contrasted with humoral alteration, mainly through the efforts of the physicians in Paris during the first half of the nineteenth century.

The diagnostic skills of shrewd and experienced eighteenth- and early nineteenth-century physicians were no doubt fairly good. They recognized that certain rashes, certain throat findings, certain fevers, and even certain body odors indicated specific diseases. But as they lacked even the rudimentary knowledge of pathology, physiology, biochemistry, and bacteriology in the modern sense (the beginnings of these sciences were fifty to seventy-five years distant), early nineteenth-century treatment remained purely theoretical rather than scientific. Without appreciation of the value of statistical studies and without clinical laboratories, the practice of medicine had no scientific basis. Contemporary medical theorists built nosologies in which they categorized diseases into families based on some assumed or symptomatic similarity, such as diarrheal diseases and fevers; the latter were the real villains of the medical drama. They thereupon deduced that the same therapies would be suitable for all diseases within each family. In this way, physicians established a relationship, albeit tenuous, among diseases, theories, and therapies.

When one realizes the enormous handicaps these physicians faced in treating the ill child, one is forced to appreciate their courage. They were inadequately trained to battle disease, and as Cecil K. Drinker (1887–1956)[25] aptly put it, "they went into the contest bare-handed." It was not until 1808 that Jean Nicolas Corvisart's (1755–1821) translation rescued from an ill-merited oblivion Leopold Auenbrugger's (1722–1809) study of percussion published almost a half-century earlier, following which the value of percussion was universally recognized and it was soon used in medical clinics all over Europe. The stethoscope was invented in 1816 by René Théophile Laennec (1781–1826); its value in physical diagnostic was first reported in 1819 with the publication of his *De l'Auscultation Médiate*. The publication of this book revolutionized the study of diseases of the chest. The second edition (1826) was even more important because it gave not only the various clinical signs elicited in the chest but added also the pathological anatomy, diagnosis, and treatment of each disease encountered. It was not until 1868 that the importance of the clinical thermometer in clinical practice was exhaustively demonstrated by Carl Reinhold Wunderlich (1815–1877)[82] in his encyclopedic study on the relation of body heat to disease *Das Verhalten der Eigenwärme in Krankheiten* (1868). The book reached a much wider audience when its English translation, entitled *Medical Thermometry*, was published by the New Sydenham Society in 1871. Fielding H. Garrison (1870–1935)[29] has said of Wunderlich that "he found fever a disease and left it a symptom." An eminent American surgeon, William W. Keen (1837–1932),[71] has testified that there were probably not half a dozen clinical thermometers employed in the largest Union army throughout the Civil War. Although Sir John Floyer (1649–1734) produced his "physician's pulse-watch" in the early eighteenth century, it was largely ignored by the profession at large until about 1830, when the great French clinician Louis began to use a watch with a second hand to count the pulse.

The first decades of the nineteenth century were part of a period of transition from art to science in medicine, but with as yet little increase in practical benefit to the patient. The practitioner still used chiefly opium, quinine, calomel, rhubarb, magnesia, tartar emetic, castor oil, ipecac, squill, and mercury, supplemented with turpentine, cubebs, iodide of potassium, and gentian. All forms of illness were ascribed to one or two conditions such as peccant material in the blood or the existence of excessive tension or laxity in the nervous and vascular system. A glance at the etiological sections in American books and journals between 1800 and 1850—in fact until 1880—shows that the old miasmic atmosphere theories were still of paramount importance. The familiar explanations of the cause of epidemic diseases recur with monotonous regularity, involving miasmata, ozone, sewer gas, and similar items.

However, until the development of modern medical science there was always a certain divergence between lay and professional attitudes toward epidemic diseases. The general public, if religious, continued to accept the theory of divine punishment, even as late as the early nineteenth century. If more rationally minded, they clung, in spite of contrary medical opinion, to the theory of contagion. Contagion was universally admitted in measles and smallpox. In typhoid fever, dysentery, malaria, and yellow fever, on the other hand, the physician gave it a minor place if any at all; this attitude continued until the dawn of the bacteriological era.[72] It was not until the 1880's that the germ theory was accepted by leaders of American medicine. The lack of interest in the germ theory on the part of the medical profession was a striking example of American neglect of research in basic science during much of the nineteenth century.[71] Experimental proof of specificity of infectious diseases was to become an achievement of the greatest importance to medicine.

Infant Mortality

In Boston between 1840 and 1845, 40 percent of all deaths were among children under 5 years of age. In Massachusetts during the 1850's, the life expectancy for males was 38.7 years; for females 40.9 years. In the nation at large the age for males was about 35.[66]

In 1850 mortality statistics showed no improvement over those of 1790. Proportionately as many children under 5 years of age died in 1850 as in 1789 and the percentage of total deaths for all age groups showed that more children and youths between the ages of 5 and 19 died in the mid-nineteenth century than at the end of the eighteenth century.[24]

Early death was still a common tragedy but as puritanism declined, there was a subtle change in the way parents responded to the deaths of their children. This is evident by studying headstones in graveyards. Seventeenth- and eighteenth-century children's headstones, were merely scaled-down adult stones and were decorated, if at all, by a death's-head or a trumpet-blowing angel ("this Trump of Doom") or whatever other symbol was prevalent at the time. Later gravestones were likely to bear a cherub, lamb, or flower to indicate that a child lay there.[16]

The nation's greatest medical problems throughout the nineteenth century lay in the growing cities, which provided concentrations of poverty and disease such as Americans had never known before. Disease in the city was visible and violent. Most children lived in substandard housing with abysmal sanitation and often were fed contaminated food and milk. House privies and water closets drained into underground vaults where the sewage soaked into the ground or was hauled away. In many poorer sections of our cities, sewage often ran into drain ditches which emptied in the nearest stream. Urban mortality rates rose as city population increased. For example, New York had a death rate of about 21 per

1,000 in 1810 and 37 per 1,000 in 1857, or an increase of 76 percent. Savannah, in a malarial pocket, had a death rate during the 1820's and 1830's of 70 per 1,000.[34]

About 1820 the United States entered a new epidemic period in which yellow fever, smallpox, typhoid fever, and especially cholera swept through cities and rural communities. Tuberculosis was also responsible for an increasing mortality; among children diarrhea and enteritis—particularly during the summer months—were the chief causes of death. Cholera infantum, or summer diarrhea, was especially prevalent among bottle-fed infants. The milk offered to infants in New York was graphically described in Robert Hartley's (1796–1881)[36] *An Essay on Milk,* published in 1842. At that date five-sixths of the milk consumed in New York was from cows housed in city sheds, which often adjoined a distillery, and fed entirely upon distillery wastes. This milk was known as "swill milk" and was filthy beyond belief (Fig. 4–2).

Care of Dependent Children

In the early nineteenth century, binding out or apprenticeship continued to be, as it had been in the eighteenth century, the preferred way for caring for children who for one reason or another were dependent on the public for support. But by the nineteenth century the age at which children were bound out had risen, which meant that the period during which the community was responsible for their care lengthened. And primarily because of the growing humanitarian concern for dependent children, they were maintained as public charges until at least their eighth year and often until they were twelve.

The indenture was a formal agreement which defined the reciprocal obligations of the family and of the apprentice, who was to receive vocational training while he received care in a foster family. It was not always easy to find enough families willing to assume the responsibilities of caring for an apprentice, especially one who was too young for productive work. Indenture and apprenticeship ended about 1875 because of several factors. Perhaps the most important reason was that they were now prohibited by municipal and state laws[12] but, in addi-

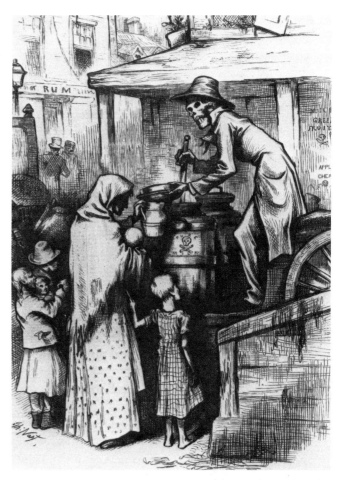

Figure 4–2. Swill milk. (Wood engraving after a drawing by Thomas Nast, in Harper's Weekly, *August 17, 1878, p. 648.)*

tion, the climate had shifted by this time to new forms of care for dependent children such as the asylum or orphanage.[65]

In the larger Eastern cities the problem of poor relief grew rapidly, especially with the waves of immigrants and the increasing number of native-born paupers. To care for these, almshouses were maintained. By the nineteenth century, the almshouses housed hundreds of paupers; many of these were children, who were not always segregated from the older paupers, the insane, and the terminally ill. The almshouse fulfilled the function of offering care in those cases where neither outdoor relief nor indenture was practicable. Almshouse occupants were rarely suited for rewarding industry but much more likely were in dire need of medical attention; for that reason the almshouses of eighteenth-century colonial America actually became our first hospitals, the first institutions providing inpatient care. Physicians, surgeons, and apothecaries were employed by the almshouses and there, according to Samuel X. Radbill,[62] "nursing care, such as it was, was rendered," and "it was in these institutions that foundlings and sick children of the poor were treated, and in them, other forms of child welfare were carried out."

The Philadelphia Almshouse, established in 1732, was known after 1835 as the Philadelphia Hospital and after 1902 as the Philadelphia General Hospital. It is the oldest house of healing in the United States. But it was much more—a lying-in hospital, a foundling hospital for infants, and a place where the insane were cared for humanely. Orphanages and asylums grew rapidly during the nineteenth century and not just as an alternative to indenture and outdoor relief. There was a widespread belief that caring for the child in the orphanage would give the community the chance to instill in the child, away from parental influence, the proper morals and conduct to become a disciplined, diligent citizen. The institution was thought of not merely as a refuge but as a place for transforming the child's character to fit the needs of a work-oriented society.[65] While there were only eight child-care institutions in the United States before 1800, ninety were built between 1825 and 1850 alone.

The first American orphanage was established when the Ursuline nuns in New Orleans in 1728 cared for children orphaned by an Indian massacre in Natchez.[12] This early orphanage, in the tradition of St. Vincent de Paul (1576–1660), received not only support from the Ursuline order but also modest governmental support. The oldest orphanage still in existence in the United States is the Bethesda Orphan House, which was established in Savannah, Georgia, in 1739 by the English evangelist George Whitefield (1714–1770), whose talent in raising funds made this institution possible. Whitefield[62] noted on Tuesday, January 29, 1740: "Took in three German orphans, the most pitiful objects, I think, I ever saw. . . . This day I began the cotton manufacture, and agreed with a woman to teach the little ones to card and spin."

Besides the proliferation of private and sectarian orphanages for dependent normal children, the nineteenth century, especially after 1830, witnessed the establishment of institutions for special groups of children, including the Connecticut Asylum for the Education and Instruction of Deaf and Dumb Persons in 1817, the New York Institution for the Instruction of the Deaf and Dumb in 1818, the New England Asylum for the Blind in 1832, and the Massachusetts School for Idiotic and Feeble-Minded Youth in 1850.

By the mid-nineteenth century, almshouses and orphan asylums represented the extremes of care for dependent children; the former reflected the effort and neglect of public bodies, while the latter symbolized the achievement and limitation of private philanthropy.

The health problems of dependent children in institutions were staggering. The diet in almost all orphanages and almshouses was deplorable even by the standards of that time. Infectious diseases took a terrible toll. Pneumonias and every other form of respiratory-tract infection were rife. Eczematous and furuncular eruptions were the inevitable lot of children in institutions.[62] Purulent ophthalmia, which could lead to blindness, was a constant and ominous problem. A serious outbreak occurred in 1831 in the children's department at Bellevue, the New York City hospital and almshouse.[12] A petition of the commissioners of almshouses[12] to the Common Council for the accommodation of certain children affected with sore eyes, dated May 18, 1831, contained the following description of the epidemic:

The whole number in the establishment is about 600—say 400 boys and 200 girls from infants up to ten years old. About 140 of this number are affected with various degrees of contagious purulent ophthalmia or inflammation of the eyes—many are slightly affected while a great many others (principally boys) present the painful spectacle of total blindness and most appalling swellings, and redness. 25 eyes are seriously injured. Five children [are] totally blind and many [others] in . . . one eye.

Alfred Stillé (1813–1900),[75] professor of the theory and practice of medicine at the University of Pennsylvania from 1864 to 1883, vividly described his experiences as a young intern in 1836 when he lived for six months in the children's asylum of the Philadelphia almshouse.

It was a very interesting field for me from a humanitarian as well as a medical point of view. A hundred or more children [Stillé was the only house officer] were sheltered there on their way to the early grave to which most of them were destined. Illegitimate and other outcasts formed the majority, and ophthalmia, that curse of children's asylums, made of them a blear-eyed, puny crowd, most pitiable to see. I soon became convinced of the causes that produced the crippling and mortality of these outcasts and waifs. I pointed out to the committee of the board how the disease was disseminated by the children washing in the same basins and using the same towels, and how it was maintained by their having no shaded places for exercise in the open air, and also by the insufficient food permitted them; for if the soup which they received one day was nutritious, the meat of which the soup had been made, and which formed their dinner on the following day, must necessarily be nearly devoid of nutriment. But, of course, the commitee on the children's asylum and the guardians knew better than I, and at the time, at least, nothing was done to correct this wrong.

The mortality of foundlings under a year of age in some almshouses as late as 1850 was as high as 97 percent. This stark fact alone was a strong incentive to demand hospitals for sick children of the poor.[60]

American Pediatric Texts, 1800–1850

The Maternal Physician (1811)

The first American book on the management and feeding of infants, entitled *The Maternal Physician*,[4] was published in New York City in 1811 and was written by a mother who concealed her identity. The anonymous author dedicated the book to her mother in language that must have thrilled any parent who had lived through the Revolutionary War: "That helpless babe which reposed on your affrighted bosom when you fled the vicinity of Boston on the day of the ever memorable battle of Lexington, now a wife, a mother and near the meridian of life, as a small tribute for all your maternal cares, most respectfully addresses this little volume to your perusal; candidly confessing that all which is valuable in it she derives from you."

The author's eight healthy and happy children had all (except the youngest) "passed through the usual epidemics" and "were her best apologies for presuming to give advice unasked, and perhaps undesired, to her country women." The mode of treat-

ment was based upon her own clinical experience but was augmented by frequent and liberal extracts from the principal medical authorities of the day: Underwood, Buchan, Rush, and others.

She recommended bathing the infant daily in very cold water; in this she was inspired by John Locke (1632–1704). Although she stressed the superiority of mother's milk as the only proper food for infants, she acknowledged that occasionally a substitute might be necessary, when "a little good cow's milk, diluted nearly one half with water and rendered palatable with sugar may be offered the infant." She assailed paps and "other crudities."

She cut the frenum of the tongue in all of her eight children and claimed that it "is an operation so simple and so easily executed that no mother need to hesitate for a moment about performing it herself."

For teething, she suggested giving the infant "a cork to bite on, and syrup of white poppies." However, in her opinion, infants fed exclusively on milk escaped the perils of teething, which at that time was something most parents feared greatly. She hoped that lancing the gums would become universal and advised mothers "to cut them with a very keen razor while the infant sleeps, and [she] avows that they never awaken from it."

Some of her methods of treatment, like dressing diseases of the navel with roasted raisins and grated nutmeg, and her treatment of a runny nose with injections of breast milk, will seem quaint. Her treatment of a "fever from taking cold" was as follows:

The feet and legs should be bathed in warm water, and drafts applied to the feet; and for young children, garlic drafts are to be preferred, for their peculiar virtue and being easy to the feet. This done half a tea-spoonful of oxymel of squills may be given with a little hyssop tea sweetened with honey and garlic drafts—to make—simmer the cloves of garlic in olive oil or hog's lard, then cut some brown papers about the size of a dollar, dip them and apply them to the soles of the feet, binding them on with proper bandages.

Dr. Sydenham assures us "that among all the substances which occasion a derivation or revulsion from the head, none operates more powerfully than garlic applied to the soles of the feet." I have found them equally efficacious for older children when afflicted with worm complaints.

At the end of her book the anonymous American matron listed a number of "simples" or botanical remedies with which "the beneficent creator has enriched our country and if resorted to," she wrote, "would often supersede the use of compound drugs, especially in the disorders peculiar to childhood"; thus, she continued, "every mother ought to have a general knowledge of them, so that she may prescribe them for slight complaints with ease to herself, and infinite benefit to her little family."

These remedies were widely used in the practice of early nineteenth-century domestic medicine. The matron's comments about the illnesses for which she considered these botanical agents of therapeutic value may be of interest to the present-day pediatrician because some of these remedies are still being prescribed in the dwindling rural sections of our country:

Arum or Wake-Robin (dragon root, and wild turnip)—excellent in colds and colics and windy complaints of children, and in the treatment of rheumatic pains.

Alder—bark of value in intermittent fevers and as a decoction in gargarisms for inflammations of the tonsils.

Ash Tree—sap of the black and white ash excellent for earache.

Anise Seed—good in spasmodic windy complaints of infants. A good carminative and a moderately helpful anodyne.

Angelica—An elegant carminative and especially valuable for children with flatulent complaints.

Avens Root—a powerful stomachic and for strengthening the tone of the viscera in general.

Agrimony—as a tea good for fevers, especially those of the dysenteric kind.

Bayberry Bush—the leaves and berries are good for flatulent infants [also] good when used as an ointment for burns.

Balsam of fir—almost a specific for green wounds and inward bruises.

Baum and Balm—dry, parching fevers.

Blood Root—tincture for jaundice, weakness of the stomach. Powerful styptic.

Burdock—leaves to be used as drafts in all febrile affections.

Caraway Seeds—essential oil and simple distilled water best cordial and carminative medicines I have ever used for infants.

Elder—gentle laxative. An infusion of the flowers is said to cure St. Anthony's Fire (erysipelas).

Elecampane—candied root is excellent for coughs and asthma.

Sweet, or Slippery Elm—inner bark for cutaneous eruptions.

Sweet Fennel—"he who sows fennel, sows sorrow" not seeds, are good in smallpox, measles, malignant fevers, indigestion, flatulence, colic.

Fever Bush—febrifuge hence its name.

Sweet Flagroot—powerful carminative for infants. The candied root highly esteemed as an antiseptic, and used to prevent contagion when epidemic diseases are prevalent.

Gold Thread—root is astringent bitter—an excellent in gargarisms for canker.

House Leek—leaves simmered in fresh butter, oil or lard, makes an excellent ointment for burns or any cutaneous eruptions.

Hyssop—none superior in inflammatory fevers. A very strong decoction, sweetening with honey and a small piece of spermaceti dissolved in it cured peneumonia.

Catnip—excellent herb for infants for use in infant's bowel complaints.

Spearmint—a powerful vermifuge yields a large quantity of essential oil which dropped on sugar in doses of from 1–6 drops, and given to children who are subject to worms, will frequently expel numbers of those vermin. Also improves appetite and cures nausea.

Tansy—vermifuge excellent.

Peppermint—for faintness and anorexia.

Pennyroyal—aperient and deobstruent particularly in hysteric complaints.

Sassafras—leaves, berries and seeds are good in gargles for the canker, and inflammation of the tonsils. Bark of the root bruised and boiled in milk and water, and a little Indian meal stirred into it, while cooking makes an excellent application for burns. And is said to prevent an eschar.

Thorough Wort or Stanch Blood—emetic and a cathartic. Leaves will stop the bleeding of fresh wounds.

Strawberry Bush—plant taken in infusion as a tea, is excellent for the jaundice, and the leaves bruised and applied to a fresh wound will stop bleeding. The fruit is said to dissolve incrustations of the teeth—Excellent remedy for scurvy.

Violets—Syrup of violets for infants to cure the blood (*laxative* and aperient).

George Logan (1825)

The second American treatise on the diseases of children was written by George Logan (1778–1861),[48] of Charleston, South Carolina. Logan graduated from the University of Pennsylvania in 1802, producing as his thesis *Observations on the Hepatic State of Fever*. It is of interest that his father's medical thesis was on the diseases of children. For many years Logan served as physician to the orphanage in Charleston, where he learned much about the diseases of children.

His *Practical Observations on Diseases of Children*, published in Charleston in 1825, was written because he was impelled "by a sense of duty, and not the ambition of being an author," Joseph Waring[78] described the book as offering "a common sense approach to the handling of children." Among the recommendations Logan made were vaccination at the age of ten days and the use of splints for deformed feet. There is strong emphasis on breast-feeding or wet-nursing; the use of weak milk and gruel with sugar was suggested only as a last resort. Slave women were available on the plantations and often served as wet nurses. Pediatric ailments called for ipecac, salts, castor oil, magnesia, calomel, antimony, quinine, seneca, snakeroot, and blisters. Logan claimed that tetanus came from improper care of the infant, such as the application of dirt and manure to the umbilical stump, and that nevi may have been the result of prenatal impressions, especially when they resembled fruit or animals. He found clipping the tongue seldom necessary, and he believed cyanosis was due to an open foramen ovale. The latter observation must have been entirely a clinical one, since no autopsy reports were located in Logan's writings to buttress the relation of foramen ovale and cyanosis. He recommended treating ophthalmia with zinc sulfate.

William Potts Dewees (1825)

The third and most comprehensive American textbook of pediatrics of its day, *Treatise on the Physical and Medical Treatment of Children*, was published by William Potts Dewees (1768–1841)[23] in 1825, the same year as Logan's text. This book, the first American work to deal with children's health and diseases in a scientific manner, was highly praised by physicians on both sides of the Atlantic Ocean.

Dewees, a resident of Philadelphia, was best known for his obstetrical writings and practice. He graduated from the University of Pennsylvania in 1806 and subsequently became adjunct professor of

midwifery in 1825 and professor in 1834 at the same university (Fig. 4–3). Dewees, a prolific writer, especially on obstetrical subjects, was the first American to exert a wide influence upon midwifery. His compendious *System of Midwifery* (1824) was reprinted twelve times and his *Treatise on the Physical and Medical Treatment of Children* eight times. He wrote his treatise on pediatrics because "no one on this side of the Atlantic has thought [it] proper to give the public at one view the American practice in the diseases of children." He was also bothered because "this supineness of our physicians is no less surprising than reprehensible."

Dewees believed there was a distinct need for an American text because "most of the diseases of this country have a peculiarity of character, an intensity of force, and a rapidity, altogether unknown to European climates." This is a point which might be de-

Figure 4–3. William Potts Dewees (1768–1841). (Portrait from Stephen W. Williams, American Medical Biography *{Greenfield, 1845}.)*

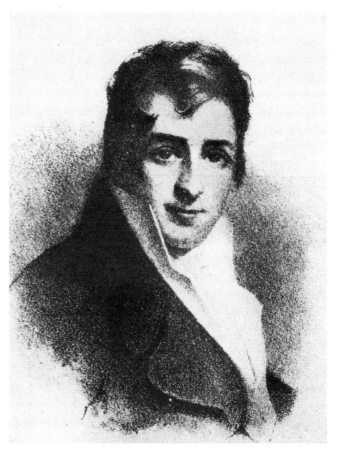

bated in light of our present understanding of the nature of diseases of childhood on both sides of the Atlantic in the early nineteenth century. Strangely, he claimed that many of the diseases described by English authorities such as Underwood "are entirely unknown in this country." Study of these so-called unknown diseases, he believed, would be "both unnecessary and mischievous and would lead to clinical confusion."

The book was divided into two parts; the first dealt primarily with the hygienic care of the newborn, while the second was concerned with the diseases of children. In describing Dewees's textbook, Radbill[61] recently wrote: "This marks the dawn of scientific American pediatric literature." Samuel S. Adams (1853–1928),[3] an early president of the American Pediatric Society, characterized the importance of Dewees's work:

This distinguished luminary in the American pediatric firmament had the temerity to boldly strike at the hitherto impenetrable barriers of the management of the infant in health and disease, and by enforcing his convictions on their physical treatment, opened a field of study that has never flagged since its inception. If Dewees had only accomplished the one reformation of delivering the child from the incarceration of the swaddle, that was sufficient to entitle him to the plaudits of succeeding pediatrists.

Fortunately, by 1825, Dewees[22a] could write that "the mischievous and preposterous custom of swaddling, is nearly abolished, in almost every part of the world; the child from its birth is now permitted more freedom for its limbs, which it exercises with much advantage to itself."

Jaundice in the newborn infant, he noted, "is but too often fatal, with whatever propriety or energy we may attempt to relieve it." Yet he advised treating the jaundiced infant "by giving small doses of castor oil; that is a small tea-spoonful every two hours, until it purges freely." However, if the infant's evacuation did not contain bile, he recommended following up "the purging the next day," by giving "calomel in very small doses, until a cathartic effect be produced."

Aphthae were thought by Dewees to be contagious and epidemic, usually symptomatic of, but not one of the causes of, infantile diarrhea. He treated aphthae with local applications of "equal parts of borax, and loaf sugar, rubbed together until very fine; a small quantity of this in the dry state is to be thrown into the mouth, and repeated every two or three hours. This mixture is quickly dissolved by the saliva of the child, and is soon carried over all of the fauces." Borax remained the treatment for thrush for the next seventy-five years; it was still being recommended by both Job Lewis Smith (1827–1897)[73] and L. Emmett Holt (1854–1924)[40] in the closing years of the nineteenth century.

Dewees, like most of his contemporaries, approved of bloodletting in the treatment of many childhood diseases. For example, in measles "if fever be high, cough and oppression severe, blood should be drawn immediately." The amount was not given nor how frequently it should be performed.

In treating cholera infantum, which he claimed was a disease peculiar to this country, he advised removing the sick infant to the country, as had Rush in the previous century. For those unable to be sent to the country, Dewees's great desideratum was "to tranquilize the stomach" and his first efforts were directed toward the removal of all irritating matter in the stomach itself [he did not say what this irritating matter was] by "encouraging the infant to puke by draughts of warm, or even cold water, where the warm will not be drunk, until no foreign substance appears in the matter thrown up." To further tranquilize the stomach he advised giving the patient "a tea-spoonful of strong coffee, without sugar or milk, every fifteen minutes." If the stomach had not been tranquilized by the strong coffee, calomel was recommended; and if the symptoms persevered, laudanum was added to the calomel, followed by bleeding or the application of leeches over the stomach. He divided the diarrheas of infancy into six varieties: feculent, bilious, mucous, chylous, lienteric, and chronic. Each was described in minute detail.

John Eberle (1833)

John Eberle (1788–1838)[26] published his *Treatise on the Diseases and Physical Education of Children* in 1833, seven years after the appearance of Dewees's book. Like Dewees, Eberle divided his book into two parts. The first was concerned with the prophylactic and physical management of children; the second dealt with the diseases of children. This division was a common American practice that was also followed in contemporary English books on the diseases of children.

Eberle was of German descent and a native of Pennsylvania. After graduating in 1809 from the University of Pennsylvania School of Medicine, he founded the *American Medical Recorder* in 1818 and served as its editor in chief for a number of years. In 1825 he was appointed professor of materia medica and of the theory and practice of medicine at the newly organized Jefferson Medical College in Philadelphia. In 1830, Eberle accepted the offer of Daniel Drake (1785–1852) to organize the faculty for the medical department of Miami University, to be located in Cincinnati as a competitor of the Medical College of Ohio. The two schools soon were consolidated and he and his colleagues found themselves members of the conjoint faculty. In 1837 Eberle accepted the chair of the theory and practice of medicine at the Transylvania School of Medicine in Lexington, Kentucky. His health failed and he died in Lexington after less than a year's residence.[45]

His pediatric treatise was in its day a popular work; it was revised and republished in 1850 by a former colleague. Eberle dealt with the diseases of children in connection with the practice of medicine, while Dewees viewed them as an appendage of obstetrics.

Eberle included a chapter on the conduct of mothers during pregnancy in the first section of the book in which he discussed the "ruinous effects" of maternal alcohol intake on "the life and health of the fetus in utero," or what we now term the fetal alcohol syndrome:

The majority of children born of decidedly intemperate mothers, are weak and sickly, and but few of them arrive at the age of adolescence. Many females appear to think, that although these and other melancholy consequences follow in the train of habitual intermperance, it is extremely improbable that any injury can result to themselves or the foetus, from the occasional use of small portions of spirituous liquors. Were it indeed absolutely certain, that the use of such potations, would always be restricted to occasional small portions, the indulgence would perhaps, rarely occasion any serious consequences. But as no prudence and resolution can be safely regarded as an entire protection against the gradual formation of the habit of intemperance, where such drinks are occasionally taken during gestation, even though it be at very considerable intervals and in very moderate quantities at

first, it is far the safest plan, to abstain wholly from every kind of spirituous liquors.

Eberle was in advance of most of his contemporaries and predecessors in rejecting the role of maternal impressions in producing congenital anomalies. He also was non-Lockean in his recommendation that the infant be bathed in warm rather than cold water. He advised against the popular practice of bathing the head of a newborn infant with brandy or some other spirituous liquor, in order "as is imagined, to invigorate its system and fortify it against the injurious effects of cold and other causes of disease." When artificial feeding was unavoidable, Eberle recommended "a mixture of two parts of fresh cow's milk, and one part of warm water, with a very small portion of sugar. . . . [This] will in general, answer the purpose better than any other article of food, that can be contrived." In regard to dentition, he believed that children who resided in crowded cities, confined to close and poorly ventilated apartments, were "much more liable to unpleasant consequences from teething, than those who enjoy the pure and salubrious air of the country." And like most of his British and American medical contemporaries, he reported that "the occurrence of convulsions from difficult dentition is very common."

Eberle devoted a long chapter to cholera infantum, which he attributed to "atmospheric heat, dentition, and the impure air of cities." His treatment was to apply leeches to the infant's temples, or to induce small blisters either behind the ears or on the back of the neck, to give small doses of calomel and ipecac, and to apply a large stimulating poultice over the abdomen. He also mentioned that in his practice "the little patient sometimes manifests a most urgent craving, for certain strong and stimulating articles of food, such as salted and smoked herring or shad, old and rancid bacon, and salted beef." Eberle cited Rush's similar observation of a craving for salty foods by infants with cholera infantum (p. 45).

Eberle's treatment of diphtheria began with "bleeding to the extent of producing fainting . . . as an indispensable measure in the treatment of this affection." And after bleeding the patient he recommended that "leeches should be . . . applied to the throat."

James Stewart (1841)

James Stewart (1799–1864),[74] an 1823 graduate of the College of Physicians and Surgeons in New York City, was said to excel in his accuracy of diagnosis. His essay "Cholera Infantum" received the highest prize of the New York Academy of Medicine, although it was simply a record of facts and experiences gathered at the bedside through a long series of years.

In 1839, he translated Billard's *The Diseases of Children* from the French with an appendix of one hundred pages of Stewart's pediatric comments. His own *Diseases of Children* was first published in 1841; a second edition appeared in 1843. In it, pathological anatomy and Laennec's innovation of auscultation were mentioned for the first time in an American pediatric text.

Stewart described the diseases of children under three divisions which he said were "founded on the functions of the human frame." First, the vital functions, "or those which are essential to life—as the circulation and respiration." Second, the natural functions "instrumental in repairing the several losses which the body sustains—as digestion, chylification and secretion, which may be suspended for a time without destruction of life." And, third, "the animal functions by which we communicate with the surrounding world—as the motor and nervous system." His system of organization, although novel, was cumbersome and led to strange bedfellows, for example, convulsions, cholera, hydrocephalus, ophthalmia, and otitis were all described under diseases of the nervous system.

His treatment of infantile convulsions called for vigorous bleeding from the arm, leeching, and cupping. He was prescient in claiming that pertussis and scarlet fever were diseases of "specific contagions." Stewart was the first American writer to record his belief in the specific origin of infectious diseases "occurring epidemically."

About the year 1850, Stewart, under the pen name "Philopedos," originated a plan for the establishment of a hospital for children in New York City. When the institution was opened on March 1, 1854, under the name of the New York Nursery and Child's Hospital,[60] it was the only hospital on this continent devoted to children. (There had been a hospital devoted exclusively to sick children in Boston as early as 1846, but financial difficulties forced it to close after a few years.)

The New York Nursery and Child's Hospital was established for the children of wet nurses who had to neglect their own children in order to nurse the children of their employers. The nurses' children nearly all took sick while under the care of the institution; the hospital part was therefore needed as an infirmary. But, in addition to these functions, the wet nurses were admitted when they needed medical care, so that it was also a lying-in and gynecological hospital. Later on, when the New York Nursery and Child's Hospital merged with Babies Hospital, it became restricted to sick children.

David Francis Condie (1844)

David Francis Condie (1796–1875)[20] published his *Practical Treatise on the Diseases of Children* in 1844, and it went through six editions between 1844 and 1868. It was the most widely accepted textbook on children's diseases in the United States until it was superseded by Job Lewis Smith's in 1869 and by Meigs and Pepper's in 1870.

Condie was born in Philadelphia and received his M.D. from the University of Pennsylvania in 1818. He spent his entire professional life in Philadelphia and is said to have always visited his patients on foot because he disapproved of physicians' driving. He believed that "those who rode in one-horse carriages were physically deficient; those who rode in two-horse carriages were mentally deficient."[45]

The introductory chapters of his book were devoted to the "management of children . . . and their physical and moral education." The necessity of pure air for infants was strongly enforced and the dangers inherent in rearing infants in the close air of a stove-warmed nursery were stressed. He advised that "until the age of puberty, preparations of milk and the farinaceous vegetables should, in fact, constitute the principal nourishment." This recommendation was made by Condie and others in the 1840's because at that time there was a rather widely accepted belief that the "carnivorous propensities of American youth were responsible for their leanness and sallowness."

Condie's book was the first to contain a detailed account of the symptomatology of the diseases of infancy and children. His emphasis on the seriousness and frequency of gangrene of the mouth (noma or cancrum oris) in infants points up how important this condition used to be. For example, in the Children's Asylum of Philadelphia in the 1830's, there were 70 out of 240 inmates affected with this disease at the same time. The mortality was staggering.[33] In the treatment of diarrhea he was ahead of his contemporaries in not using strong purgatives. He followed Rush's advice about the best treatment for cholera infantum: the removal of the patient from the "close, hot and impure atmosphere of the town" to the country.

In the third edition of his book (1850) Condie described a newly reported form of infantile convulsions:

A very peculiar form of infantile convulsions has recently been observed. It consists of repeated bobbings of the head forward, at first slight and occasional, but becoming in process of time, so frequent and powerful, as to cause a heaving of the head forwards towards the knees, succeeded by an immediate return to the upright position.... Sir Charles Clarke [1782–1857] has seen four cases of the disease, and from the peculiar bowing of the head, has named it the *Salaam Convulsion.*

This is the first mention of infantile spasms, or salaam spasms, in American pediatric literature. Condie was quite prophetic when added: "Of this strange form of convulsions, the pathology is still a subject for future investigation; and until this is ascertained, its treatment must be tentative and experimental."

The exanthemata are well covered, but he is guilty of an *error loci* in including morbus caeruleus under cutaneous rashes rather than in the section set apart for congenital malformations.

John Forsyth Meigs (1848)

John Forsyth Meigs (1818–1882),[51] of Philadelphia, published *A Practical Treatise on the Diseases of Children* in 1848. He was the son of Charles Delucena Meigs (1792–1869). Both father and son published books on pediatrics within two years: the son in 1848, and the father in 1850. John F. Meigs, the son, was born in Philadelphia in 1818, the third of ten

children (Fig. 4–4). When not yet twenty years old he received his M.D. from the University of Pennsylvania in 1838. His textbook passed through seven editions between 1848 and 1882. The first three editions were published under his name alone, and in 1870, William Pepper (1843–1898) became a coauthor for the fourth edition and remained such for the remaining three editions.

Childhood diseases were divided into five classes: diseases of the respiratory organs, digestive organs, nervous system, the eruptive fevers, and worms in the alimentary canal. Meigs's book was a distinct improvement on previous American pediatric textbooks because of this new and convenient classification of diseases according to the systems they affected. His division of diseases of the respiratory tract into those of the upper air passages, the lungs, and pleura was also novel. The ordering of the subjects into definition, synonym, forms, frequency, causes, anatomical lesions, symptoms, diagnosis, prognosis, and treatment shows the vision of the author. This system, slightly modified, was adopted by

Figure 4–4. John Forsyth Meigs (1818–1882). (Courtesy of the Countway Library of Medicine.)

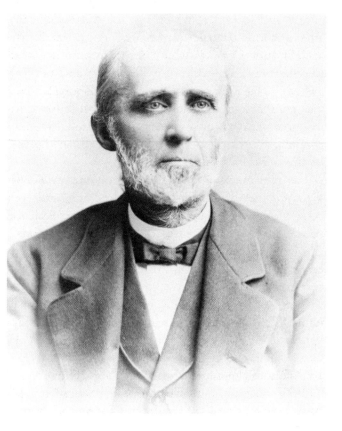

Osler[57] in writing his *Principles and Practice of Medicine* (1892).

Charles Delucena Meigs (1850)

Charles Delucena Meigs,[50] father of John Forsyth Meigs, was born in Bermuda on February 19, 1792, received his M.D. from the University of Pennsylvania in 1817, and served as professor of obstetrics and diseases of children at the Jefferson Medical College from 1841 to 1861 (Fig. 4–5). Save for his *Observations on Certain Diseases of Young Children* (1850), all of his published medical works were about obstetrics and gynecology.

His book, as its title implies, laid no claim to being a complete text of the diseases of infancy and childhood. It presented the author's view of the pathology of a few of the diseases peculiar to early childhood and his experience in treating them. The book was actually a summary of the pediatric lectures he gave to his students in 1849.

In the chapter on bowel complaints, Meigs quoted Johann Franz Simon's (1807–1843) figures (p. 134) on the chemical composition of cow's milk and human milk and from these he concluded that it was the larger quantity of casein in cow's milk that accounted for the frequent attacks of indigestion in bottle-fed infants. This erroneous hypothesis was accepted by most pediatricians until well into the present century.

An entire chapter was devoted to coryza. His plan for the treatment of this disease was, after having removed the mucous and solid crusts, to keep the interior of the nostrils constantly anointed with one of the "finer animal oils" or with what he believed particularly helpful, "the ointment of cucumbers." He also claimed that a light flannel cap "fitting closely to the infant's head" was in itself sufficient, in a large number of instances, to cure the malady.

Organization of Early Nineteenth-Century Pediatric Textbooks

The modern reader will find all of these early nineteenth-century pediatric textbooks difficult to read because their organization presented a poorly indexed and curious array in which symptoms, diseases, hygienic matters, comments on psychology, and the meconium were thrown together in what ap-

peared to be a purely arbitrary manner. Even the last edition (the ninth) of Dewees's textbook showed a similar confusion, worms being considered between croup and scarlet fever and whitlow between anal prolapse and vaginal discharge. Remittent fever included typhoid fever, some cases of infectious diarrhea, probably pyelitis and endocarditis, and in all likelihood abdominal tuberculosis—to say nothing of typhus fever and possibly some cases of pneumonia. Acute hydrocephalus meant tuberculous meningitis. Under the heading hydrocephalus, all forms of meningitis and encephalitis plus those due to congenital defects and birth injuries were described. Hopelessly confused were the conditions called croup, laryngismus stridulus, inward fits, Millar's asthma, and spasm of the glottis. Some, like John Cheyne (1777–1836)[19] in England, spoke of cynanche trachealis (diphtheria) as croup. Bretonneau in France in 1826 also conceived of croup and malignant angina (*diphthérite*) to be identical and the same as Bard's *angina suffocativa*. How confusing the croup complex became is apparent from the following attempt

Figure 4–5. Charles Delucena Meigs (1792–1869). (Courtesy of the Countway Library of Medicine).

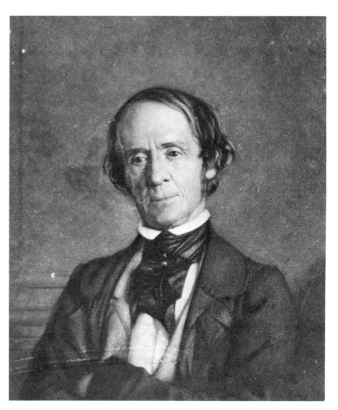

of Meigs and Pepper to explain what they meant by "spasmodic or false croup":

It is the disease commonly called in this country croup, or, by those who make the distinction between it and pseudo-membranous laryngitis or true croup, spasmodic croup. It is known also by the names of false or pseudo-croup. We prefer the term spasmodic laryngitis, because it is expressive of the essential characters of the disease. It is the stridulous laryngitis of Guersent and Valleix; the stridulous angina of Bretonneau, the acute asthma of infancy of Millar; and the spasmodic croup of Wichmann, Michaelis, and Double. It is not the laryngismus stridulus described by the English authors, Kerr, Ley, and Marsh, which is the same as the thymic or Kipp's asthma of the Germans, and spasm of the glottis of the French. It is called by Dr. Wood, in his work on the practice of medicine, catarrhal croup.

Further along, the authors struggle with "pseudo-membranous laryngitis, membranous or true croup." "It is the croup of the French writers, while, in this country, it is called by the various names of slow, creeping, true, membranous or inflammatory." Order was introduced into this chaos by Eduard Heinrich Henoch (1820–1910),[38] of Berlin, in his textbook published in 1861. After a preliminary consideration of the diseases of the newborn, Henoch then proceeded in an orderly fashion to diseases of particular systems of the body.

The unsatisfactory nosography of the period renders the use of many early nineteenth-century reports of diseases difficult, since disease classification still largely rested, as late as 1860, on a symptom-complex. Because of this there has been some disagreement as to what diseases were primarily involved during the earlier periods of the century.

One is surprised in reading these textbooks to find little or no mention of many conditions that are so well known today. Intracranial hemorrhage in the newborn was not mentioned, nor was any form of hemorrhagic disease of the newborn, except bleeding from the umbilicus. Hemophilia was not mentioned, despite John C. Otto's (1774–1844) classic paper on this disease published in 1803 (p. 86). In spite of Hezekiah Beardsley's description of pyloric stenosis in 1788 (p. 51), it was not included in any of these books. The term rheumatism was used by Condie to describe pain in the muscle but none of the textbooks contained a description of acute rheumatic fe-

ver. Since there was little interest in performing a physical examination of the chest, heart disease was scarcely considered, with the exception of cursory mention of the congenital variety of morbus caeruleus. There were many curious misconceptions, such as Eberle's ascribing the increase in the number of cases of convulsions to the vicious system of educating infants in "modern times." He was referring to the year 1833.

Some Significant American Contributions to Pediatrics, 1800–1850

Benjamin Waterhouse and Vaccination (1800)

Vaccination, the method introduced by Edward Jenner,[43] has often been described as simply inoculation with a safer virus. Benjamin Waterhouse (1754–1846) was an important figure in Boston's smallpox story, the self-appointed herald of Jennerian vaccination at a time and to a public not yet ready to accept it (Fig. 4–6). Waterhouse received samples of the new vaccine from Jenner in July, 1800, and immediately did what Zabdiel Boylston and Edward Jenner had done. He vaccinated his five-year-old son, Daniel Oliver Waterhouse, and on succeeding days three-year-old Benjamin, one-year-old Mary, seven-year-old Elizabeth, a twelve-year-old servant boy, and two adults of his household. Daniel Waterhouse was thus the first person vaccinated in the New World, as Zabdiel Boylston's son had been the first person inoculated.[81] Little Benjamin developed a slight illness on the sixth day; on the seventh and eighth, redness was noted in the area where the vaccine had been inserted; bluish pustules appeared on the tenth day, corresponding precisely to the illustration Jenner had furnished. The children's illnesses had been so mild that they had scarcely been diverted from their play. When his patients' recovery from vaccination was complete, Waterhouse asked William Aspinwell (1743–1823), head of the smallpox hospital near Boston, to inoculate them with smallpox virus to complete the test. Aspinwell agreed and admitted them to his smallpox hospital, where they were inoculated with virus taken from a hospital patient. All proved resistant.[44] News of Waterhouse's success spread so that in a very short time he was deluged with patients seeking vaccination and by physicians requesting the vaccine that Waterhouse had termed the "kine-pox."

Waterhouse was born in Newport, Rhode Island, in 1754. In 1775 he went to Great Britain, where he attended medical lectures in London and Edinburgh for three years. He then went to Leyden, where he remained for four years, receiving his medical degree in 1781. In 1782, after seven years abroad, Waterhouse returned to Boston. The following year he assisted John Warren (1753–1815) in establishing the Harvard Medical School.

Waterhouse began his long fight for vaccination in 1800, a crusade that earned him the title of the "Jenner of America." For a number of reasons, including political ones, jealousy, and controversy over fees, he was dismissed in 1812 from his chair at Harvard. But being a gifted scientific man he continued his crusade against smallpox. His pamphlet *A Prospect of Exterminating the Small-Pox* (1800–1802) was the first work on vaccination published in the United States. This remarkable contribution to the history of American medicine may well be the most important prior to the discovery of anesthesia.

President Thomas Jefferson (1743–1826) showed great interest in vaccination; in 1802, after having received a supply of cowpox vaccine from Waterhouse, he arranged for the vaccination of "about seventy or eighty of my own family; my sons in law about as many in theirs, and including our neighbors who wished to avail themselves of the opportunity, our whole experiment extended to about two hundred persons."[11] Thanks to Jefferson's support, vaccination spread throughout Virginia and other parts of the United States. The President himself, while at Monticello, performed many vaccinations. In a letter to Jenner in 1806 he wrote: "Future generations will know by history only that the loathsome smallpox existed and by you has been extirpated."[11]

The legislative history of vaccination is a long and often bitter one. The first law making vaccination compulsory in America was passed in 1855 but was not strictly enforced until 1872.

Benjamin Waterhouse and Cautions to Young Persons Concerning Health (1805)

About the year 1804, Waterhouse began to note a certain deterioration in the health of the young med-

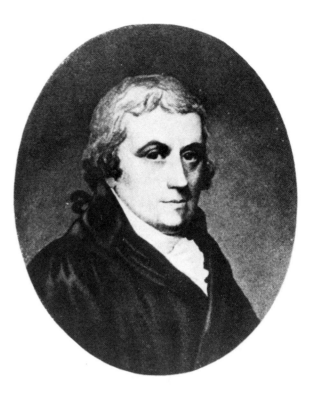

Figure 4–6. Benjamin Waterhouse (1754–1846), professor of the theory and practice of physic at Harvard Medical School. (Engraved by S. Harris; courtesy of the Boston Athenaeum.)

ical students he was teaching at the Harvard Medical School. This he attributed to their sedentary life plus overuse of wine, ardent spirits, and tobacco.[79] "Unruly wine and ardent spirits," he wrote, "have supplanted sober cider." Chewing and smoking tobacco, too, were condemned. "I have been a Professor in this University twenty-three years," he wrote, "and can say, as a physician, that I have never observed so many pallid faces, and so many marks of declining health; nor ever knew so many hectical habits and consumptive affections, as of late years; and I trace this alarming inroad on your young constitutions principally to the pernicious custom of smoking cigars."

These and other "cautions to young persons concerning health" were given in a public lecture delivered at the close of a medical course on November 20, 1804. The following year the lecture entitled *Cautions to Young Persons Concerning Health* was published as a pamphlet of 32 pages. It was to become the most popular of any of Waterhouse's writings and it was enthusiastically received by both Jefferson and Rush. (This displeased Waterhouse because he considered A Prospect of Exterminating the Small-Pox his most important publication by far.) Few writings of the time had as wide an audience and through this little pamphlet, which was translated widely, Waterhouse already well known to the medical profession, became a national and even international figure.

John C. Otto on Hemophilia (1803)

An anonymous German author[46] in 1793 published a description of a bleeding disease affecting males and not females. The report appeared in an obscure German text; for this reason credit for the first clinical report of the hereditary nature of hemophilia is usually given to the Philadelphia physician John C. Otto,[58] whose similar account, published ten years later, received widespread attention. His paper was one of the first significant contributions to North American medicine.

It cannot be stated how long true hemophilia had been known before Otto's description of it. Certain commandments in the Talmud concerning circumcision of boys whose brothers had died from bleeding after the operation would suggest that the risk was understood. There was even mention of three sisters whose firstborn sons had bled to death after circumcision; this suggests a certain insight into the hereditary character of hemophilia among the ancient Jews.

Otto was born in 1774 near Woodbury, New Jersey. He graduated from the College of New Jersey (Princeton) in 1792 and received his M.D. from the University of Pennsylvania in 1796. As a student he had worked in Benjamin Rush's office, becoming the favorite pupil and friend of this eminent physician. When Rush died in 1813, Otto succeeded him as physician to the Pennsylvania Hospital.

Otto's account of hemophilia, written in his twenty-ninth year, contained a description of all the essential clinical features of this disease. He noted that the disease was transmitted in families and that "although the females are exempt they are still capable of transmitting it to their male children." He further observed, "It is a surprising circumstance that the males only are subject to this strange affection, and that all of them are not liable to it." Otto's account of hemophilia is probably the first complete description ever given of this disease, yet its genetic implications were overlooked by American physicians for nearly a century thereafter.

Elisha North on Cerebrospinal Meningitis (1911)

Elisha North's (1771–1843)[54] book of 249 pages published in 1811, entitled A Treatise on a Malignant Epidemic Commonly Called Spotted Fever, was described by Jacobi[42] as "worthy of the name of a classic." This was the first book ever published on cerebrospinal meningitis, and in it North recommended the use of the clinical thermometer, not in general use until the time of Wunderlich (1868).

In 1807 a new and peculiar disease, spotted fever, or epidemic cerebrospinal meningitis, occurred in Connecticut and demanded North's attention. "It had come upon Goshen, Connecticut," he wrote, "like a flood of mighty waters, bringing along with it the horrors of a most dreadful plague." Its first appearance in the state occurred in Winchester on April 10, 1807, completely mystifying and baffling all the physicians who tried to cope with it. They not only found difficulty in giving it an adequate name but they were also unable to classify it. Equally baffling to them was how to treat it. North wondered "whether the spotted fever may be considered as only a variety of cynanche maligna or scarlatina; and be arranged under the order phlegmasia or exanthemata; or whether it ought to be regarded as only a variety of the malignant petechial fever of [older] authors; or whether it is a new species of disease, to be added to the list of human calamities."

North's description of the epidemic resembled those of the bacteremic cases seen in World Wars I and II. He described "a great surprising sudden loss of strength . . . violent pain in the head and many times of the limbs . . . syncope . . . coma . . . mania . . . delirium . . . and petechiae." Petechiae were so commonly noted during the first season in which the disease prevailed that it was considered to be one of its most striking characteristics, giving rise to the name "petechial fever" or "spotted fever," which has been generally, though very improperly, applied to the disease. North described the spots as being commonly between "the size of a pin head and a six cent bit." In discussing "the more unusual symptoms of the fever," he wrote: "there are a dilatation, and, in some, a contraction of the pupils of the eyes, redness and suffusion of the eyes; blindness in some, in others double or treble vision; a drawing back of the head, with a kind of clonic spasm of the muscles of the neck." It would appear that these cases, which resemble the present-day sporadic type of cerebrospinal meningitis, were relatively less common than the acute (?bacteremic) form.

As to the cause of the epidemic, North was eighteenth-century in his views: "The spotted fever is asthenic in nature. Hence, the remote and predisponent causes must be such as debilitate the system." He made no suggestion of contagion. It would be difficult for us to be absolutely sure of the nature of this "spotted fever" were there not appended autopsy notes of two cases by Dr. L. Danielson and Dr. E. Mann: "The second examination was made twelve hours after death, on the body of a girl of five years old. . . . Between the dura and the pia mater was effused a fluid resembling pus."

A major problem in tracing the historical aspects of cerebrospinal meningitis was that for nearly a century the only recognized form was the epidemic. Most of the reported outbreaks occurred in small towns and in garrisons; they were described incompletely by local physicians, whose accounts were usually published in local medical journals.[42] Little was added to the knowledge of this disease until the discovery of the meningococcus *Neisseria meningitidis*, the causative agent of cerebrospinal meningitis, by Anton Weichselbaum (1845–1920) in 1887.

North's treatment consisted in giving an emetic, generally ipecac, at the commencement of the disease, followed by a cathartic of senna, rhubarb, or some other mild purge. He then applied a blister to the back to cure the headache. For pain he suggested elixir of paregoric or tincture of opium in sufficient doses to ease pain and remove distress. To control the fever, a tea of Virginia snakeroot and Peruvian bark was given. The patient's feet were kept warm with sinapisms or bottles of warm water. For a common drink, warm teas of sage, pennyroyal, hemlock, or rob of elder were prescribed. If called to see a patient in "the sinking state of fever," North ordered "the patient to bed, having first bathed his feet in warm water"; he then applied "blisters to the nape of the neck and prescribed tincture of opium, hot brandy slings, heated wine and warm teas."

John Brodhead Beck on Infanticide (1817)

The relations of pediatrics to forensic medicine are very close. Nothing demonstrates this more than the immense literature in every language on infanticide. John Brodhead Beck's (1794–1851)[5] small brochure on infanticide, published in 1817, is still considered one of the most significant contributions to this subject in the English language. In fact, this little brochure covered the subject so thoroughly that many later writers have done little more than reproduce it. The little work was subsequently incorporated by its author's brother Theodoric Romeyn Beck (1791–1855)[7] into the latter's enduring *Elements of Medical Jurisprudence* (1823).

Beck graduated from Columbia College in 1813 with the highest honors of his class and received his M.D. from the College of Physicians and Surgeons in 1817. In 1826 he became professor of materia medica and botany in the College of Physicians and Surgeons and later was appointed professor of medical jurisprudence in the same institution, holding these two professorships for many years.

John Brodhead Beck and Infant Therapeutics (1849)

In 1849 Beck published a small book entitled *Essays on Infant Therapeutics*,[6] in which he discussed the effects of opium, emetics, mercury, blisters, and bloodletting on the young child. He warned against the excessive use of opium and discussed the use of mercury, vesicatories, and depletion with a good deal of knowledge and emphasis. The modern reader will find these essays almost entirely anecdotal, with very little scientific explanation for the use of the drugs discussed. However, Beck's little book does have the distinction of being the first one written about infant therapeutics in America.

Thomas Hopkins Gallaudet and the Deaf Child (1817)

The emerging concern for the unfortunate, although it was more for their educational problems than the medical aspects of their handicaps, nevertheless was one of the glories of that century. Thomas Hopkins Gallaudet (1787–1851),[27] educator of the deaf, was among the first Americans to be moved by the new humanitarian concern for the welfare of the young that developed in the early part of the century. His interest in the deaf child began about 1815 when he became acquainted with Alice Cogswell, who had lost her hearing from "spotted fever" when she was two years old and to whom he tried to teach the names of certain objects. Alice's father, Thomas Cogswell, and a number of friends raised a sum of money to send Gallaudet to Europe to "acquire the art of instructing the deaf and dumb" used in schools for the deaf there. Gallaudet by this time, because of ill health, had declined to accept a ministerial position, for which he had prepared himself at the Andover Theological Seminary.

He first went to England but was disappointed by his reception there. The Institut Royal des Sourds-Muets in Paris, however, guided by the Abbé Sicard, welcomed him enthusiastically, and there Gallaudet studied for about three months. He returned to the United States in 1816 with Laurent Clerc, a gifted teacher of the deaf and dumb at the Paris institution, and with his help raised money for the first free American school for the deaf, established in Hartford in 1817 and named the Connecticut Asylum for the Education and Instruction of Deaf and Dumb Persons. The interest shown in this school was great. In 1817, with the exception of the Pennsylvania Hospital (1751), a small hospital for the insane in Williamsburg, Virginia, and the almshouses, no public charitable institutions existed in our country. On April 15, 1817, the date some consider the birthday of organized philanthropic effort in America, the school was opened with seven pupils. Gallaudet served as the school's superintendent until 1830. During these thirteen years, despite his failing health and other discouraging events, he was able to train a number of teachers who later were to become the heads of similar schools.

Gallaudet's effort was not confined to the education of the deaf. He helped to establish normal schools in Connecticut and interested himself in the education of black youths. He was a dedicated supporter of higher education for women and stressed the need of well-trained women in the professions.

Gallaudet's[22] sermon delivered at the opening of the Connecticut asylum had this moving comment about the deaf and dumb: "But there is a *sickness more dreadful than that of the body; there are chains more galling than those of the dungeon—the immortal mind preying upon itself*, and so imprisoned as not to be able to unfold its intellectual and moral powers, and to attain to the comprehension and enjoyment of those objects, which the Creator has designed as the sources of its highest expectations and hopes. Such must often be the condition of the uninstructed deaf and dumb! How imperfectly can they account for the wonders that surround them."

One of Gallaudet's first pupils at the Hartford School was Sophia Fowler, who soon after her graduation became his wife. Their oldest son, Thomas (1822–1902), became the well-known Episcopalian missionary to the deaf. Their youngest son, Edward Miner (1837–1917), with the help of Amos Kendall (1789–1869), an American journalist, and some friends, established a school for the deaf in Washington in 1864. Thirty years later this school became Gallaudet College, named in honor of Thomas Hopkins Gallaudet, to whose grateful memory deaf citizens throughout the country erected a monument by Daniel Chester French (1850–1931), now on the grounds of the college.[22]

Samuel Gridley Howe and the Blind Child (1832)

Samuel Gridley Howe (1801–1876),[69] educator and reformer, champion of peoples and persons laboring under disability, was born in Boston on November 10, 1801. Howe graduated from Brown University in 1821 and then entered the Harvard Medical School, receiving his M.D. in 1824 (Fig. 4–7). Soon thereafter he sailed to Greece like a crusader to aid that country's revolution against the Turks. For six years he fought, was a surgeon of the Greek fleet, and then helped in the reconstruction that followed. In 1831, having returned to Boston, he eagerly accepted an offer to direct a newly founded school, the New England Asylum for the Education of the Blind, which was to be the first formal attempt to educate the blind in the United States.

In August, 1832, Howe started the school in his father's house in Boston with seven pupils, ranging in age from six to twenty, and with a staff of three, consisting of Howe and two teachers of the blind he had hired in Europe. Howe did everything himself, from planning the curriculum to rounding up the students. His first two pupils were six-year-old Abby and eight-year-old Sophia Carter of Andover, Massachusetts. Howe is said to have gone about blind-

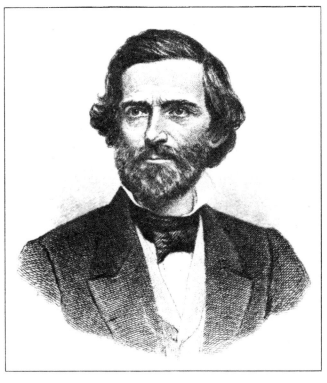

Figure 4–7. Samuel Gridley Howe (1801–1876), M.D., Harvard Medical School, 1824. (Courtesy of the Countway Library of Medicine.)

folded at first, to better understand the world of the blind.

Having trained his pupils by teaching methods created by himself and according to his maxim, "Obstacles are things to be overcome," Howe was able in 1833 to obtain private funds and the gift of the mansion of Thomas Handasyd Perkins (1764–1854) to house the increasing number of pupils. By 1835 the Perkins mansion had become too small to accommodate the forty-two students and a large staff of teachers, forcing Howe to find a more suitable site. Learning of the availability of a hotel in South Boston known as the Mount Washington House, he exchanged the smaller Perkins mansion for it in 1838 (Fig. 4–8). The move was made in May, 1839, and the school was renamed the Perkins Institution in honor of its patron. Perkins, as it was familiarly known, remained in South Boston until 1912.

Howe was eminently successful in educating blind

children to lead happy and useful lives. Famous as he was for his work with the blind, he became even more famous for his work with the deaf-blind. His triumph was the case of Laura Bridgman (1829–1889), who came down with an attack of scarlet fever during an epidemic in Hanover, New Hampshire, when she was a year and a half of age. Her two older sisters and brother died during the epidemic; as Laura convalesced, her parents realized that her sight and hearing had been totally destroyed and that her senses of taste and smell were seriously impaired. In 1837 Howe read a newspaper account about her written by a member of the Medical Department of Dartmouth College and he immediately decided to admit her to his asylum, if her parents concurred, and then to try a plan for the education of a deaf and blind child. Laura entered the institution on October 4, 1837, where she was to live for the rest of her life. Howe's great experiment in education had now begun. His success in communicating with Miss Bridgman roused the enthusiasm of Charles Dickens during his visit to America in 1842. Laura Bridgman's impact on her time was immense, and through her the world became aware of a class of handicapped children critically in need of attention and care.

Howe did not limit himself to the care and training of the blind child, but during his life he worked for many other causes. He supported Horace Mann (1796–1859) in the crusade for common and normal schools, pioneered in the education of mentally retarded children, worked for prison reform, and aided

Figure 4–8. The Perkins Institution for the Blind in South Boston, formerly the Mount Washington House.

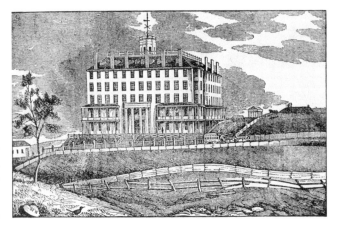

Dorothea Dix (1820–1887) in improving the care of the insane.

In his own special field, the education of the handicapped, Howe continued to do significant work, adding instruction of the feebleminded to his many accomplishments. After proving that they could benefit from schooling, he led a movement that resulted in the organization of the Massachusetts School for Idiotic and Feeble-Minded Youth (1850), now known as the Fernald School, named for its first superintendent, Walter E. Fernald (1859–1924). In its field it was to become as prominent as Perkins.

David Hosack and German Measles (1814)

Physicians of the seventeenth and eighteenth centuries probably observed cases of rubella, but it was not until the early nineteenth century that it was finally distinguished from measles and scarlet fever and considered as a distinct entity.[64]

David Hosack (1769–1835)[41] observed an epidemic of an eruptive disease in New York in 1813 resembling measles. His description fits that of rubella and was a far better one than any other report of this disease until Henry R. Veale's (1832–1908)[77] in 1866. Hosack wrote:

An eruptive disease in many respects resembling the measles, has prevailed to a considerable extent during the last three months. Such was the resemblance it bore to the measles in its invasion, the character and extent of the eruption, that by many it was called the French measles. It, however, differed from the measles (rubeola vulgaris) in several particulars. The fever preceding the eruption, was very inconsiderable in degree, and of short duration, not more than twenty-four hours; and in some few cases the eruption appeared without any preceding fever; the eruption itself generally disappeared at the end of the second or beginning of the third day; the eyes were rarely affected with it as in measles, and in no cases as in the latter disease, was it attended with cough or oppression, excepting such as are attendant upon most febrile complaints. In several cases this disease occurred in children, who some time afterwards, were attacked with the measles, attended with all its characteristic symptoms, and in other instances, adults who were certainly known to have had the measles in early life, were the subjects of this eruptive complaint.

Hosack[41] further noted:

It is not the same species of disease that has been noticed by Dr. Robert Willan [1757–1812] under the appellation of *rubeola sine catarrho*. . . . It is probably the same species of rubeola that has been observed by Rosen, Morton, Tozzetti, Robordiere, and Professor Spielman, and which has given rise to the opinion, that the real measles, rubeola vulgaris, may be taken a second time; an error into which Dr. Willan himself appears to have fallen.

William Wood Gerhard and the First American Clinical Description of Tuberculous Meningitis (1834)

It was said of William Wood Gerhard (1809–1872), of Philadelphia, that no man of his day enjoyed so high a reputation as a clinical teacher.[52] He had had the enormous advantage of having studied under August François Chomel (1788–1858), Gabriel Andral (1797–1876), and Louis, the particular favorite of the American students in Paris. Gerhard was not only trained in pathology, anatomy, and physical diagnosis, but also in the diseases of children. Osler[52] considered him to be "the most distinguished of the American pupils in Paris between 1830 and 1840."

Gerhard's report of the clinical and pathologic findings of thirty children with cerebral affections studied during a year's observation at the Children's Hospital of Paris contained the first accurate clinical description of tuberculous meningitis in the American medical literature.[30] The study by Robert Whytt (1714–1766),[80] of Edinburgh, had antedated Gerhard's report of the clinical course of tuberculous meningitis by more than sixty years. However, Gerhard's detailed clinical and pathological study was the first American description of this disease in children and it may still be read with profit by modern students.

Many children who had died of a cerebral disease were known to have been of "a scrofulous temperament" prior to Gerhard's time, but it was his clinical study of children with "cerebral affections" that first clearly showed that "the substance formed beneath the arachnoid was ... tuberculous, consisting of round, hard, semi-transparent or opaque yellowish bodies, which presented the usual characters of tuberculous matter." Gerhard then discovered that "this disposition of the tuberculous granulations, closely resembles the appearance of a lung infiltrated with tuberculous matter, through which miliary tubercles are disseminated."[30]

The spell of Louis's[49] *méthode numérique*, or statistical approach to medicine, remained with Gerhard for his entire professional life, as is evident in all of his published papers, which were meticulous in the detail of clinical observations and in their dispassionate devotion to fact. Gerhard's papers were light-years ahead of most of those, largely anecdotal in style, which were published in American medical journals of the 1830's and 1840's. Gerhard, on the other hand, held himself to publishing only those cases that were "rigorously confined to fact." Such papers were exceedingly rare in American medical literature during the entire nineteenth century. Superb examples of Gerhard's clinical and statistical approach to clinical problems were his classic papers, published in 1836 and 1837, in which he proved by clinical and anatomical studies performed on the patients he had cared for in the wards of the Pennsylvania Hospital that typhus and typhoid fever were two distinct and separate diseases.[32] In his paper "Pneumonia in Children" (1834), Gerhard[31] for the first time recorded the findings on auscultation and percussion in the pulmonary diseases of children.

John H. Griscom and the Health Hazards of Urban Children (1845)

John H. Griscom (1809–1874), of New York City, a pioneer sanitarian, was one of the first to investigate and to describe in vivid terms the relationship between child health and sanitary conditions. He, along with Lemuel Shattuck (1793–1859) and Stephen Smith (1823–1922), was largely responsible for the development of the public health movement of the latter half of the nineteenth century. Each of them called attention to the appalling human costs of urbanization and to the ignorance of the rudimentary laws of sanitation; Griscom and Smith made this clear primarily by describing living conditions of poor families crowded into tenements, and Shattuck aroused public interest by his report urging that physiology and sanitary science be taught to every child in the public schools.

Griscom's *Sanitary Condition of the Laboring Population of New York City* (1845)[35] was inspired by Sir Edwin Chadwick's (1800–1890)[18] similar study of the laboring population of Great Britain (1843). These two reports may be said to have initiated the public health era in Britain and America. Chadwick,

Smith, and Griscom had deep-rooted convictions that health was directly affected by the state of the physical and social environment and that disease was initimately related to filthy environmental conditions caused by lack of drainage, water supply, and the means for removing refuse from houses and streets.

Griscom's efforts set in motion legislative processes, albeit hesitant at first, which were to have enormous influences in ameliorating the health of our children, both rich and poor. He did so by his careful documentation of the reasons for the inordinate amount of sickness and death, especially among the destitute children in New York City. It surprises us today that in Griscom's day, few besides him had tried to warn the public of the health hazards of bad housing and that no serious effort had been made to rescue the destitute forced to live in hovels from their impending fate.

Children Treated with Heroic or Drastic Measures

The use, or rather the abuse, of drugs in pediatric practice was commonplace, especially during the first half of the nineteenth century. The sanguinary period of heroic treatment with reliance on excessive bloodletting, purging, and puking was in the ascendancy during the first few decades of the nineteenth century. The physician believed that by their "vigorous" treatment they were ridding the body of evil humors and purifying the blood. No class of remedies was more generally resorted to in the management of childhood diseases than cathartics; these were followed closely by emetics.[1] Credit—or perhaps discredit—is given to American physicians for the putative value of calomel in the treatment of diphtheria (croup) and in many other pediatric diseases. The doses recommended were enormous. One girl, aged seven years, took 133 grains (8.62 gm) within sixty-odd hours, and two days later "appeared as if she had never had a complaint."[33]

An example of frightful drug abuse in treating children, which could easily have been matched by many other similar case reports, was the following therapeutic regimen proudly reported by its author in 1837:[47]

R. D., a 2½-year-old boy, came down with *catarrhus a contagione* of influenza on January 14, 1836. The next day he was given 10 grains of calomel in combination with 4 grains of scammony and nauseating portion of *vinum antimonii* while the fever continued for four days.

Six days later he was given twenty grains of aloes and hot baths were ordered; the following day an infusion of senna and calomel was also given. A blister which had been drawn on the back of the neck was kept discharging by frequent renewals. Nauseating portions of antimony wine were reordered, as were frequent doses of mercurial cathartics assisted by an infusion of senna.

During the following week he was given frequent half grain doses of tartar emetic and an attempt was made to open the temporal artery but this failed because the patient would not cooperate. He was bathed in hot water and the tartar emetic increased until five grains were given within a period of an hour.

And the wonder of it all was that the patient recovered, which once again attests to the unquenchable recuperative strength of the human body despite a terrible therapeutic onslaught. Nowhere in the case report was any mention made of the patient's vital signs or of the findings on physical examination—if one was even done.

They must have been stout youngsters in those days to withstand the attacks of their physicians. They took their bleedings and blisterings as well as their cathartics and some lived through it. In treating patients who had croup, it was not unusual for the physician to withdraw enough blood to induce syncope (usually from six to eight ounces), to follow this by placing three or four leeches on the trachea, and finally to apply a full-sized blister to the chest.

In the midst of such unphysiologic practices, a few could see the dangers. Beck[6] objected to indiscriminate bleeding, even by leeches, because he felt that infants needed blood and could not always repair its loss. Underwood remarked that "nature alone will ofttimes effect wonders for infants if she be not officiously counteracted." His difficulty and that of countless others, even down to this day, lay in a proper definition of "officiously."

Another physician,[17] writing in 1831 on the treatment of scarlet fever, advised bleeding and the application of leeches to the head and neck, followed by massive doses of calomel; embrocations of equal parts of spirits of turpentine, ammonia water, and olive oil for the throat; plus shaving of the head. The scalp was to be constantly covered "with a single fold of linen wet with acetic acid and ice-cold water."

He also wrote that "in many cases the fond affections of a mother for the golden locks of her darling, placed an insuperable barrier to this part of the treatment, and ultimately endangered, *if not sacrificed the life of her offspring*" (italics mine). And on the first symptoms indicating the approach of coma he recommended that a blister be applied to the head or the nape of the neck, extending along the spine.[17]

A principle accepted by most nineteenth-century physicians was that anything that produced desired changes in the patient's gross pathological symptoms was acting on the disease and thus was a useful form of therapy. For example, almost anything that reduced the patient's fever was considered desirable, even though the reduction in fever might be completely unrelated to any change in the patient's illness and might even be harmful in the long run. Many physicians argued that a therapy which had a profound physiological effect of any kind on the patient must per se be beneficial. For example, in a paper about the effects of blisters on children induced by plasters, a very common treatment for many childhood illnesses, the physician-author noted that blisters affected children far more severely than adults, sometimes producing convulsions, gangrene, and even death. Therefore, he concluded from this that blisters "ought to hold a high rank" as remedial agents in the diseases of children, although he also criticized their "indiscriminate application" by many physicians.[6]

Thomas Jefferson, among a few others, urged physicians to wait for the therapeutic effects of nature whenever they were not entirely confident of their therapy and even to use placebos as "a pious fraud" if "the appearance of doing something be necessary to keep alive the hope and spirits of the patient."[11] Jefferson realized that few physicians heeded his advice, and drastic therapy continued almost unabated. The effect on the patient, however, was so violent that, according to Jefferson, "the inexperienced and presumptuous band of medical tyros let loose upon the world, destroys more of human life in one year, than all the Robinhoods, Cartouches, and Macheaths do in a century." Jefferson was including children in his estimate; the primary targets of his onslaught were bloodletting and calomel.[66]

While in the short run heroic therapy might have produced demonstrable physiological changes, it was more often detrimental in the long run to the patient's health, as a few contemporary physicians such as Jacob Bigelow (1787–1879) and J. Marion Sims (1813–1883) realized. Bigelow[9] in his classic paper on self-limited diseases, delivered before the Massachusetts Medical Society on May 27, 1835, stressed that certain diseases ran a course to recovery or death that could not be altered significantly by the efforts of physicians. Oliver Wendell Holmes[39] believed that Bigelow's paper "did more than any other work or essay in our own language to rescue the practice of medicine from the slavery of the drugging system which was part of the inheritance of the profession."

The early nineteenth-century physician was extremely partial to drugs that "cleanse the stomach and bowels." Emetics and cathartics, far more drastic and with more dramatic and immediate results than our twentieth-century favorites, were de rigueur as a primary form of therapy for almost all diseases. The emetics were cyclonic in their action; the cathartics so drastic that one country physician recalled they were equal in their action "to a regular oil-well gush."[53] Late in the eighteenth century, calomel gained great popularity when Rush prescribed a dose of ten grains and ten of jalap (another powerful purgative) in treating adult patients during the 1793 Philadelphia yellow fever epidemic. (He prescribed three grains of each for infants and children.)

Beck,[6] writing on the effects of mercury on the young subject in 1849, warned of the indiscriminate use of calomel in pediatric practice, yet he described it as "an agent of immense power." He warned the physician not to use salivation as a criterion by which to judge the effect of calomel on the child's illness because, even in large quantities, "it was not so likely to produce salivation in children as in adults." While claiming that "no one appreciates the importance of mercury as a remedy in the diseases of children . . . more highly than myself" because "its judicious use has been . . . the instrument of saving multitudes of lives," he was one of the first to acknowledge that "it is unquestionably resorted to in a great number [of diseases] where it positively does harm." However, nowhere does he give any pharmacologic reason for using calomel in the treatment of pediatric diseases. Perhaps this was because he knew

so little about the drug's action; only one poorly designed study of the pharmacologic effect of calomel given to three dogs was cited. In this experiment Beck[6] claimed that calomel acted as "a sedative" on the mucous membrane of the stomach and intestines of the three dogs to whom it had been administered.

Bloodletting in Children

The first few decades of the nineteenth century marked what Fielding Garrison[28] called "a prow-wave of extensive and intensive bloodletting." Bloodletting was based on the symptomatic therapy of the period. If the patient had a fever, antiphlogistic treatment was needed, and bleeding during the early part of nineteenth century was the chief antiphlogistic therapy.[28] Scarcely any disease was permitted to pass through the hands of the physician without use of the lancet; even the nonprofessionals often carried a lancet in their pockets, and whenever the patient was indisposed for any reason they would often tie up his arm and let the blood flow.

Bleeding *ad deliquium* was almost a routine treatment for infants and children suffering from croup and all inflammatory fevers because it was firmly believed that (especially for croup), syncope was "the essential point of the cure, [and] without it no relief can be effected."[6] However, by the 1840's some physicians, while not at all opposed to bloodletting in children, felt that "among enlightened practitioners . . . the practice ought to be, *never* . . . bleed to syncope, but to stop as soon as paleness of the lips and cheeks come on." Bloodletting during the first-half of the century was also universally recommended in the treatment of acute peritonitis.[14] The precise amount of blood to be drawn was a matter of much discussion, but most accepted Beck's caution: "A general standard founded upon the age of the patient is really good for nothing, except as a 'mere approximation.' "[6]

Frequent comments were made that the physician who did not use bloodletting in the treatment of sick children did not understand his profession or the duty which he owed his patients. It was not at all unusual for the physician to take his lancet out of his pocket even before removing his hat and before examining the patient.[59] A physician writing of medical practice before 1850 recalled that the lancets were not always clean, yet he never heard of any septic condition as a result of the bleeding.[59] But by the 1840's, albeit slowly, an increasing number of physicians were recommending that great caution be exercised in the repetition of bloodletting, despite the opinions of eminent authorities such as Benjamin Rush,[68] who in his *Defense of Bloodletting* wrote: "I could mention many more instances in which bloodletting has snatched from the grave children under three or four months old, by being used three to five times in the ordinary course of their acute diseases."

Bloodletting was seriously questioned by Louis's[49] "numerical method" of clinical studies when he obtained results "so little in accordance with the general opinion" that he hesitated to publish them. Louis's role in bringing about the final abandonment of bloodletting in America came partly through his writings, partly through his many influential American pupils, such as George Cheyne Shattuck, Jr., (1813–1893), Holmes, Henry I. Bowditch (1808–1892), Gerhard, and Stillé, and partly through a duplicate study made in Boston by James Jackson (1777–1867).

Leeches

Bloodletting by the use of leeches was also a common pediatric practice, leeches substituting for the lancet. Buchan[15] petulantly wrote that "children are generally bled with leeches. This, though sometimes necessary, is a very troublesome and uncertain practice, because it is impossible to estimate the quantity of blood taken by leeches." Two other disadvantages were that the bleeding from the wounds produced by the leeches' bites was "often very difficult to stop, and the wounds are not easily healed." For these reasons Buchan[15] wrote: "Would those who practice bleeding take a little more pains, and accustom themselves to bleed children, they would not find it such a difficult operation as they imagine."

Beck[6] also was opposed to the use of leeches in bleeding children for the same reasons given by Buchan. Beck also complained: "From the manner in which leeches are ordered by some physicians, in the diseases of children, one would be led to suppose that no harm could ever result from them." He also believed that physicians were overusing leeches because "not unfrequently they are used without being actually necessary."

Beck[6] believed that blisters, mercury, and bloodletting were useful and important therapeutic measures. Nonetheless, his study of their use in pediatric practice led him to conclude that all three were potentially dangerous, sometimes lethal, abused beyond belief by reckless and foolhardy physicians, and —although this was never explicitly stated—of little demonstrable benefit in treating disease. Blisters, or skin irritants, sometimes applied successively over the same place, were widely used in the treatment of inflammatory affections in children. A blister was raised on the affected part of the body with a plaster and then broken; the pus flowing from the blister was thought to contain harmful matter. The sores made by the blisters were often irritated to make the effect more intense; this delayed healing and at times produced gangrene or ulcers. A disturbing thing about blistering was that, like calomel, it was thought to do little harm even if it did no good. For this reason it was frequently used in treating children.

Another counterirritant, less commonly used than a blister, was the seton, a strip of silk or linen drawn through a wound in the skin to make a suppurating sore. The discharge of pus was considered beneficial.

Opium

Early nineteenth-century American physicians commonly believed Sydenham's[76] panegyric about opium —that it was a *donum Dei* and that the "art of physic would be defective and imperfect without it." Opiates were used almost universally for teething, worms, diarrhea, or for almost any other pediatric problem. But by mid-century many had grave doubts about the use of opium and its derivatives because of their toxicity in infancy and childhood. But mothers and nurses had no trouble obtaining proprietary preparations containing opium, such as Godfrey's Cordial* and Dalby's Carminative†; these were advertised as good for colic and all manner of pain in the bowels, fluxes, fevers, smallpox, measles, cough, colds, and dentition. They were occasionally given merely to quiet fretful infants who upset parents or

*Godfrey's Cordial, a nineteenth-century English proprietary preparation, was chiefly a mixture of infusion of sassafras, treacle, and tincture of opium. The quantity of opium was about "½ grain of opium to an ounce."

†Dalby's Carminative, also a nineteenth-century English proprietary preparation, was a compound of several essential oils and aromatic tincture in peppermint water, containing tincture of opium. It was said to have had about "⅛ grain of opium to an ounce."

nursemaids: unfortunately, such use too often quieted them permanently. There are many nineteenth-century case reports of opium being misused for this purpose. A typical example of this kind was given by Beck[6] of a child fourteen months old whose appearance "was haggard and aged who appeared no larger than an infant of one or two months." For almost its entire life "it had been kept upon paregoric." The mother resorted to this method of keeping the infant quiet while she attended to her work. Many of the medicated lozenges and candies sold over the counter during this time owed most, if not all, of their so-called therapeutic properties to the opium they contained.

Emetics

During the first half of the nineteenth century there was no class of remedies, with the exception of cathartics, more generally resorted to in the management of childhood diseases than emetics, and many physicians believed that no other remedies were more useful. Tartar emetic (antimony and potassium tartrate) and ipecac were two favored emetics; the latter, although long used by the natives of Brazil in the treatment of diarrhea, was not introduced into Europe until 1658, when it was sold as a secret remedy to the French government. By the 1840's ipecac had largely supplanted tartar emetic in this country as a far safer agent, largely due to the writings of Beck. But despite his warnings many parents continued to dose their children with an extremely popular patent medicine known as the Hive Syrup of Dr. Coxe, unaware that an ounce of it contained a grain of tartar emetic. Beck[6] noted that it was given on the slightest occasion to infants and almost always without even consulting a physician. The dangers of tartar emetic, especially when given to patients with whooping cough, for whom it was frequently prescribed, were well known to George Armstrong, the founder of the first dispensary for children in England. He wrote that "it is a most notorious fact, that the hooping-cough is far more fatal in London than in the country; and I believe that this arises from the very free use of antimonials in London."[6]

By 1840 the emetic properties of ipecac, in preference to tartar emetic, were employed in a wide variety of conditions such as intermittent fever, continued fever, rheumatism, dysentery, epilepsy, asthma, pertussis, chronic diarrhea, and jaundice and whenever it was thought necessary to evacuate the stomach.

Child Labor

Industrial child labor began in America at the end of the eighteenth century. Until the last quarter of the nineteenth century child labor was considered both economically and ethically valuable. The cotton industry in New England brought the industrial revolution to America and with it the introduction of children as an industrial work force. Advocates of the newly developing industries used the existing and largely accepted views of the sanctity of work and fear of idleness as persuasive arguments in favor of the new factories' employing children as laborers. The machine and child labor, unfortunately, were made for each other. The machine performed the heavier work[12] previously requiring adult craftsmen. The light work, often requiring deft little fingers, could be done more efficiently by children. The idea of children working in mills shocked very few people, since children had always worked at home.

In 1820 about half of all textile workers in Massachusetts, Connecticut, and Rhode Island were children, and in 1832, boys under twelve comprised 43 percent of cotton mill workers. Hours of work for them were as long as ten to twelve hours a day, six days a week; the pay was abysmally low, ranging from twenty-five to fifty cents a week. In Paterson, New Jersey, in 1835, six hundred children under sixteen worked from sunrise to sunset in the summer, with a half-hour for breakfast and three-quarters of an hour for dinner. In winter the children worked from dawn to 8 P.M. with no time off for breakfast, which they ate by candlelight before work began. Provisions for the care of the health of factory children were almost nonexistent.[8] Sanitary facilities in most factories and mills were primitive.

During the eighteenth century and the early years of the nineteenth century, child labor on the family farm or in the home was not a major concern of humanitarian reformers. Children were expected to work and their labor was thought to be socially productive and individually salutary. But child labor in factories was an entirely different problem because factory work offered little or no time for trade education and left no time for formal schooling. It was this interference with the child's education that led to the earliest public concern about child labor rather than protecting the working child from industrial hazards or exploitation.

The earliest of the compulsory school attendance laws, the Massachusetts statute of 1836, declared that children under fifteen could be employed in manufacturing only if they had received three months of schooling in the year preceeding their employment.[12] An attempt to make that law apply to agriculture and the mechanical trades as well as to manufacturing failed. Moreover, these laws were so poorly enforced that Horace Mann[12] wrote: "It is obvious that children of ten, twelve, or fourteen years of age may be steadily worked in our manufactories, without any schooling, and this cruel deprivation may be preserved for six, eight, or ten years, and yet during all this period, no very alarming outbreak will occur to rouse the public mind from its guilty slumber."

But bad as child labor was, it was a strong catalyst in arousing a dormant public to consider, perhaps for the first time, the child qua child. This set in motion efforts to meet the particular needs of the child and by the century's end many substantial advances in the welfare, education, and health of children had begun to be realized.

References

1. Abt, I. A. A survey of pediatrics during the past 100 years. *Illinois Med. J.* 77:485, 1940.
2. Ackerknecht, E. H. *Medicine at the Paris Hospital, 1794–1848.* Baltimore: Johns Hopkins Press, 1967.
3. Adams, S. S. The evolution of pediatric literature in the United States. *Trans. Am. Pediatr. Soc.* 9:5, 1897.
4. Anon. *The Maternal Physician: A Treatise on the Nurture and Management of Infants from the Birth until Two Years Old, by an American Matron.* New York: Isaac Riley, 1811.
5. Beck, J. B. *An Inaugural Dissertation on Infanticide.* New York: J. Seymour, 1817.
6. Beck, J. B. *Essays on Infant Therapeutics.* New York: W. E. Dean, 1849.
7. Beck, T. R. *Elements of Medical Jurisprudence* (2 vols.). Albany, N.Y.: Websters & Skinners, 1823.
8. Bettmann, O. L. *The Good Old Days—They Were Terrible.* New York: Random House, 1974.
9. Bigelow, J. *A Discourse on Self-Limited Diseases.* Boston: N. Hale, 1835.
10. Billard, C. M. *Traité des Maladies des Enfans Nouveau-Nés et à la Mammelle.* Paris: J. B. Baillière, 1828.
11. Blanton, W. B. *Medicine in Virginia in the Eighteenth Century.* Richmond: Garrett and Massie, 1931.
12. Bremner, R. H. (ed.) *Children and Youth in America,* vol 1. Cambridge, Mass: Harvard University Press, 1970.
13. Brieger, G. H. (ed.) *Medical America in the Nineteenth Century.* Baltimore: Johns Hopkins Press, 1972.
14. Bryan, L. S., Jr. Blood-letting in American medicine, 1830–1892. *Bull. Hist. Med.* 38:516, 1964.
15. Buchan, W. *Domestic Medicine.* Philadelphia: Richard Folwell, 1801.
16. Cable, M. *The Little Darlings: A History of Child Rearing in America.* New York: Scribner's, 1975.
17. Callaghan, D. Account of the epidemic of scarlatina anginosa which prevailed in Pittsburgh, Penn., in 1830. *Am. J. Med. Sci.* 8:71, 1831.
18. Chadwick, E. *Report on the Sanitary Conditions of the Labouring Population of Great Britain.* London: W. Clowes & Sons, 1843.
19. Cheyne, J. *The Pathology of the Membranes of the Larynx and Bronchia.* Edinburgh: Mundell, Doig & Stevenson, 1809.
20. Condie, D. F. *Practical Treatise on the Diseases of Children.* Philadelphia: Lea and Blanchard, 1844.
21. Cone, T. E., Jr. Dr. Henry Pickering Bowditch on the growth of children: An unappreciated classical study. *Trans. Stud. Coll. Physicians Phila.* (4th ser.) 42:67, 1974.
22. Deland, F. *The Story of Lip-Reading.* Washington, D.C.: Volta Bureau, 1968.
22a. Dewees, W. P. *Treatise on the Physical and Medical Treatment of Children.* Philadelphia: H. C. Carey and I. Lea, 1825.
23. Dewees, W. P. *Treatise on the Physical and Medical Treatment of Children* (10th ed.). Philadelphia: Blanchard and Lea, 1853.
24. Doull, J. A. The Bacteriologic Era (1876–1920). In Franklin H. Top (ed.), *The History of American Epidemiology.* St. Louis: Mosby, 1952.
25. Drinker, C. *Not So Long Ago.* New York: Oxford University Press, 1937.
26. Eberle, J. *Treatise on the Diseases and Physical Education in Children.* Cincinnati: Corey and Fairbank, 1833.
27. Gallaudet, T. H. In *Dictionary of American Biography,* by William A. Robinson, New York: Charles Scribner's Sons, 1931.
28. Garrison, F. H. The history of blood letting. *N.Y. Med. J.* 97:500, 1913.

29. Garrison, F. H. *An Introduction to the History of Medicine*. Philadelphia: Saunders, 1913.

30. Gerhard, W. W. Cerebral affections of children. *Am. J. Med. Sci.* 13:313, 1833; 14:99, 1834.

31. Gerhard, W. W. On the pneumonia of children. *Am. J. Med. Sci.* 14:328, 1834.

32. Gerhard, W. W. On the typhus fever which occurred in Philadelphia in the spring and summer of 1836. *Am. J. Med. Sci.* 19:239; 20:289, 1836.

33. Gittings, J. C. Pediatrics one hundred years ago. *Trans. Am. Pediatr. Soc.* 40:9, 1928.

34. Glaab, C. N., and Brown, T. *A History of Urban America*. New York: Macmillan, 1967.

35. Griscom, J. H. *The Sanitary Condition of the Laboring Population of New York*. New York: Harper, 1845.

36. Hartley, R. M. *An Historical, Scientific and Practical Essay on Milk*. New York: Leavitt, 1842.

37. Hempstead, G. S. B. Reminiscences of the physicians of the first quarter of the present century, with a review of some features of their practice. *Cincinnati Lancet Clinic* 1:33, 53, 66, 1878.

38. Henoch, E. *Beiträge zur Kinderheilkunde*. Berlin: A. Hirschwald, 1861.

39. Holmes, O. W. The Medical Profession in Massachusetts. In *Medical Essays*, p. 351. Boston: Houghton Mifflin, 1911.

40. Holt, L. E. *Diseases of Infancy and Childhood*. New York: Appleton, 1897.

41. Hosack, D. Quarterly report of the diseases which prevailed in New-York, during the months of April, May, and June 1813. *Am. Med. Philosophical Register* 41:156, 1814.

42. Jacobi, A. History of Cerebro-Spinal Meningitis. In W. J. Robinson (ed.). *Collectanea Jacobi*. New York: Critic and Guide Co., 1909.

43. Jenner, E. *An Inquiry Into the Causes and Effects of the Variolae Vaccinae*. London: S. Low, 1798.

44. Kahn, C. History of smallpox and prevention. *Am. J. Dis. Child.* 106:597, 1963.

45. Kelly, H. A., and Burrage, W. L. *American Medical Biographies*. Baltimore: Norman Remington, 1920.

46. Kerr, C. B. The fortunes of haemophiliacs in the 19th century. *Med. Hist.* 7:359–370, 1963.

47. Lewis, J. T. On the diseases and management of children. *Transylvania J. Med.* 10:51, 1837.

48. Logan, G. *Practical Observations on Diseases of Children*. Charleston, S.C.: A. E. Miller, 1825.

49. Louis, P. Ch. A. *Researches on the Effects of Bloodletting in Some Inflammatory Diseases*. Transl. by C. G. Putnam, preface and appendix by James Jackson. Boston: Hilliard, Gray, 1836.

50. Meigs, C. D. *Observations on Certain of the Diseases of Young Children*. Philadelphia: Lea and Blanchard, 1850.

51. Meigs, J. F. *A Practical Treatise on the Diseases of Children*. Philadelphia: Lindsay & Blakiston, 1848.

52. Middleton, W. S. William Wood Gerhard. *Ann. Med. Hist.* (n.s.) 7:1, 1935.

53. Monroe, G. J. Old-time practice. *Cincinnati Lancet Clinic* (n.s.) 46:362, 1901.

54. North, E. *A Treatise on a Malignant Epidemic, Commonly Called Spotted Fever*. New York: T. & J. Swards, 1811.

55. Numbers, R. L. Do-It-Yourself the Sectarian Way. In G. B. Risse, R. L. Numbers, and J. W. Leavitt (eds.), *Medicine Without Doctors*. New York: Science History Publications, 1977.

56. Nye, R. B. *Society and Culture in America, 1830–1860*. New York: Harper & Row, 1974.

57. Osler, W. *The Principles and Practice of Medicine*. New York: Appleton, 1892.

58. Otto, J. C. An account of an haemorrhagic disposition existing in certain families. *Med. Reposit.* 6:1, 1803.

59. Pruitt, J. W. The olden time. *Eclectic Med. J.* 38:532, 1878.

60. Radbill, S. X. A history of children's hospitals. *Am. J. Dis. Child.* 90:411, 1955.

61. Radbill, S. X. Centuries of child welfare in Philadelphia. *Phila. Med.* 71:359, 1975.

62. Radbill, S. X. Reared in adversity: Institutional children in the 18th century. *Am. J. Dis. Child.* 130:751, 1976.

63. Report of the Committee on Education. *Trans. Am. Med. Assoc.* 1:235, 1848.

64. Rosen, G. Acute Communicable Diseases. In W. R. Bett (ed.), *The History and Conquest of Common Diseases*. Norman: University of Oklahoma Press, 1954.

65. Rothman, D. J. *The Discovery of the Asylum*. Boston: Little, Brown, 1971.

66. Rothstein, W. G. *American Physicians in the 19th Century*. Baltimore: Johns Hopkins Press, 1972.

67. Rush, B. *An Account of the Bilious Remitting Yellow Fever as it Appeared in the City of Philadelphia in the Year 1793*. Philadelphia: T. Dobson, 1794.

68. Rush, B. Defense of bloodletting. *Med. Obs. & Inqs.*, vol. IV, p. 353. Philadelphia: T. Dobson, 1796.

69. Schwartz, H. *Samuel Gridley Howe—Social Reformer*. Cambridge, Mass.: Harvard University Press, 1956.

70. Seibert, H. The progress of ideas regarding the causation and control of infant mortality. *Bull. Hist. Med.* 8:546, 1940.

71. Shryock, R. H. *Medicine in America: Historical Essay*. Baltimore: Johns Hopkins Press, 1966.

72. Smillie, W. G. The Periods of Great Epidemics in the

United States. In F. H. Top (ed.), *The History of American Epidemiology*. St. Louis: Mosby, 1952.

73. Smith, J. L. *A Treatise on the Diseases of Infancy and Childhood*. Philadelphia: Henry C. Lea, 1869.

74. Stewart, J. *A Practical Treatise on the Diseases of Children*. New York: Wiley & Putnam, 1841.

75. Stillé, A. Reminiscences of the Philadelphia Hospital. In D. Hayes Agnew, et. al., *History and Reminiscences of the Philadelphia Almshouse and Philadelphia Hospital*. Philadelphia: Detra & Blackburn, 1890.

76. Sydenham, T. *Works of Thomas Sydenham*, with notes by Benjamin Rush. Philadelphia: T. & T. Kite, 1809.

77. Veale, H. R. L. History of an epidemic of rötheln, with observations on its pathology. *Edinb. Med. J.* 12:404, 1866.

78. Waring, J. I. *History of Medicine in South Carolina, 1670–1825*, vol. 1. Charleston, S.C.: South Carolina Medical Association, 1964.

79. Waterhouse, B. *Cautions to young persons concerning health in a public lecture*. Delivered at the close of the medical course in the chapel at Cambridge, Nov. 20, 1804. Cambridge, Mass.: University Press, 1805.

80. Whytt, R. *Observations on the Dropsy in the Brain*. Edinburgh: J. Balfour, 1768.

81. Winslow, O. E. *A Destroying Angel: The Conquest of Smallpox in Colonial America*. Boston: Houghton Mifflin, 1974.

82. Wunderlich, C. R. A. *Das Verhalten der Eigenwärme in Krankheiten*. Leipzig: O. Wigand, 1868.

So much less has been done in the proper and scientific study of children than at other periods of life, that it is no wonder that we have entered upon the especial investigation of and research in this branch of anthropology with the keen interest of explorers in an almost unknown country. Of still further interest, also, when we discover not only that there is a vast expanse of unknown, but that much which was supposed to be known is in reality a poor subterfuge of unreal facts forming structures of misleading results, which in the scientific medicine of adults would not for a second be tolerated; in fact would be laughed to scorn as relics of the dark ages of necromancy. This same misnamed medical knowledge, however, when representing the infant and child, has been accepted with but little question.

Thomas Morgan Rotch (1891)

The second half of the nineteenth century holds particular interest for the modern pediatrician because it was the period in which pediatrics emerged as a distinct branch of medicine and not as the unwanted foster child of internal medicine. Great philanthropic energy went into the provision of special facilities for children who were formerly treated much the same as adults. By mid-century hospitals were established for the reception and care of foundlings and for sick and crippled children. By the end of the century there were more than two dozen children's hospitals scattered across the United States, and out of 119 medical schools suitable for study, 64, or 54 percent, had a special chair of pediatrics.

It was a period of enormous population growth, from slightly more than 23 million in 1850, with 42 percent of the population under fifteen years of age, to almost 76 million in 1900, with 34 percent under fifteen years of age. In 1900, there were almost 16 million families in the United States with an average size of 4.6 persons per family, a decrease of about one person per family since the first census of 1790, when the average family numbered 5.7 persons. But despite the unprecedented medical advances of the latter half of the century, infant mortality during the years 1895–1899, at least in Massachusetts, was about 17 per cent higher than in the period 1851–1854; it was 153.2 per 1,000 live births for the former period, and 131.11 per 1,000 live births for the latter.

That the infant mortality rate was so high initially excited little or no comment or surprise.[35] But by the latter half of the nineteenth century the humanitarian spirit, sparked in the previous century especially by William Cadogan, took firm hold in the United States and from it sprang a general desire for a betterment of social and hygenic conditions for the infant and child. There eventually developed a certain noble rivalry among the health departments of our large cities to lower the infant mortality rate. This ambition to better all previous records is characteristically American, and it brought about truly remarkable results. A patriotic nerve was pricked by an 1857 report asking, "Why should infant mortality in American cities be greater than even in Paris, 8 percent above Glasgow, 10 percent above Liverpool, and nearly 13 percent greater than in London? Why should it be increasing here and diminishing there?"[66]

Lemuel Shattuck[73] the celebrated nineteenth-century public health reformer, calculated that between the years 1811 and 1838 there was an "increasing and alarming mortality" in children under five years of age who lived in Boston; the mortality of 1838 in this age group was greater than in any other year in this period.

Shattuck tried to discover some of the causes for this "increasing and alarming mortality."

More luxury and effeminancy in both sexes prevail now than formerly; and this may have had some influence in producing constitutional debility, and the consequent feeble health of children.

The nursing and feeding of children with improper food is another cause. The influence of bad air in confined, badly located, and filthy houses, is another and perhaps the greatest. Epidemic diseases [between 1811 and 1841] which are particularly prevalent among children have increased. It will hereafter be shown that scarlet fever has prevailed very much in the last nine years [1831 to 1839], and has increased the mortality. In the period 1811 to 1820, this disease produced 13 per 1,000 of the whole deaths. In 1831 to 1838, it produced 489. Other infantile diseases have also increased. These considerations would, perhaps, sufficiently account for the increased mortality under 5 years of age.

Emerging Interest in Child Health

In the years between the end of the Civil War and the turn of the century the subject of child health became distinctly defined. Urbanization, industrialization, and immigration would become the broad social factors which reshaped American life during these years. The public health movement and the growing number of state boards of health helped to bring problems relating to children into clearer view. In 1872 the American Public Health Association was founded by Stephen Smith, and by 1877 fourteen states had established health departments. Ironically, the first organized efforts for the protection of children from abuse developed as an outgrowth of humane work for animals.

On April 9, 1874 Henry Bergh (1811–1888), founder (1866) and president of the Society for the Prevention of Cruelty to Animals (ASPCA) petitioned Judge Lawrence of the Supreme Court of New York to issue a warrant to remove "little Mary Ellen," an eight-year-old girl, from her foster parents, who were accused of brutally beating her. Bergh became involved, according to the *New York Times* of April 10, 1874, because "the charitable lady" who had discovered Mary Ellen's dreadful plight "had gone to several institutions in the vain hope of having them take the child under their care; that as a last resort she applied to Mr. Bergh, who, though the case was not within the scope of the special act to prevent cruelty to animals, recognized it as being clearly within the general laws of humanity and promptly gave it his attention." He then decided that "the child being an animal," the American Society for the Prevention of Cruelty to Animals (ASPCA) would offer her protection.

Mary Ellen's foster mother was subsequently found guilty of felonious assault and was sentenced to one year's imprisonment at hard labor. Mary Ellen was placed in an institution known as the Sheltering Arms. Her case of child abuse was widely reported in the contemporary newspapers. And it alone led to the formation of the Society for the Prevention of Cruelty to Children (SPCC) which was organized in December, 1874, with Elbridge T. Gerry (1837–1927), lawyer and philanthropist, legal adviser to the American Society for the Prevention of Cruelty to Animals, as its first president. Beginning with the SPCC, societies devoted exclusively to child protection or jointly to animal and child protection increased rapidly. By 1900 the number of such societies exceeded two hundred fifty.

Stephen Smith, surgeon, pioneer in the American

public health movement, and brother of Job Lewis Smith, in 1868 became the first Commissioner of Health for New York City, holding that position until 1875. In 1879 President Rutherford B. Hayes (1822–1893) appointed him to be one of seven civilian members of a newly created National Board of Health. Unfortunately, this forerunner of a cabinet department of health lasted only four years, when states' rights pressure forced its demise.[10] Needless to say, the dramatic improvement in mortality from the age-old childhood illnesses during the last century would have been greatly hampered had it not been for the leadership and knowledge of public health officials such as Smith.

By the 1890's the pediatric and public health leaders of the day had learned to work together. For example, an early evidence of legislative action taken directly for the health of children was an appropriation of ten thousand dollars by the New York State legislature in 1879 to provide a corps of physicians to visit poor homes in the tenement districts of New York City to treat sick infants. Concurrently, a tremendous growth of medical literature dealing with infants and children accelerated the interchange of ideas and data.

Better sewerage, pure water, clean milk, cleaner streets, food inspection, attention to ventilation, and education about matters of general hygiene were to become of far greater importance in overcoming the unfavorable effects of city life on the health of infants and children than the ministrations of the individual physician to the sick child.[35]

One fact sadly accepted by nineteenth-century physicians was that the first years of a child's life were the most treacherous. For example, in almost all cities during this period more than a third of all infants born died under the age of five years.[35] Most of these deaths were attributed to improper feeding. To learn how to overcome this terrible infant mortality became the *raison d'être* of pediatrics for the sixty years between 1870 and 1930 (p. 131). The "milk question" became of pivotal significance as a vital element in infant feeding and mortality.

Medical Practice and the Importance of the German School of Pediatrics

During the last half of the last century clinical thermometry came into use, although not routinely in pediatric practice until the beginning of the twentieth century. The clinical thermometer was followed by cellular pathology and bacteriology, by Pasteur and Koch's discovery of the role of bacteria in causing disease, by surgical antisepsis, by the production of diphtheria antitoxin, by microphotography, by biologic and blood chemistry, and by the electric lightbulb and the roentgen ray.

By this time German medicine had broken the metaphysical trammels of the philosophy of nature (*Naturphilosophie*), usually called "romantic medicine," which had bound it in the early part of the century. In Vienna, Carl Rokitansky (1804–1878) and Josef Skoda (1805–1881) had advanced far along the path first opened in France; Johann Schoenlein (1793–1864) was developing the modern German clinic; the golden age of physiology marked by the work of Claude Bernard (1813–1878) in France and of Johannes Müller (1801–1858) and Carl F. Ludwig (1816–1895) and others in Germany had begun, and Rudolf Virchow (1821–1902) had proclaimed his cellular theory of life and disease. Laboratories, that great contribution of Germany to scientific teaching and investigation, were established and rapidly developed between 1850 and 1880, first for physiology, then for chemistry, pathology, pharmacology, and hygiene. Mainly through her laboratories Germany secured that leadership in medical science which turned to her universities a stream of foreign students, many of whom were from the United States. Eduard Henoch, director of the Pediatric Clinic and the Polyclinic at the Charité in Berlin from 1872 to 1893 and the pioneer of modern pediatrics in Germany, was a superb teacher of pediatrics; many American pediatricians attended his clinics and were inspired by his instruction.[1] Jacobi wrote that Henoch's lectures on pediatrics belonged "to the most exquisite specimens of literature."[28] Upon his retirement in 1893 his chair was offered to Jacobi, who, however, declined it. The chair was occupied by Otto Heubner (1843–1926) and subsequently by Adalbert Czerny (1863–1941).[28]

By the second half of the nineteenth century, the principal writers on pediatrics were mainly Germans, replacing the French who had dominated the century's first half. The German school of pediatrics was largely responsible for developing the laboratory approach to pediatrics. German pediatricians were also the first to formulate an exact classification of the diseases of infants and to discover the calorimetric method of infant feeding.

The leaders in this effort were Alois Bednar (1816–1888), Carl Hennig (1825–1911), Carl Gerhardt (1833–1902), Eduard Henoch, Philipp Biedert (1847–1916), Adolf Baginsky (1843–1918), Gottfried Ritter von Rittershain (1820–1883), Alois Epstein (1849–1918), and Max Kassowitz (1842–1913).

Pediatrics Emerges as a Specialty

Abraham Jacobi

As a specialty, pediatrics, or "pediatry" or "pedology" as it was called in the nineteenth century, was introduced to America by Abraham Jacobi, a German clinician, who had fled his native country because of his involvement in the revolution of 1848 (Fig. 5–1). While in Berlin for his state examination he was arrested on a charge of *lèse majesté* and imprisoned for two years. Escaping first to England, he finally arrived in New York in 1853. Samuel S. Adams[2] said of him, "Jacobi pressed the button which set pediatrics in motion." In 1860 Jacobi established the first children's clinic in the New York Medical College; his academic title was professor of infantile pathology and therapeutics. This was the first time in this country that a teacher appointed for that branch of medicine gave any systematic instruction in the diseases of children. Jacobi said that it was "the first beginning of medical bedside instruction in America."

Years later he wrote:[41]

If some one were anxious to learn how I with my knowledge of pathology and therapeutics, which indeed was rather infantile, became a professor, this is how it happened. A friend of mine, who has a tablet of his own in the history of American obstetrics, had taken a chair in the reorganized school. So my dear Charles Budd wished me to go in with him, and [he] came as a committee to offer me a place in the faculty. When I used what I had of common sense and replied that I did not feel competent, he tried his great art on himself. He *delivered* himself, with a forcible tongue, of so many uncomplimentary remarks about me, that I accepted his terms at once.

And so academic pediatrics was born in this country!

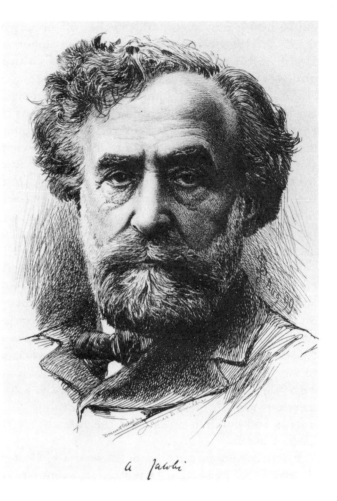

a Jacobi

Figure 5–1. Abraham Jacobi (1830–1919).

Jacobi taught pediatrics in New York City from 1857 to 1899; his teaching experience actually began in 1857 when he participated fleetingly in the spring course at the College of Physicians and Surgeons. He drolly described his first lecture: "I nearly broke down, more or less deservedly. My subjects were the diseases of the young larynx and laryngismus stridulus. *Nolens volens* I exhibited in my own person an attack of laryngismus. We all survived."[41]

When the New York Medical College ceased to exist in 1865, Jacobi then established a children's clinic in the University Medical College. In 1870 he was appointed clinical professor of the diseases of children in the College of Physicians and Surgeons of Columbia University, but his academic title did not provide a seat on the faculty. (It would be almost two decades later before the first full professorship of pediatrics, with a vote on the faculty, was offered to Thomas Morgan Rotch (1849–1914) at the Harvard Medical School.) It could be accurately said that the entire history of American pediatrics during the second half of the nineteenth century is reflected in Jacobi and his writings.[91]

Although small in stature, he had both tremendous drive and exceptional organizing ability. In his day there was hardly a medical institution in New York City that cared for children in which Jacobi had not had a hand. He was the organizer of the children's service of the Mt. Sinai Hospital of New York. He was one of the founders of the German Hospital (now Lenox Hill) and the organizer of its children's service. It was largely due to him that the section on pediatrics of the American Medical Association (1880) and that of the New York Academy of Medicine (1885) were established. One of Jacobi's outstanding contributions was his ardent struggle against conventional but unsound practices. In an ironic tone he wrote of himself that "the revolutionary spirit of my youth and a warm temperament which boiled at a low temperature, made me overlook the slow pace at which reforms are established." He was violently opposed to the indiscriminate use of "calomel and always calomel," the great panacea for the treatment of children, and he was daring enough to suggest keeping infants undressed on hot days, for which he claimed he was reprimanded even from the pulpit.[50]

After Jacobi resigned his teaching position at the College of Physicians and Surgeons, he was succeeded by L. Emmett Holt, who would become in his day as forceful a leader and teacher of pediatrics as Jacobi had been.

Job Lewis Smith

Another giant among the remarkable group of men who literally created American pediatrics in the second half of the century was Job Lewis Smith (Fig. 5–2); he came from upper New York State to New York City under the aegis of his famous brother Stephen and his equally famous preceptor, Austin Flint (1812–1886).[21] Job Lewis Smith received his M.D. from the New York College of Physicians and Surgeons in 1853. Immediately after receiving his degree, he began to practice in what was then considered the far uptown section of New York City. In the area just north of his professional office there were hundreds of shanties. His description[20] of

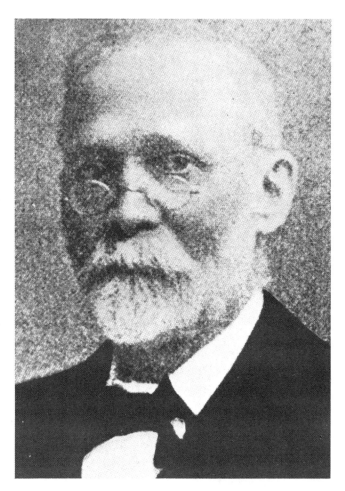

Figure 5–2. Job Lewis Smith (1827–1897).

a typical shanty makes it clear why childhood and adult diseases were so prevalent: "Some shanties have but one room. . . . It is evident that to the occupants of the shanty domiciliary and personal cleanliness is almost impossible. In one small room are found the family, chairs usually dirty and broken, cooking utensils, stove, often a bed, a dog or cat and sometimes more or less poultry. . . . There is no sink or drainage, and the slops are thrown on the ground."

Smith was appointed clinical professor of morbid anatomy in the newly organized Bellevue Hospital Medical College in 1867. In this capacity he taught the diseases of children both in the outpatient department at Bellevue Hospital and at the autopsy table. In 1876 he was appointed clinical professor of the diseases of children at Bellevue, sixteen years after the first special chair of pediatrics had been created for Jacobi at the New York Medical College.

Like Jacobi, Smith never confined himself exclusively to the care of children; with both men, this was a matter of deliberate choice. Later in life Smith[20] wrote: "Any specialist, in my opinion, is a better specialist for being a good general practitioner." Had it not been for Jacobi, who surpassed him in his influence on American pediatrics, Smith would have been known as the father of American pediatrics. Smith's principal publication was his textbook, which passed through eight editions between 1869 and 1896. His book was not only the favorite of the medical students of his day but also the mainstay of the general practitioner. His textbook reflected his enormous clinical experience coupled with his personal experience in the practice of pathology (p. 124).

Pediatrics was officially ranked as a specialty in 1880 when the Section on Diseases of Children was formed at a meeting of the American Medical Association in Richmond, Virginia. Jacobi was chosen president. In 1888 the American Pediatric Society, the first medical specialty society in the United States, was founded with Jacobi as its first president. Smith was the second, Rotch the third, and Osler its fourth president.

Thomas Morgan Rotch

In 1871 the medical curriculum at the Harvard Medical School was radically altered. Francis Minot (1821–1899) was assistant professor of the theory and practice of medicine and clinical lecturer on the diseases of women and children. This was the first time that the diseases of children were mentioned in the Harvard Medical School announcement. The instruction consisted of a few didactic lectures on the "eruptive fevers." In 1873 Charles P. Putnam (1844–1914) was appointed lecturer on the diseases of children. He gave a clinical lecture weekly during the second year at the Boston Dispensary for Women and Children. In 1874 Minot ceased to be lecturer, leaving Putnam as the only instructor. When Putnam resigned in 1879, Rotch was appointed special clinical instructor (Fig. 5–3). In 1888 he was promoted to assistant professor of diseases of children and in 1893 to full professor with a chair on the faculty. In 1903 the title was changed to professor of pediatrics.[55] This was the first real professorship of pediatrics in this country except for an

appointment of short duration at Boston University in 1890.[55] The second American full-time incumbent of such a position was Samuel S. Adams at Georgetown University Medical School in Washington.

Rotch was born in Philadelphia December 9, 1849, and received his M.D. from the Harvard Medical School in 1874. He was the pioneer pediatrician in Boston, concentrating his studies on the early years of life that had the highest death rate.

Luther Emmett Holt

Jacobi for most of the second half of the nineteenth century and L. Emmett Holt in the last few years of that century were the undisputed leaders in advancing the science and art of pediatrics. Both, during their later years, devoted their thoughts and energies to the problems of public child hygiene and preventive pediatrics. Both were described as men "imbued

Figure 5–3. Thomas Morgan Rotch (1849–1914).

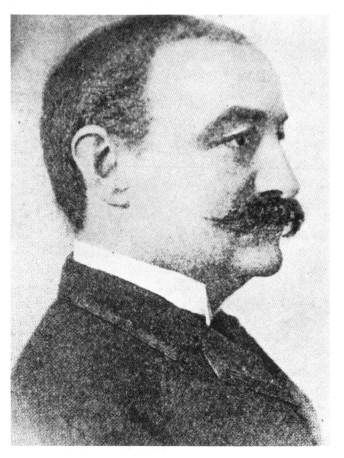

with a love of humanity and of children in particular, and with a strong abiding faith that their ideals for healthy and happy childhood could be made realities for America's children."[49]

Holt was born in Webster, New York, in 1855; he came to New York City in 1876 to accept a vacancy for a student intern at the Hospital for the Ruptured and Crippled at an annual salary of four hundred dollars (Fig. 5–4). It was here that he came under the guidance of Virgil Gibney (1847–1927), who became professor of orthopedics at the College of Physicians and Surgeons. In gratitude to Gibney, Holt would later dedicate his famous textbook to him.[33] Holt graduated from the College of Physicians and Surgeons in 1880 and subsequently accepted a surgical internship at Bellevue Hospital. However, the following year he decided against a career in surgery and opened an office for the practice of medicine. He became professor of diseases of children in the New York Polyclinic from 1890 to 1901 and was appointed professor of diseases of children at the College of Physicians and Surgeons in 1902. In 1894 he published his enormously popular little book on the care and feeding of children (p. 127). His textbook *The Diseases of Infancy and Childhood*, published in 1896 (p. 127), became a classic. Holt's influence on American pediatrics was enormous, and perhaps even more than Jacobi he deserves to be thought of as the father of modern scientific American pediatrics.

As the director of the Babies Hospital from 1889 to 1923, Holt guided it to become the most celebrated pediatric hospital in the United States during the first two decades of this century. The New York Babies Hospital, founded in 1887, was the first hospital (as opposed to a foundling asylum) in the United States exclusively for the care of infants. At the time the Babies Hospital was opened there were less than half a dozen general hospitals in this country with wards for infants.

Louis Starr (1849–1925) initiated the first systematic instruction in pediatrics in Philadelphia in 1880 when he was appointed instructor of diseases of children at the University of Pennsylvania. Isaac A. Abt (1867–1955) was the pioneer teacher of pediatrics in Chicago.

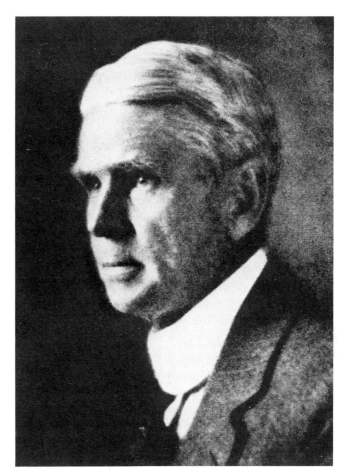

Figure 5–4. L. Emmett Holt (1855–1924).

Health Problems of Infants and Children

During the second half of the nineteenth century urban living for the poor was unbelievably degrading. Between 1868 and 1875 an estimated half a million of New York's one million population lived in slums. As many as eight persons shared a living room 10 by 12 feet and a bedroom 6 by 8 feet. One Lower East Side tenement was packed with 101 adults and 91 children.[6] A report of the New York Sanitary Association in 1857 stated that New York City had the highest death rate (36.8 per 1,000 population) of any of the large cities of the world.[67]

In the previous dozen years nearly two and a half million immigrants had poured into New York. Many of them were penniless, diseased, and starving Irish peasant families fleeing from the potato famine of the mid-1840's. They reached New York in a terrible state of malnutrition and were crowded into dark, damp, unheated basement tenements, under indescribably filthy and foul conditions, where they died in appalling numbers. Deaths from diarrheal diseases in infancy are said to have increased by 250 percent[75] during this twelve-year period. Smallpox, typhus fever, cholera, diphtheria, scarlet fever, and cerebrospinal meningitis each year killed thousands of children.

Unfortunately, the technological advances of the Gilded Age were not accompanied by corresponding advances in medicine; public hygiene, especially in the urban areas, was dismal, with a shocking effect especially on the health of infants and young children of the poor. New York City had no effective sanitary protection whatever prior to about 1860. Between the years 1854 and 1856, 62.5 percent of the total number of deaths occurred under the age of five years, 50 percent under two years, and 27.5 percent under one year of age. In Boston during the nine-year period between 1832 and 1840, 43 percent of the deaths occurred in children under five years of age.[73] In Chicago during the twenty-five-year period between 1850 and 1875, 51.5 percent of the deaths occurred in children less than five years of age.[1] As late as 1894 in Milwaukee nearly one-half of all deaths occurred in children under five years of age.[11]

It is likely, as Bolduan[7] claimed in his historical essay on the public health of New York City, that it was "a reasonably clean and tidy town during the first quarter of the nineteenth century." The general death rate from all causes was about 25 per 1,000 and the infant mortality ranged between 120 and 140 per 1,000 live births. The last half of the century would see a radical change for the worse in the cleanliness and tidiness of New York City.

The second quarter brought profound changes. Population growth became accelerated, factories multiplied, immigration from Europe increased rapidly, standards of living were lowered, the housing situation became acute, and conditions became more and more unsanitary. By 1850 the infant mortality rate had climbed to 180 per 1,000 live births. In 1851 an epidemic of smallpox caused 562 deaths, many of them infants and children. Three years later cholera claimed over 2,500 victims. Smallpox continued to ravage the city, causing 664 deaths in 1865, 1,662 in 1872, and 1,889 deaths in 1875.

A basic urban problem was polluted air, which permeated most sections of the city. Windows were often permanently shut against outside air that was fouled by a mixture of soot, factory smells, and animal stenches. Indoors, because of poor ventilation, the air was no better. Sewer gas from shoddy plumbing was a constant health problem.

As for personal care, the Victorians were not prone to bathe. Our love of the bathroom is a modern fetish. In 1882, for example, only 2 percent of homes in New York City had water connections.[6] Some doctors considered bathing a needless waste of time. However, bathing the baby was generally approved, although it was a splashy ordeal requiring hot water from the kitchen stove.

Endemic diseases fed by the filth and overcrowding of the cities ran their course. The hospitals, especially the charitable ones in the cities, during the period 1860–1900 were not too different from almshouses where patients often languished in appalling squalor. A sensational case, reported in the New York Tribune of April 25, 1860, focused attention on the condition in the wards of Bellevue Hospital in New York.[10] A young Irishwoman gave birth to a baby on a Sunday night. The next morning the infant was found dead next to the mother, who had been too weak to prevent rats from devouring the infant's nose, upper lip, toes and half of the left foot (Fig. 5–5).

The rich and the middle classes feared hospitals as pesthouses and kept their ill children at home.[34] Summer diarrhea was a terrible scourge even in the homes of the better-off, especially among bottle-fed infants, and was responsible for at least 20 percent, and often an even higher percentage of the deaths of infants two years old and younger (Table 5–1).

Milk and other perishable foods, in the absence of reliable refrigeration, were subject to the whims of the weather. Milk was commonly adulterated, as well as contaminated with pathogenic bacteria. The milk might come from diseased cows, improperly fed, often with swill from neighboring distilleries, and they were housed in filthy dairies (p. 141).

It was not until 1896 that the New York City Board of Health adopted a section of the sanitary code prohibiting the sale of milk except under a permit.[7] Contamination of drinking water from improper drainage and sewage was a constant menace to life and health, and the ever-present mosquitoes, thriving in the marshlands, caused malarial infections of adults and children alike. Malaria was also

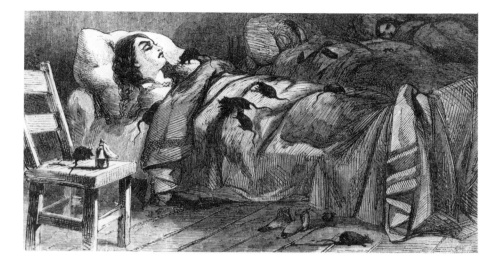

Figure 5–5. Ward in Bellevue Hospital, New York, with rats overrunning patients' beds. (The Bettmann Archive, Inc.)

commonly encountered in children seen at the Boston Children's Hospital during the 1870's and 1880's due to the brackish water in the fens located close to the hospital.

Common and Epidemic Diseases

Epidemic diseases in the 1850's were called "zymotic diseases" from the Greek word *zymos*, meaning fermentation. These diseases were thought to be due to fermentation of tissues, always as the result of an external stimulus. The so-called zymotic diseases were also known as "miasmatic" diseases. They included smallpox, measles, scarlet fever, diphtheria (croup), whooping cough, typhoid fever, diarrhea (all kinds), cholera infantum, and cerebrospinal meningitis. Tuberculosis was considered a constitutional, or diathetic, disease, as was cancer.

The external stimuli believed to cause zymotic diseases were almost always considered to be cosmic in origin and were thought to be transmitted through the air. The miasma could be produced by man himself, by the products of his household, by any type of decaying vegetable or animal matter, or by cosmic phenomena. Noah Webster (1758–1843)[89] in his encyclopedic *A Brief History of Epidemic and Pestilential Diseases* (1799) tried to correlate the relationship of cosmic forces such as meteor showers, volcanic eruptions, earthquakes, and other environmental factors with the production of serious epidemics and pestilential diseases. He believed epidemics were the

Table 5–1. Deaths from Diarrheal Diseases in U.S.A.—1880 Census

	Age (years)			
	1	2	1–5	All ages
Diarrheal diseases*	27,398	12,941	47,870	63,391
All causes	175,184	58,816	302,624	750,843
% of diarrheal deaths at all ages	43	20	75	100
Diarrheal deaths as percentage of deaths from all causes in each age group	15.6	21.9	15.8	8.4

*Diarrheal diseases were recorded under five categories: diarrhea, dysentery, enteritis, cholera morbus, and cholera infantum.
Source: H. K. Faber and R. McIntosh. *History of the American Pediatric Society.* New York: McGraw-Hill, 1966. Reprinted by permission.

result of an accumulation of a number of unfavorable environmental factors which combined to affect large numbers of people at the same time and so produce overwhelming disaster. This bizarre theory was accepted by many medical men for more than half a century.

There were over three hundred thousand deaths in 1850 and over 40 percent of these deaths were said to be due to zymotic diseases.[75] These diseases were far more serious in the younger age group; in children of five to nine years of age, 56 percent of the deaths were from the so-called zymotic diseases (Table 5–2). There was no accurate measure of infant mortality in 1850, since there were no accurate records of birth, but even the incomplete data give one some idea of the appalling ratio of infant deaths to total deaths. This ratio was 17 percent in 1850 as compared with 2.5 percent of total deaths in 1975. The deaths from zymotic diseases in 1850 by causes are shown in Table 5–3. Cholera leads the list because 1850 was a bad cholera year, but the deaths from other intestinal infections held a high rank. Table 5–4 gives a tabulation of all causes of death of infants; intestinal infections led all the rest.

The discovery of bacteria led to a radical change in the concept of diseases, particularly the infectious ones. Etiology, rather than pathologic-anatomic criteria became the principal factor for classification. Osler[17] considered the final differentiation of "the continued fever" to be the most conspicuous contribution of the century.

Table 5–2. Deaths from Zymotic Diseases—1850 Census*

Age (years)	% of Total Deaths for Age Group
Less than 1	32
1–4	54
5–9	56
10–19	45
20–49	39
Males	44
Females	33
50–79	25
Total deaths	323,023
Deaths from zymotic disease	131,813
% of deaths from zymotic disease	40

*Zymotic diseases do not include tuberculosis or pneumonia.
Source: Adapted from C. E. A. Winslow, Wilson G. Smillie, James A. Doull, and John E. Gordon. *The History of American Epidemiology.* Franklin H. Top (ed.). St. Louis: Mosby, 1952. Reprinted by permission.

Table 5–3. Deaths from Zymotic and Other Diseases — 1850 Census

Zymotic diseases	
Cholera	31,506
Dysentery and diarrhea	26,922
Fever—remittent, intermittent, intestinal	19,220
Typhoid fever	13,099
Croup (diphtheria)	10,706
Scarlet fever	9,584
Cholera infantum and cholera morbus	5,528
Whooping cough	5,280
Measles	2,983
Erysipelas	2,786
Smallpox	2,352
Nonzymotic diseases	
Consumption (pulmonary tuberculosis)	33,516
Lobar pneumonia	12,130
Cephalitis in children under five (chiefly cerebrospinal meningitis)	6,422
Convulsions and teething (chiefly in children under two)	6,072

Source: C.-E. A. Winslow, Wilson G. Smillie, James A. Doull, and John E. Gordon. *The History of American Epidemiology.* Franklin H. Top (ed.). St. Louis: Mosby, 1952. Reprinted by permission.

Table 5–4. Deaths from Intestinal Infections in Children under One Year of Age—Census of 1850.*

Cholera infantum	1,111
Cholera morbus	908
Diarrhea	1,467
Dysentery	3,311
Cholera	1,417
Enteritis	645
Teething	836
Typhoid fever	391
Total	10,085
Total deaths in children under one year	54,265
Deaths from zymotic diseases in children under one year	20,064

*Does not include 2,844 deaths from convulsions due in great part to intestinal infections.
Source: C.-E. A. Winslow, Wilson G. Smillie, James A. Doull, and John E. Gordon. *The History of American Epidemiology.* Franklin H. Top (ed.). St. Louis: Mosby, 1952. Reprinted by permission.

Diphtheria

Jacobi[40] claimed that diphtheria occurred infrequently on the Atlantic coast of North America until 1857, at which time it became epidemic. The first death from diphtheria was not reported in New York City until February 15, 1852. As late as 1858 there were only five deaths from diphtheria reported for the year in New York City, but from about 1860 on diphtheria became "one of the most terrible scourges of early life."[94] For example, the annual mortality from this disease in Massachusetts between 1860 and 1880 was as high as 200 per 100,000 population.[11] Between 1866 and 1890 there were 43,000 deaths attributed to diphtheria in New York City. Job Smith[77] claimed that "in New York what has been gained in saving life by suppression of small-pox has been counterbalanced by the mortality produced by diphtheria." The earliest records of diphtheria mortality in Illinois date from 1860, in which year 70 out of 100,000 population died of the disease; in 1880, 122 per 100,000 died, and this seemed to have been the peak of the diphtheria death rate in Illinois, according to Isaac Abt.[1] In New York City in 1881 more than 1 percent of the children under ten years of age died from diphtheria; the mortality from diphtheria in New York City during the early 1890's was four times greater than that from scarlet fever. Before the advent of diphtheria antitoxin the mortality was terrible: 40 to 70 percent in some reports.[11]

Diphtheria prevailed epidemically, endemically, and sporadically during the second half of the nineteenth century. In most large cities it was endemic, occasional cases occurring throughout the year, and with periods in which outbreaks of considerable severity occurred. An important factor in furthering the intensity of the studies of diphtheria was the pandemic which broke out at various points in Europe and North America between 1856 and 1858. During the earlier part of the nineteenth century, France, Norway, and Denmark had been the only countries severely affected by diphtheria epidemics, but after the fifth decade of the century the disease was to be found in all civilized communities of the temperate zone.[27,94] Though the incidence and severity of the disease varied widely during this period; it was overwhelmingly a disease of childhood. And for most of the nineteenth century it was believed that some atmospheric condition or miasma was responsible for its appearance.

Sewer gas was often blamed as the cause of typhoid fever, pneumonia, croup, malaria, and diphtheria. It was not until the mid-1880's that this concept was effectively refuted. This delay, which was the result of a lack of interest in the germ theory on the part of our medical profession, was a striking example of American neglect of basic research for almost the entire nineteenth century.[74]

Theodor A. E. Klebs (1834–1913), of Zurich, a pioneer in bacteriology, discovered the diphtheria bacillus in 1883. Its relationship to the disease was demonstrated by Friedrich Loeffler (1852–1915) in 1884. He was also able to reproduce the characteristic membrane by swabbing the mucous membranes of various animals with pure cultures of the bacillus. In 1888 Pierre P. E. Roux (1853–1933) and Alexandre E. J. Yersin (1863–1943) demonstrated the existence of the extracellular toxin responsible for the disease. Two years later Emil von Behring (1854–1917) and Shibasaburo Kitasato (1856–1931) discovered diphtheria antitoxins and their immunizing powers; finally, in 1894, Roux and André L. Martin (1853–1921) established the value of Behring's specific antitoxin in the treatment of human diphtheria and showed how it could be produced on a large scale by using horses, thus affording an ample supply for human use.

One of the earliest American bacteriological laboratories was set up in New York about 1885 by T. Mitchell Prudden (1849–1924). In 1889 Prudden[63] reported that he had cultivated streptococci, rather than the Klebs-Loeffler bacilli, from the throats of twenty-two children diagnosed by competent clinicians as having diphtheria as a complication of measles or scarlet fever. Obviously, the clinical diagnosis of diphtheria in the prebacteriological era was often in error.

TREATMENT. While bacteriology was beginning to revolutionize the diagnosis and treatment of diphtheria, an important discovery for the relief of respiratory difficulty in laryngeal diphtheria was published in 1885 by Joseph O'Dwyer (1841–1898),[57] a New York pediatrician and a founding member of the American Pediatric Society. About 1880 O'Dwyer had considered the possibility of intubation, which had been completely neglected after the rebuffs the French pediatrician Eugène Bouchut (1818–1891) had received from the French Academy of Medicine in 1858 for his unsuccessful attempts at the procedure. O'Dwyer developed a successful technique as well as special instruments for intubation of the larynx. His claims, based upon the successful intubation of hundreds of cases of diphtheria, were recognized in 1887 by the New

York Academy of Medicine. Intubation, once a dramatic but now a forgotten advance in pediatrics, ended the practice of tracheotomy. With the use of intubation, O'Dwyer in 1882 was able to report the first recovery of a patient with diphtheritic croup in the New York Foundling Hospital in its thirteen years of existence.[9] Tracheotomy in most hands had previously proven an almost complete failure.

Dillon Brown (1861–1909)[12] in 1889 described his use of the O'Dwyer tubes in three hundred fifty cases of intubation apparently all for laryngeal diphthheria. Of the last fifty cases in his series, thirteen, or 26 percent, recovered. This was a significant improvement, because in that era nearly all patients with untreated laryngeal diphtheria died. O'Dwyer's intubation remained the method of choice in hospital practice throughout the first two decades of the present century, but by the 1920's it was largely forgotten.

Jacobi[40] wrote that "whenever the records of diphtheria will be written up, there will be four names at the head of those who deserve the places of honor." He cited Bretonneau, Armand Trousseau (1801–1867), Behring, and O'Dwyer.

Before the introduction of antitoxin, physicians were desperate in their search for effective pharmacologic means of treating diphtheria. A large number of medicinal agents were used, none of which had any proven value. Chlorate of potash or soda and tincture of iron perchloride were the two remedies most widely used in this country. The latter was prescribed because of its putative astringent and antiseptic properties. August Seibert (1854–1929)[71] claimed to have had favorable results in the treatment of pharyngeal diphtheria by "injecting fresh chlorine water through the diphtheritic pseudomembrane into the inflamed mucosa below." He injected "about fifteen drops into each spot and according to the extension of the process as many as six or eight injections are made at each sitting." He claimed that in his last fifty cases so treated, the disease was checked in forty-two. If this treatment was so successful, one wonders why it did not become more widely accepted. Others believed that spraying hydrogen peroxide on the diphtheritic membrane was of value. Alcohol, in the form of strong wine, brandy, or rum, was regarded as of the utmost importance. It was to be given at the first sign of "loss of vigor." Jacobi[40] urged that "alcoholic stimulants ought to be given early and often, and in large quantities, thoroughly diluted." He advised as much as nine ounces or more of brandy or whiskey daily.

The first real breakthrough in the treatment of diphtheria was the introduction of diphtheria antitoxin for passive immunization in 1894 and of toxin-antitoxin for active immunization in 1913.

A landmark contribution in the history of diphtheria was *The Report of the American Pediatric Society's Collective Investigation into the Use of Antitoxin in the Treatment of Diphtheria in Private Practice* (1896), produced through the efforts of a committee of four: Holt, William P. Northrup (1851–1935), O'Dwyer and Adams.[22] The committee, by corresponding with 615 physicians from 114 cities and towns, collected a series of 5,794 treated cases of diphtheria authenticated either by positive culture (83 percent) or by acceptable clinical data (17 percent). The general mortality rate of those treated was 12.3 percent, or, omitting those who died within the first day of the disease, 8.8 percent. Of the 4,120 receiving antitoxin within the first three days, the mortality rate was 7.3 percent; of the 1,148 children who received it on or after the fourth day, the mortality was 27 percent. The most striking beneficial effects of the antitoxin were noted in the 1,256 cases of laryngeal diphtheria. In half of these, recovery took place without intubation or tracheotomy. "Of the 533 cases in which intubation was performed the mortality was 25.9 percent, or less than half as great as has ever been reported by any other method of treatment." For comparison, the committee cited an 1892 report of 5,546 intubation cases in which the mortality was 69.5 percent, and another report, published in 1890, with a mortality rate of 51.6 percent.[12]

Death following the administration of antitoxin occurred in 3 of the 5,794 children, but the committee, taking into account the probable crudity of the horse serum of the time, did not believe the number of serious reactions to be a contraindication to the use of antitoxin. The late-nineteenth-century medical literature contained several case reports of sudden death within minutes of injecting diphtheria antitoxin (?anaphylactoid reaction). (Anaphylaxis was not fully described until 1902 with the publication by Paul Portier and Charles R. Richet [1850–1935][62] of their paper on the phenomenon; the name itself was coined by Richet.)

A second report by the American Pediatric Society in 1897 of the results in 1,704 cases of laryngeal diphtheria treated with antitoxin disproved the allegation that the favorable results were due to the mildness of the disease; laryngeal diphtheria was always extremely serious. The mortality rate of those receiving antitoxin was 21 percent.[22] In the pre-antitoxin period the mortality had been as high as 69.5 percent. Laryngeal diphtheria for that reason furnished the crucial test of serum treatment. Three benefits of antitoxin were noted: first, in the number of cases that recovered without operation (tracheotomy or intubation); second, in the percentage of recoveries in the operative cases; and third, in the shortening of the time the intubation tube was needed.

By the end of the century much of the fear of diphtheria had ebbed, but the antitoxin which was so effective in the treatment of established disease was an agent for passive immunization and provided only temporary protection. Clearly, some safe method of producing active immunization was needed. Bacteriologists recognized this quite early and in 1913 the first effective diphtheria prophylactic was produced. Unfortunately, this toxin-antitoxin was not absolutely safe, and it was not until 1923 that an effective and safe antigen toxoid for the protection of man was produced by Gaston L. Ramon (1886–1963)[65] at the Pasteur Institute.

In 1893 an important event in the history of infectious diseases in America occurred when the Health Department of New York City established a small diagnostic laboratory with Hermann M. Biggs (1859–1923), as director, and William H. Park (1863–1939), a nose and throat specialist, in charge of the bacteriologic study of diphtheria.[92] Within a short time Park had devised a small diagnostic kit for making throat cultures, and then the laboratory inaugurated the plan of having supplies of these diagnostic outfits available to physicians in conveniently located drugstores. Throat cultures left by physicians at these drugstores were collected daily by a messenger from the laboratory. After incubation overnight, they were examined early the next day and the results were telephoned to the attending physicians. Their diagnostic procedures in suspected cases of diphtheria led the venerable Koch to say, "You put us to shame in this work."[94] Park's laboratory was the first outside Europe to produce diphtheria antitoxin.

Scarlet Fever

Sometime in the early years of the nineteenth century—probably about 1803—scarlet fever in children became milder than it had been throughout most of the eighteenth century, although it was still a common disease. There is no question that an increase occurred in its severity about 1830. In 1840 the number of deaths nearly doubled and scarlet fever became, as Charles Creighton,[16] the father of modern British epidemiology, noted, "the leading cause of death among the infectious diseases of childhood." It remained so in Europe, in Great Britain, and in the United States until the last decades of the nineteenth century, at which time the mortality from scarlet fever was 55 percent for children under two years of age and 20 to 30 percent for children under five.[36] By 1915 the average mortality from scarlet fever in children under five years of age was still between 20 and 30 percent.[68]

In New York City, scarlet fever was rare between 1805 and 1822. During these eighteen years there were only 43 recorded deaths from this disease. After 1822 it gradually assumed an epidemic character and by the end of 1847 had caused 4,874 deaths.[68] In 1865, when the Council on Hygiene and Public Health of the Citizens' Association reported on the sanitary condition of New York, scarlet fever was noted as a prevalent and often fatal disease.[68] In 1844 there were 306 deaths due to scarlet fever in Chicago. Characteristic of the disease was the wide variation in annual death rates. For example, during the period 1850–1859, scarlet fever showed a maximum mortality rate of 272 per 100,000 and a minimum of 6.[81] During the year 1889 at the Willard Parker and Riverside Hospitals (New York) the death rate from scarlet fever reached 12.3 percent. At the Municipal Hospital (Philadelphia) in 1897 the death rate was 11.8 percent. In children between one and five years at this institution the mortality reached 21.8 percent.[11]

A review of the mortality rate of scarlet fever in children two to four years of age living in Providence, Rhode Island, attested to the wide variation in the mortality rate of this disease. From 1865 to 1924 this rate decreased from 691 to 28.3 per

100,000.[61] But since the attack rate did not show a corresponding decline, the number of deaths cannot be attributed to a lower prevalence or to changes in the population but must have been caused by a lessening severity of the disease. From 1886 to 1888 one in every five cases of scarlet fever died, while from 1923 to 1924 only one in every one hundred fourteen cases ended fatally.[61] A similar trend was also noted in England and Wales.[27] These trends may be interpreted in terms of our understanding of bacterial virulence, as well as social and economic developments since the middle of the nineteenth century.

At first scarlet fever was overshadowed by diphtheria as a cause of death among children, but toward the end of the century the former disease overtook the lead of diphtheria. Smith,[76] writing in 1872, claimed that scarlet fever in New York City "on account of its greater frequency, and its large percentage of fatal cases causes more death than any other contagious affection. Though not more common than measles, it is attended, with us, by more than double its mortality."

The nineteenth-century physician feared the complications of scarlet fever. These included clonic convulsions, suppuration of the cervical lymph nodes (occasionally they became gangrenous), gangrene of the mouth, articular rheumatism (the definitive relationship of hemolytic streptococcal throat infection and rheumatic fever was not established until 1930), pericardial and peritoneal inflammation, and nephritis with marked albuminuria; the last-named disease was often also attributed to chilling of the body in a cold room, to an open window, or to the child's sitting on cold stones. The first suggestion of the streptococcal origin of scarlet fever was published in 1889.[47] Some fifty years of research, however, were needed before the true nature of the mechanism by which the disease was produced became apparent. However, as early as 1893, André Bergé,[19] of Paris, claimed that "scarlet fever is a local infection" caused by a streptococcus which "grows in the crypts of the tonsils where it secretes an "erythemogenic" toxin, the diffusion of which produces the exanthem." Yet for the next three decades, bacteriologists searched in vain for this toxin.

TREATMENT. The nineteenth-century physician had no effective means of treating scarlet fever, except possibly for bed rest. Almost all textbook authors advised keeping the child in bed for at least three weeks and maintaining the patient on a fluid diet for at least two weeks. Milk was considered the best diet for scarlet fever patients, and many recommended diluting it with Vichy water or limewater. For the burning and soreness of the throat, potassium chlorate was tried and found valueless, as was hydrogen peroxide. To reduce fever, quinine was favored (acetylsalicylic acid was not introduced into medicine until 1899); for fevers that remained continuously elevated over 104° F, cold packs or cold sponging were recommended.

The method of applying cold used at the Willard Parker Hospital for Contagious Diseases in New York was as follows:

The patient is placed upon blankets, but the legs, feet, arms, and hands are wrapped in warm, dry blankets, and hot kettles are enclosed in the wrappings. An ice-bag is placed to the head. The face and trunk are freely sponged in warm water and alcohol, evaporation being hastened by fanning, so long as it cools the patient, clears the cerebrum, gives force and rhythm to the heart, and leaves the patient to a quiet sleep. The warmth to the extremities seems to exert a favorable influence upon the heart's action and to favor a free superficial circulation.[15]

Summer Diarrheas of Infants (Cholera Infantum)

As has been noted, more than a quarter of the children born in the civilized world of the second half of the nineteenth century died before their fifth birthday, and nearly one-half of these deaths were caused by the summer diarrheas.[84] Rush had devised the term cholera infantum, which came eventually to embrace the group of affections classed under the general heading of summer diarrheas of infants. It received its name because of the violence of its symptoms, which closely resembled those in Asiatic cholera. Some nineteenth-century physicians called all summer diarrheas cholera infantum but most authors employed it to designate only the most violent form in which there were frequent, explosive, watery or perhaps serous stools, accompanied by vomiting with rapid and great emaciation. As the century progressed, the term cholera infantum became increasingly restricted, being used to denote only the most serious form of choleriform summer diarrhea and not as a generic name for all summer diarrheas. A few authorities, such as Victor C. Vaughan (1851–1929)[85] substituted the term acute milk infection for cholera infantum.

Although Rush, as we have seen, had written a classic paper about cholera infantum in 1777, serious and sustained interest in the condition did not develop until the latter decades of the nineteenth century, especially with the opening of the bacteriological era about 1876. William D. Booker (1844–1921),[8] the first professor (clinical) of pediatrics at the Johns Hopkins University School of Medicine and one of the first to perform elaborate bacteriological studies of the stools in diarrhea of infants, described the early history of this disease as follows:

About the middle of the Eighteenth Century there occurred in the towns and cities along the Atlantic coast of the United States of America, a serious disease among infants which had not been observed before. It was characterized more especially by vomiting and diarrhoea, and was confined almost exclusively to children in the first two years of life. Its incidence was limited to the summer months, and it appeared each year in an epidemic form with such regularity that it was looked for as an annual visitor—the dread of parents and the opprobrium of physicians. It was thought to be peculiar to America, and was viewed in the light of one of those physical occurrences which occasionally give rise to diseases before unknown, while others from causes equally unscrutable, disappear. . . . The disease was not recognized in Europe; it was unknown to the aborigines of our continent; and the first settlers of the colonies left us no record of its existence.

Rush's[70] paper, only six pages long, was remarkable for the amount of information it contained and for the accurate description of the clinical features of the disease. Rush, contrary to most others of his time, denied the etiologic importance of dentition, worms, and summer fruits in cholera infantum.

James Jackson,[37] of Boston, in 1812 was the first to report the postmortem findings in infants dying of cholera infantum. He considered the principal "remote causes" of the disease to be dentition, season of the year, improper food, restraint from exercise in the open air, and an impure atmosphere. C. D. Meigs[53] in 1820 also believed that dentition was an important etiological factor and that the development of cholera infantum depended principally on a loss of the healthy function of the liver. Logan[51] in his textbook (1825) attributed the disease to "pain

and irritation of teething, season of the year, neglect of cleanliness, and local circumstances," which produced "an increased and vitiated state of bilious secretion, acrimony and other disturbances of the first passages." By the late 1890's most writers agreed with Rotch[69] that "cholera infantum is an infectious disease caused by a specific organism not yet discovered." The so-called specific organism was never discovered.

The zenith of summer diarrhea occurred in the later years of the nineteenth century. It was almost exclusively confined to infants who were artificially fed. Since its maximum frequency and severity coincided with the hottest weather, it was universally believed that atmospheric heat played a key role in causing the disease. The summer heat was thought to exhaust the tone of the skin and the energy of the stomach; rendering the infant's system more susceptible to impressions exercised by external agents and diminishing its resistance to them. At least three-quarters of the deaths from diarrheal diseases occurred during the first five years of life (Table 5–1).

The stools in cholera infantum were usually so thin and watery that they soaked into the diaper almost like urine and in some cases produced scarcely more of a stain. Almost all writers described the odor of the stools as being musty and offensive rather than fecal. Vomiting was persistent and urine output often ceased. The loss of strength and emaciation were more rapid than in any other type of diarrhea.[85] Those who wrote about this disease described the infant as having sunken eyes with eyelids and mouth permanently opened, dry skin, and emaciation so marked that the skin lay in folds. (It is of interest that the word *dehydration* was not used during the nineteenth century to describe the infant's condition.) Vaughan[85] wrote that "the flesh rapidly disappeared and that there was no other disease, with the exception of Asiatic cholera, in which the wasting proceeded more speedily and exhaustion resulted more quickly." Not until the last decade of the century did a few writers suggest the use of parenteral fluid replacement, and then only as a last resort, although hypodermoclysis and intravenous fluid replacement had been recommended previously in the treatment of Asiatic cholera. Rotch[69] wrote: "In extreme cases the subcutaneous injection of normal salt solution can be tried. Care should be taken not to introduce in fifteen minutes more than

37.5 cc (1 drachm) for every pound of the child's weight."

Hypodermoclysis was first introduced by Arnaldo Cantani (1837–1893), of Italy, as a means of treating terminal stages of "serous diarrhea and of algidity of collapse."[72] Cantani's formula for an adult consisted of two quarts of boiled water, two and a half ounces of pure sodium chloride, and a dram and a half of sodium carbonate. The recommended amount for an adult was one to two and a half quarts. No mention was made of the appropriate amount for children. The temperature of the solution when injected by hypodermoclysis was to be 100.4° F, unless the rectal temperature was very low, and in this case it should be raised as high as 109.4° F.[72]

Intravenous fluid therapy for severe diarrhea was practiced in Europe toward the end of the nineteenth century, but I could find no reference to the use of intravenous therapy in American pediatric literature of that period. The standard European preparation contained one part of sodium bicarbonate and six parts of sodium chloride in one liter of boiled water. The recommended temperature of the injected fluid was between 100.4° F and 104° F; the quantity administered averaged two quarts for adults.[72]

Holt[33] in the first edition of his textbook (1897) recommended hypodermoclysis with "a saline solution" (common salt forty-five grains, sterilized water one pint) in the treatment of severe cholera infantum. He did not mention the intravenous route. The fluid was to be injected "into the cellular tissue of the abdomen, buttocks, thighs, or back. To be efficient at least half a pint should be given in the course of every twelve hours." Although Holt further claimed that "a very much larger quantity can often be used with advantage," the amount of the "much larger quantity" was not specified. He also described a simple apparatus for making the injection, in which the needle from a hypodermic syringe was attached to a few inches of rubber tubing and this was then attached to the nozzle of a bulb syringe.

The four drugs that almost all physicians relied on in the treatment of summer diarrhea were calomel, for its antifermentative and antiseptic action; castor oil, to rid the body of all "irritative" material; bismuth, as a diarrheal sedative; and opium, to relieve tenesmus.[46] But almost everyone from Rush's time until the early twentieth century had found drug therapy wanting. Many fell back on Rush's advice about the value of taking the sick infant to the country. (The suburban areas must have been far more rural in the 1890's than today; one author[83] advised that the poor city mother take her child "in the cool of the morning and evening on the trolley-cars into the suburbs for the invigorating influence of fresh country air.")

Whooping Cough

According to Smith[76] and Holt,[33] whooping cough killed at least a quarter of all affected infants under one year of age. The records of the city of New York in the 1890's showed that about five hundred children under two years died annually of pertussis and that of these 65 percent were less than a year of age. In 1889 pertussis was the fifth most common cause of death in the first year of life in New York City (Table 5–5). Several writers of the period noted that females were somewhat more liable to be attacked than males.[77]

In New York City, during the half-century ending with 1853, a total of 4,840 children died of pertussis; that is, one death from this disease for seventy-five deaths from all other causes.[77] The age of the patient was the most important prognostic factor in pertussis. Holt[33] and others found that after the fourth year it was rare to encounter either a fatal outcome or serious complications. But during infancy, and particularly during the first year, there were few dis-

Table 5–5. The Ten Chief Causes of Death in the First Year of Life in New York City—1889.*

Cause	Percent
Diarrheal disease	31.0
Bronchitis and pneumonia	16.6
Prematurity	6.9
Tuberculosis	3.8
Whooping cough	3.2
Other neonatal conditions	2.8
Diphtheria and croup	2.3
Injury at birth	1.2
Syphilis	0.9
Congenital malformations	0.8

*N = 10,527.
Source: Adapted from L. E. Holt, Jr., R. McIntosh, and H. L. Barnett. Pediatrics (13th ed.). New York: Appleton-Century Crofts, 1962.

eases more to be dreaded.[33] This was especially true on account of the connection of whooping cough with the three most fatal nineteenth-century conditions of infantile life—bronchopneumonia, diarrheal disease, and convulsions. The prognosis was found to be far worse in infants three months of age or less than in older infants; the prognosis was particularly bad in delicate infants, in those who were rachitic, in those who were prone to bronchitis, in those who had suffered previously from pneumonia, and especially in those with a strong "family tendency" to tuberculosis.[33]

In foundling asylums and hospitals for infants, pertussis was ranked among the most fatal diseases; in some epidemics the mortality in such institutions was as high as 50 percent.[11] Two-thirds of the deaths were due to bronchopneumonia and the next most frequent cause was diarrheal disease. Convulsions were the mode of death in either of these complications or occurred apart from them. And as a predisposing cause of tuberculosis, pertussis was considered second only to measles.[33]

TREATMENT. Because drugs accomplished so little, resort was made to every possible hygienic aid, especially fresh air. In pleasant weather the child was to live almost continuously out of doors. Of the many drugs prescribed, bromoform (a compound analagous to chloroform) was considered among the most effective. It was never prescribed in solution but always alone, to be taken by dropping it on a little sugar in a spoon, beginning with a dose of one drop every four hours and increasing the dose by one drop each day until some effect was produced. Also recommended was belladonna, which was considered valuable as an antispasmodic. Cannabis indica was widely used and was, according to J. P. Crozer Griffith (1856–1941),[29] "probably one of the most reliable means of treatment." Other drugs frequently prescribed for pertussis were pilocarpine, lobelia, resorcin, hyoscine, turpentine, ouabain, asafetida, antipyrine, chloral hydrate, and opium.

Measles

This disease was viewed with great anxiety during the latter part of the nineteenth century. It took a terrible toll, especially in institutions; for example, during the year 1897 in the Municipal Hospital of Philadelphia, 39 percent of the cases of measles admitted died.[80] In children ranging between the ages of one and five years, the death rate reached as high as 48 percent.[11] Jacobi[42] had pointed out in the 1860's that during certain epidemics the mortality from measles amounted to almost 35 percent. In New York City in the early 1890's, statistics showed that 1,150 children under two years of age died of measles, scarlet fever, and diphtheria; 305, or more than a quarter of these deaths, were caused by measles.[11]

In the 1880's and 1890's the prognosis depended on the age and state of health of the patient, the character of the epidemic, and the season of the year in which it occurred. Most of the deaths from measles were in children under three years of age; Holt,[33] writing in 1897, claimed that "in institutions containing little children, no epidemic disease is so fatal." He reported that during the 1892 epidemic of measles in the Nursery and Child's Hospital in New York City the mortality for infants less than a year of age was 33 percent. Between a year and two years of age, the mortality rate rose to 50 percent, and for infants between two and three years of age, it declined to 30 percent. The average mortality from measles among all children under two years of age was about 20 percent, but as with the other infectious diseases, the mortality from measles was much higher in institutions.

The important prognostic symptoms were thought to be the initial temperature and the character of the eruption. An initial temperature above 102° F, or one which remained high until the eruption appeared, was considered ominous. So too was a temperature that rose after a full eruption or that did not fall as the rash faded.

Of fifty-one fatal cases of measles in infants from one to two years of age in the 1892 epidemic analyzed by Holt, the cause of death was bronchopneumonia in forty-five, ileocolitis in four, and membranous laryngitis in two.[33] More than half the deaths in these fifty-one infants occurred during the second week of the disease; the earliest was on the fifth day of the disease.

TREATMENT. In the treatment of measles, Holt[33] and others recommended that the sickroom be darkened, because "the eyes are very sensitive to light." Frank E. Waxham (1852–1911)[88] advised placing the patient "in a large, well-ventilated apartment, which should be shaded from bright light but not *completely darkened*." Floyd M. Crandall (1858–1919)[15] wrote that "the room should be kept very dark, and no direct light should be permitted to fall on the eyes." Starr[80] recommended that the room be moderately darkened, and that "the patient's bed be so placed that the patient's face will not be turned directly toward a window. . . . The patient must be put to bed and confined there until not only the rash itself, but all traces of the remaining yellow-red stains have disappeared—about the eighth or tenth day of the disease."

The medicinal treatment included potassium citrate as a febrifuge and as an expectorant. In "malignant measles," a term widely used in the nineteenth century, whiskey or brandy plus quinine and digitalis were strongly recommended. Mustard baths and hot packs were considered of great service to "bring out the rash." For the mustard bath, which was said to have been more suitable for children under three years of age, the water was heated to 100° F and contained about one teaspoonful of powdered mustard to the gallon. The patient was immersed up to the neck for three minutes, then quickly dried and placed in bed between blankets, or wrapped in a blanket and dried later.

Cerebrospinal Meningitis

Epidemics of this disease during the nineteenth century led Jacobi[39] to assert that the United States "more than any other country has been invaded by this plague." The epidemic in Connecticut during the first decade of the century resulted in Elisha North's classic work, already noted (p. 86). Although meningococcal meningitis has probably afflicted man for centuries, its occurrence was not known for sure prior to 1805 when an epidemic in Geneva was so well described by Gaspard Vieusseux (1746–1814)[86] that it can be readily identified.

During the period from 1842 to 1850 there were several widespread epidemics in the United States: in Tennessee (1845), Alabama (1845), Illinois (1846), Arkansas (1847), and Mississippi and Missouri (1847). From 1850 to 1856 the country was free from the disease. However, during the Civil War the disease was far-reaching, especially among young soldiers. The meningococcus has been a noto-rious camp follower; the most extensive and serious epidemics have appeared in times of war. From 1860 to 1874, epidemics occurred in almost every state, especially during the winter and spring. After 1876 the disease occurred only sporadically but never died out. Occasionally for a period of years the mortality was low; then suddenly it would rise. For instance, in the Boston City Hospital, from 1880 to 1896, only thirty-nine cases died. But during the first month of the 1897 epidemic, there were forty-two fatal cases.[39]

As late as the last decade of the century, many American physicians were still not sure of the contagious nature of meningitis. Jacobi[39] commented: "Whether, as in malaria and yellow fever, an intermediary agent of infection such as the mosquito, or as in recurrent fever the bedbug, remains to be proven," and he then described this experience of Edward Gamaliel Janeway (1841–1911): "The coffin containing the body of a woman who had died of cerebro-spinal meningitis was opened, and a strand of her hair cut off. This strand was taken home by a woman, and frequently handled by her as well as by a child living in the same house. Both this woman and the child developed meningitis, and nobody else was affected."

TREATMENT. Prior to the introduction of serum treatment for meningococcal meningitis in 1908 by Simon Flexner (1863–1946) and James Jobling (1876–1961),[23] the mortality in children was as high as 80 percent. This pushed physicians to extreme measures, such as leeches to the nape of the neck, large doses of calomel, and repeated bleeding; obviously, none proved to be effective. After Heinrich I. Quincke (1842–1922)[64] popularized lumbar puncture in 1891, draining off some of the spinal fluid was recommended to relieve the patient's headache and lethargy, at least for a short time, but it did not shorten the course of the disease or reduce the fatality rate. At the end of the nineteenth century the only helpful measures were sedatives and opiates.

Lumbar puncture for diagnostic purposes was first reported in this country in 1896 by August Caillé (1854–1935).[13] Arthur H. Wentworth (1864–1947),[90] in the same year, described a series of thirty cases of lumbar puncture in children, some with and others without meningitis, in which the cerebrospinal fluid was examined. He showed that the normal fluid was as perfectly clear as distilled water; that cloudiness was caused by cells, the character of which varied with the type of meningitis; and that inoculation of the fluid into guinea pigs was the surest diagnostic method for tuberculosis. He also demonstrated that the amount of protein in normal fluid was 1/50 of one percent (= 20 mg%) or less; and it varied from 1/30 to 1/10 of one percent (= 33 to 100 mg%) in meningitis.

The first lumbar puncture performed at the Children's Hospital in Boston by Wentworth[90] on a two-year-old who had "marked cerebral symptoms" proved to be a harrowing experience.

We punctured the spinal canal, using for the purpose the needle from an antitoxin syringe, and withdrew six cubic centimeters of a clear fluid which looked like distilled water. No tubercle bacilli were found....

Immediately after tapping the canal the child became restless, throwing herself about the bed, clutching at her hair and giving vent to short cries. The pulse rose to over 250 in the minute, the respiration was superficial, and the skin was cool and slightly livid. Subcutaneous injections of brandy and ether were given, heaters applied, and the foot of the bed raised. This condition persisted about the same for three-quarters of an hour, and then the child became quieter.

During the attack I felt considerable uneasiness because I was unprepared for such a result and did not know but that it would terminate fatally. I now believe that the symptoms were due to headache, caused by the removal of fluid, and that her life was not endangered.

TREATMENT. The first breakthrough—as noted—in the treatment of epidemic meningococcal meningitis did not occur until 1908, when Flexner and Jobling[23] reported on the use of antimeningococcal serum (prepared in the horse by inoculation of *Diplococcus intracellularis* and its products) in about 400 bacteriologically proven pediatric cases. The overall mortality rate in 393 of these cases was about 25 percent. It was also evident that the sooner after onset of the disease the serum was administered, the lower was the mortality rate: first to third day, 16.5 percent; fourth to seventh, 23.8 percent; and later than the seventh day, 35 percent. Of equal importance was that few of the survivors had the crippling sequelae that were so frequent in untreated survivors. Harold K. Faber (1884–1979) and Rustin McIntosh (b. 1894)[22] have noted that although "the data for untreated patients were not entirely comparable, and

no attempt at alteration of treated or untreated patients was made," it appeared that "the serum had a marked beneficial effect and that the mortality without specific serum in other places and other epidemics was usually about 75 percent."

Tuberculosis

In the prebacteriologic era, tuberculosis was considered to be a hereditary disease.[50] It was unquestionably the single greatest cause of disease and death in the Western world during the nineteenth century.[58] An idea of the importance of tuberculosis as a public health problem in the early nineteenth century can be deduced from community mortality data. From 1768 to 1773 in Salem, Massachusetts, pulmonary tuberculosis accounted for 117 of 642 deaths (18.2 percent) from all causes and by the first decade of the nineteenth century the proportion had risen to 25 percent.[52]

The diagnosis of tuberculosis before the days of Koch and his discovery of the tubercle bacillus (announced March 24, 1882) rested on clinical features and anatomically on the presence of tubercles. This explains why a relationship between tuberculosis and scrofulosis was not established before the end of the nineteenth century. "Scrofulosis," then so frequently diagnosed, did not represent a disease entity. Rather, it was thought to be a "diathesis" of hereditary nature, which predisposed the child to characteristic manifestations of skin, mucous membranes, and glands, and, at times, of the inner organs as well. Scrofulosis included both tuberculosis and certain other entities completely unrelated to tuberculosis. By 1890 the term was much less frequently used than formerly. One of the reasons for this was that it came to be looked upon by the public as a term of reproach, inasmuch as it denoted a disease associated with "workhouse" and "pauper" children, and it was also associated in the minds of parents with unsightly swellings and scars in the neck.[58] Koch's discovery of the tubercle bacillus, which he showed was present alike in the "gray granulations" regarded as pathognomonic of tuberculosis and in the caseous gland masses in the neck which were called scrofulous, put an end to the word *scrofulosis*.

Although it has been long known that, in the quaint language of Sir Thomas Browne (1605–1682),[58] "consumptive and tabid roots sprout early," the awareness of the widespread prevalence of tuberculosis in the early periods of life was not appreciated until the nineteenth century. In the United States at the beginning of the present century tuberculosis vied with pneumonia as the chief cause of death in those over eighteen years of age. In the year 1900, of every 1,000 Americans, 2 died of tuberculosis and 20 were ill with the disease.[52] With the establishment of outpatient departments in general hospitals and in hospitals for children, it became apparent that tuberculosis of the lungs, glands, skin, and bones made up a considerable percentage of all cases seen in these facilities. In fact, at the beginning of the present century, tuberculosis was discovered in about a quarter of the infants on whom a postmortem examination had been performed at the New York Babies Hospital.[87]

In 1898, an American veterinarian, Theobald Smith (1859–1934),[78] described for the first time the cultural and pathognomonic differences between human and bovine tuberculosis. He thus opened up an additional wide field of prophylaxis, especially in regard to milk infected with bovine tubercle bacilli.

Another great scientific achievement of the nineteenth century that helped enormously in making the conquest of tuberculosis possible was the discovery of x-rays in 1895 by Wilhelm C. Roentgen (1845–1923).

TREATMENT. The treatment of tuberculosis, both in children and in adults, in the absence of effective drugs was, according to Osler,[58] "the maintenance of nutrition at the highest possible grade." To accomplish this, three measures were practiced.

The first called for a life in the fresh air and sunshine with forced rest. The importance of environment was shown in Edward L. Trudeau's (1848–1915)[82] experiments with rabbits inoculated with the tubercle bacillus. Those kept in a damp, dark place succumbed rapidly; those permitted to run wild recovered or showed very slight lesions. This rudimentary experiment was believed to offer scientific proof that patients with tuberculosis would be helped by living in places where they might constantly inhale fresh air and be exposed to sunlight. It was for this reason that the Trudeau sanitarium established in 1884 at Saranac Lake in the Adirondack Mountains of New York State and a similar sanitarium established a few years later at Colorado Springs, Colorado, were so popular in the treatment of tuberculosis.

Next in importance to fresh air and sunshine was nutrition. The accepted belief was that one of the greatest values of the open-air treatment was that it greatly improved the patient's appetite and digestion. A high-protein diet, consisting of broth, eggs, milk, and meat, was highly recommended. For children milk was thought to be especially beneficial. In the early part of the nineteenth century the diet of patients with tuberculosis had been severely restricted. Gradually, however, physicians recognized that the "consumption" of the flesh should be combated by giving the patient plenty of food.

Third, the use of such remedies as cod-liver oil, hypophosphites, and arsenic were prescribed to "improve the general nutrition."[58] Other measures suggested were "rubbing, bathing, and frictions," all of which were thought to stimulate and improve the general metabolism.

Specific Therapy. In 1890 Koch[48] announced that he had developed a glycerine extract of cultures of tubercle bacilli (tuberculin) that would cure tuberculosis. But despite initial enthusiasm for its curative value by such well-known physicians as Trudeau and Lord Lister (1827–1912), it was soon apparent that tuberculin had no therapeutic value and its long-continued vogue during the 1890's was one of the regrettable episodes of medical history.

Osler,[58] along with others, felt that creosote had "a beneficial action on the tuberculous processes." It was administered by mouth either in *perles* or in a mixture. It was also given in the form of inhalations, the *vapor creasoti,* which consisted of creosote 80 minims, light carbonate of magnesium 30 grains, water to one ounce; a teaspoonful in a pint of water heated to 140° F.

Syphilis

The three great plagues of the nineteenth century were tuberculosis, alcoholism, and syphillis.

Congenital syphilis, or "hereditary" syphilis as it was usually called in the nineteenth century, was one of the major pediatric problems of that period. The term "hereditary" applied to congenital syphilis was acceptable and was widely used until about forty years ago. It was based on the prevalent misconception that treponema became attached to the sperm and thus conveyed infection to the ovum. For example, Henry D. Chapin (1857–1942)[14] claimed that "without mercurial treatment the spermatozoa can transmit the syphilitic poison during the first year after primary infection, and there is great danger to the fetus from syphilitic contagion up to the fourth year." It was also believed that if the father had infected the mother, as frequently happened, there would be double "syphilization" of the offspring, which most likely would be stillborn or, if born, would soon succumb to an aggravated form of the disease. Max Kassowitz,[45] an eminent Austrian pediatrician, averred that "the paternal inheritance of syphilis may be ranked among the best-established scientific facts and that the continued opposition of unbelievers can no more change it than, for example, can the protective power of vaccinia against smallpox be rendered doubtful because annually whole libraries are written and printed against it."

By 1917 the belief in the transmission of syphilis to the fetus from the father without the intermediate infection of the mother had begun to be questioned. Holt[36] cautioned that "this question must be placed among those not yet definitely settled." The doctrine that syphilis might be transferred from a syphilitic fetus found very wide but not universal acceptance. The process was known as *choc en retour*, retroinfection or syphilis by conception. It was invoked to explain those cases in which the wife had become syphilitic without a discoverable chancre.

Congenital syphilis produced widespread disease, lesions being found in the skin, lungs, liver, spleen, kidneys, pancreas, teeth, and bones. The symptoms were broadly variable and the infant might even appear normal at birth. At birth, infected infants often had bullae either on the palms or on the soles of feet, or some infants had the papulopustular form of syphilid. In some cases the bridge of the nose was sharply depressed (saddle-nose). Such infants often were bothered with a troublesome coryza, or snuffles; this was one of the earliest and most constant of local symptoms in infantile syphilis. The lips frequently had a shiny, glossy appearance and after a time distinct rhagades were frequently seen. At times the liver and spleen were markedly enlarged. Osteochondritis and dactylitis were hallmarks of congenital syphilis. The majority of infants bore the marks of the disease into adult life. There was a widespread belief that rickets was especially prevalent and severe among infants born with congenital syphilis.

PROGNOSIS. Kassowitz[45] claimed that one-third of all syphilitic children died before their birth and that among those who were born alive, 34 percent died in the first six months of life. Jean Fournier (1832–1914),[14] the great French venereologist, placed the mortality, when the infection was derived from the father alone, at 28 percent; from the mother alone, 60 percent, and when from both parents, 68.5 percent. The earlier the symptoms appeared after birth, the severer was the type of the disease and the worse the prognosis.[14] Breast-fed infants had a better chance than those artificially fed. Many perinatal deaths from syphilis were probably unrecorded, being simply reported as stillbirths, premature births, or congenital debility. Toward the end of the nineteenth century, syphilis was considered as probably the largest cause of stillbirths, and some reports claimed that 70 percent of macerated fetuses showed unmistakable signs of syphilis.[14]

TREATMENT. Mercurial treatment of congenital syphilis was variously given by mouth, by inunctions, or by subcutaneous injections. Internal medication was preferred. But if diarrhea occurred, an inunction of mercurial ointment mixed with from four to eight times its quantity of petroleum jelly or rose ointment was performed on the inside of the thighs or in the axillae, using a portion about the size of a small hickory nut, or the ointment could be applied on a flannel roller and bandaged about the child once a day. Before the ointment was applied, the skin was thoroughly cleansed with soap and tepid water.

Internal medication consisted of mercury with chalk (gray powder), given in doses of one-fourth of a grain to one or two grains twice a day. Jacobi[38] preferred calomel on account of the rapidity of its action, in doses from 1/20 to 1/6 grain three times a day. Where the bones were involved, or when there was evidence of gumma in any part of the body, potassium iodide was prescribed. If the rhagades, especially those about the anus, bled, a weak topical solution of silver nitrate was recommended. The severe rhinitis that was commonly encountered was treated by washing out the nasal passages once a day with a 1 : 2,000 solution of corrosive sublimate.

Rickets

Rickets, until very recently an extremely common disease of growing children, seems to have appeared in England about 1620. Two English medical writers were the first to recognize and describe the disorder and its symptoms. The most important of these studies appeared in 1645 and 1650, and neither author believed the disease to be a new one. Rickets spread rapidly throughout Europe during the Industrial Revolution, with the ever-increasing numbers of poor families forced to live in the narrow, sunless alleys of factory towns and urban slums.

By 1880 rickets had become one of the most common diseases of American children, especially among those who lived in the crowded, poorly ventilated, and sunless tenements of Northeastern cities.

John S. Parry (1843–1876),[60] of Philadelphia, in 1872 noted:

The medical literature of this country is singularly deficient in regard to this disease. Our leading medical journals contain few original articles upon the subject, and it is often passed without notice in the systematic works on the practice of medicine and the diseases of children; while the frequency of the disease, the grave deformities which it produces, and its indirect termination in death in numerous instances make it a subject of great interest and importance.

Parry took issue with the prevalent opinion among American physicians that rickets was largely a disease of the Old World, where it was said to be exceedingly common. A few American authors who had written about rickets prior to the 1870's claimed that it was far less commonly seen in this country than in Europe. Of interest is that neither Dewees nor Eberle even mentioned rickets in their textbooks. Condie, who described rickets under the name "scrofulous disease of the bones," as late as 1868 wrote that the disease "is fortunately one of comparatively rare occurrence." Louis Bauer (1814–1898),[4] often considered "the first exponent of American orthopaedics," wrote that rickets "is one of the rarest maladies on the Western Continent." Meigs and Pepper, in the fifth edition of their textbook (1870), also believed that "rickets must be a vastly more common affection among the poorer classes in London than among the same classes in our large American cities."

A physician who was a staff member of the Columbia Hospital Dispensary in Washington, D.C., between 1868 and 1872 claimed that of the 1,028 children seen in the dispensary only 11 were found to have rickets. This would suggest that the prevalence of rickets at this hospital was only 1 percent. However, by the 1880's rickets took on a new reputation as being anything but rare in American children. Parry[60] maintained that rickets was not confined to children in hospitals and that it was not among the poor alone that rickets was found, because he had "repeatedly met with typical examples of this disease among children whose parents were able to provide them with every luxury, and more; like [Sir William] Jenner I have seen fully-developed rickets . . . among children well cared for and living in the country." (In 1860 Jenner[43] had written that "rachitis is the most common, the most important and in its effects, the most fatal of the diseases affecting children.")

Parry reasoned that "he could only account for this difference of opinion [about the prevalence of rickets] between other American writers and himself by their failure to appreciate the characteristic symptoms of the early stages of affection." He wrote:

The only means by which the statements of American authors upon practical medicine and the diseases of children can be accounted for, is by concluding that, while they recognize the grave forms of the disease, they fail to appreciate the very characteristic symptoms of the early stages of the affection. The writer having had his attention drawn to this subject several years ago, has been irresistibly forced to the conclusion that rachitis is scarcely less frequent in Philadelphia than it is in the large cities of Great Britain and the Continent of Europe.

Henry C. Haven (c. 1852–1915)[31] found that "rickets was diagnosed in about 5 percent of the 1516 patients under 7 years of age seen at the West End Dispensary for Children [Boston] during the period 1883–1886." And "in a total of 90 black children under 7 years of age, 38 had rickets, an incidence of 43 percent." Twelve years later John Lovett Morse (1865–1940),[54] also of Boston, observed the incidence of rickets to be much higher than Haven's figures. He wrote:

Four hundred consecutive infants under two years of age, medical out-patients at the Infant's Hospital [Boston] were examined for evidence of rickets. *Eighty percent* [italics mine] showed more or less marked signs. A rosary was present in every case. Only those enlargements were considered as a rosary which could be felt both parallel and vertical to the long axis of the rib. It was the only symptom in 40 per cent. The single associated symptom was most often delayed dentition, next, enlargement of the cranial eminences. Delayed dentition occurred in more than 50 per cent. Large fontanelles, large eminences, retraction of the diaphragm and enlargement of the epiphyses of the extremities were each present in about 15 per cent but were symptoms of later development. About 40 per cent of the cases were Russian and Polish Jews. Only 12 per cent came from the southern races.

Job Lewis Smith[77] reported that rickets was a frequent disease among the poor in New York City. In the New York Infant Asylum he found that "one in every nine children presented marked rachitic symptoms." But Smith also felt that "mild cases of rickets are often overlooked, since physicians may not be summoned to attend them, while if they be summoned, many who have not given particular attention to this disease, are apt to err in diagnosis, and to refer the symptoms to some other than the true cause."

Charles G. Jennings (1856–1935)[44] in 1885 also claimed that the so-called rarity of rickets was only apparent. On the basis of his experience at St. Mary's Dispensary in Buffalo, New York, he noted, "My attention was drawn to the disease [rickets] by the frequency with which I observed it, even in an advanced stage, among the children presented for treatment." Jennings also commented, as had many others, that the disease was not limited to children of poor parents.

John H. Fruitnight (1851–1900),[25] in describing the health conditions in New York City in 1893, wrote that "rachitis has become one of the most important and most common of the diathetic diseases met with in the humbler classes of our population."

Irving M. Snow (1859–1932)[79] attempted unsuccessfully to explain the great frequency of rickets among Neapolitan children in American cities, noting that two-thirds of these children developed rickets in spite of their being breast-fed. Snow leaned toward adverse environmental conditions as the principal cause of rickets.

Both Fruitnight and Jacobi frequently commented —as did almost all American pediatricians between 1880 and 1920—that with our rapidly increasing immigrant population, rickets had become an enormous problem, especially in the large Northern cities. Two main schools of thought developed: one taught that rickets was caused by improper food; the second attributed rickets to "bad air," lack of sunshine, and poor housing. Rowland G. Freeman (1859–1945)[24] did not believe that food was ever a cause of rickets because the "worst case of rickets I ever saw was in a baby fed on good breast-milk; and so fed for about a year." He claimed that "our bad cases of rickets [in New York City] all occur in people that come from tropical climates." He went on to say that "rickets does not develop during warm months. . . . My own feeling is that rickets is entirely a disease of bad air. It may be, perhaps, somewhat modified by feeding, but only secondarily." On the other hand, Joseph E. Winters (1848–1922)[93] just as emphatically declared that "the sole etiologic factor of rickets in infants and young animals is wrong food. Malhygiene never causes rickets when feeding is correct."

There was still a third school that leaned toward the possible role of syphilis as a factor in the cause of rickets. For example, Jacobi[38] wrote in 1896: "Thus there are a great many cases of early rhachitis [Jacobi preferred *rhachitis* to *rickets*] which are due to the influence of mitigated syphilis in the parents. Indeed, some of the microscopical bone-lesions of the two diseases, as they are met with in the newlyborn, are difficult to distinguish from each other. Such cases can be greatly benefited by an antisyphilitic (mercurial) treatment which must be continued through a period of many months."

Jacobi was, of course, in error in this instance, but many others also believed that syphilis was an important etiological factor in rickets. Bernard J. A. Marfan (1858–1942), for example, had believed that there was a syphilitic type of rickets, characterized by marked precocity of the symptoms, exceptional involvement of the cranial bones, anemia, and splenomegaly.

Alfred F. Hess (1875–1933)[32] wrote that "rickets is the most common nutritional disease occurring among the children of the temperate zone. Fully three-fourths of the infants in the great cities, such as New York, show rachitic signs of some degree."

TREATMENT. Although cod-liver oil had been recommended for the treatment of rickets by John Bennett (1812–1875),[5] of Edinburgh, in 1841, for some reason it fell into disuse in America during the latter part of the nineteenth century despite its efficacy in treating rickets as documented by such reputable and well-known American pediatricians as A. V. Meigs, Starr, Holt, and Koplik. As the nineteenth century was ending, several American and English pediatricians and pharmacologists wrote that cod-liver oil was of little or no use in the treatment of rickets and that its only value was that it supplied an easily digested and assimilated fat.

Scurvy

The first American description of cases of infantile scurvy was presented to the American Pediatric Society in 1891 by Northrup,[56] a physician to the New York Foundling Hospital. He had collected a small series of eleven cases of infantile scurvy over a period of about three years, although he saw thousands of children each year. Here, as later, much of the blame for the disorder was placed on the use of proprietary foods as a positive factor, while the negative factor—a deficiency of antiscorbutic substance in the diet—was underemphasized. Nevertheless, it was clear enough to Northrup that oranges rapidly cured the disease. A dramatic example is given in the first case he reported.

The diagnosis of this case is scorbutus; what confirmation of this diagnosis can be offered? The answer is, the success in treatment. The child was removed at once to the country, its proprietary mixture was stopped and in its place were given fresh cow's milk, expressed juice of beef, baked potatoes, also citrate of iron with excess of citric acid. The one thing which this scurvy case seemed to crave, for which it reached out, which it seized with ravenous avidity, was the *orange*. The child could hardly be restrained till it held the fruit in its grasp; and then proceeded to souse its lips and nose in the juice. Improvement began at once; in five days its gums were markedly better, in ten entirely normal.

Being suspicious that scurvy might occur occasionally in general practice, Northrup began to look for additional cases. By 1894 he had collected over a hundred cases of infantile scurvy reported in the world literature up to that time.[56]

PROPRIETARY INFANT FOODS AND SCURVY. Most students of infantile scurvy in the late 1890's had commented on the large numbers of cases reported in the United States and in England. This was attributed, as Sir Thomas Barlow (1845–1945)[3] had already suggested, to the widespread use of proprietary foods and the reluctance of well-to-do mothers in these two countries to breast-feed their infants. Most "pediatrists" of the period held that scurvy in infants and children was caused by the use of artificially prepared foods and boiled milk, and the lack of fresh food in the infant's diet. The almost complete absence of scurvy in breast-fed infants tended to confirm their belief. Furthermore, they found that when these same infants were weaned and given proprietary foods or condensed milk and water to the exclusion of fresh cow's milk, they developed scurvy.

Barlow in England and Northrup in the United States were convinced that children of the poor suffered less from scurvy than the children of the rich because, according to Barlow:[3] "Poor parents cannot afford to buy proprietary food which the rich parents buy, and the poor parents, even if they use condensed milk, give their children a mixed diet at a much earlier period." "Poverty," according to Clifford G. Grulee (1880–1962),[30] writing in 1923, "makes rickets; wealth unwisely used makes scurvy."

At the sixth meeting of the American Pediatric Society, held in 1894, Fruitnight[26] presented seven cases of infantile scurvy he had observed in his practice. He also raised a hotly debated issue: "Has scurvy ever occurred in breast-fed infants?" Many claimed that breast milk afforded protection against scurvy but he dissented: "This is an error, for if as in one of my cases, lactation be too prolonged, the natural and progressive chemical changes in the mother's milk coincident with its aging may . . . conduce to the development of a scorbutic attack." Although Fruitnight was aware of the character and value of antiscorbutic foods, as were most pediatricians of his day, he had not reached the point of advising them for prophylactic purposes in the infant's normal diet. His conclusion makes this clear. "If there be any doubt of the diagnosis of a given case, recourse should be had to the therapeutic test of an antiscorbutic regimen, which will, by its results, in a comparatively short space of time, determine the question beyond cavil."

As Faber and McIntosh[22] have so aptly pointed out: "This is another example of the blame for infantile scurvy being placed by pediatricians of the day on artificial foods *per se*, rather than on a deficiency of antiscorbutic substance. The concept that a disease might be caused by something left out of the diet rather than by what was in the diet took a long time before it was accepted."

Infantile Scurvy and the American Pediatric Society (1898)

In 1898, the American Pediatric Society issued its *Collective Investigation on Infantile Scurvy in North America.*[22] This was a nationwide survey on the cause of infantile scurvy. By correspondence, accounts of 378 cases had been received from 138 observers, and this information was tabulated according to age, sex, season of onset, previous and concurrent illness, symptoms, dietary history, duration of the disease, and effects of treatment. Great stress was placed upon the role of proprietary foods —Mellin's Food, in particular—and the sterilization or pasteurization of milk. Strangely, although the use or nonuse of fruit juice was carefully recorded in relation to the cure of the disease, the kind of fruit juice was never specified. Further, although the data suggested that at least 80 percent of recoveries occurred when fruit juice was given, the significance of this received no comment.

The report indicated that scurvy was most apt to develop between the ages of seven and fourteen months, inclusive. Of the 378 cases, 83 percent occurred in private practice; this pointed to the greater tendency of the disease to occur among the rich or the well-to-do. The child's previous health was usually good and there was no proof that digestive disease itself bore any etiological relation to scurvy. Family history exerted little or no influence. However, the most important etiological factor, according to all but one of the physicians involved with this investigation, was a dietetic one. The committee paid particular attention to this point and found that in 214 of the 378 cases (57 percent) the children were fed on proprietary foods. This was the period of excessive use of such foods, often recommended by the physician. Pain on motion or handling was

present in 314; leg pains were reported in more than half the cases. The gums were diseased in 313, with sponginess being present in 249 of the cases. Cutaneous hemorrhages were reported in 182 cases. Rickets of varying degrees of severity occurred in 45 percent of the cases, but in the committee's opinion "there was no evidence that the association of rickets and scurvy was at all intimate."

The committee left the question of treatment up in the air:

Treatment—Not so much could be learned of the value of treatment as could be desired on account of the fact that in nearly all cases we have a combination of diet and of medicinal measures, including the use of fruit juices [the kinds are not mentioned], and it is impossible to determine absolutely which was the active curative agent.

The conclusions to be drawn from this combined study of etiology and treatment seem justifiable to the following extent:

(1) That the development of the disease follows in each case the prolonged employment of some diet unsuitable to the individual child, and that often a change of diet which at first thought would seem to be unsuitable may be followed by prompt recovery.

(2) That in spite of this fact regarding individual cases, the combined report of collected cases makes it probable that in these there were certain forms of diet which were particularly prone to be followed by the development of scurvy. First in point of numbers here are to be mentioned the various proprietary foods.

(3) In fine, that in general the cases reported seem to indicate that the farther food is removed in character from the natural food of a child the more likely its use is to be followed by the development of scurvy.

Caillé[22] issued a minority report:

(1) From a study of this report and from due consideration of other known facts, scurvy appears to be a chronic ptomaine poisoning due to the absorption of toxins.

(2) It follows the prolonged use of improper food and abnormal intestinal fermentation is a predisposing factor.

(3) Sterilizing, pasteurizing, or cooking of milk food is not *per se* responsible for the scurvy condition.

(4) A change of food and the administration of fruit juice and treatment of any underlying cause is the rational therapeutic procedure in scurvy.

The majority report was adopted by a vote of 18 to 1.

Discussion centered about the question of

whether sterilization of milk favored the development of scurvy. Edward M. Buckingham (c.1850–1916)[22] emphatically remarked: "For my own part, I believe that sterilization produces scurvy, and the only reason it does not do so oftener is because of the imperfect way milk is sterilized. A great deal of milk masquerades under the name sterilized milk that is not sterilized." His view was hotly contested but, as Faber and McIntosh[22] appropriately commented, "with arguments that today seem without merit."

American Pediatric Texts (1850–1900)

Job Lewis Smith (1869)

Smith's *Treatise on the Diseases of Infancy and Childhood,* published in 1869, passed through eight editions in the next twenty-seven years. With scarcely an exception, medical schools throughout the United States adopted it as a textbook until the late 1890's. It was a masterful publication dealing with the diseases of children in their entirety and as a specialty; even today it can be read with profit because its shrewd observations of disease were drawn entirely from personal experience balanced with the author's intimate contact with the scientific literature of his day. The eight editions were not just reprints; each followed faithfully but critically the essential changes in pediatric opinion.

By comparing the first edition of 1869 with the eighth and last edition of 1896, one can appreciate the dramatic changes in pediatrics during those years. The first edition contained the first American record of thermometry as applied to children. Throughout each edition Smith remained true to the pledge he had made in the first edition of depending much more for the material in his book on "his own clinical observations and the inspection of the cadaver than on the writings and opinions of others."

The effect of maternal emotions on the development of the fetus was not completely rejected by Smith, who conceded that "the multitude of facts which have accumulated justify the belief that deformity or other abnormal development of the foetus is, sometimes, due to the emotions of the mother." He cited these two cases:

It is the popular belief, and the belief of many physicians, that vivid mental impressions sometimes have a direct effect on the development of the foetus. Many cases are on record in which infants were born with marks or deformities, corresponding in character with the objects which had been seen and had made a strong impression on the maternal mind at some period of gestation.... I have met the following cases. An Irish woman of strong emotions and superstitious was passing along a street in the first months of her gestation, when she was accosted by a beggar, who raised her hand, destitute of thumb and fingers, and in "God's name" asked for alms. The woman passed on: but reflecting in whose name money was asked, felt that she had committed a great sin in refusing assistance. She returned to the place where she had met the beggar, and on different days, but never afterwards saw her. Harrassed by the thought of her imaginary sin, so that for weeks, according to her statement, she was made wretched by it, she approached her confinement. A female infant was born, otherwise perfect, but lacking the fingers and thumb of one hand. The deformed limb was on the same side, and seemed to the mother to resemble precisely that of the beggar.

In May 1868, I removed a supernumerary thumb from an infant whose mother, a baker's wife, gave me the following history: No one of the family, and no ancestor, to her knowledge, presented this deformity. In the early months of her gestation she sold bread from the counter, and nearly every day a child with double thumb came in for a penny roll, presenting the penny between the thumb and the finger. After the third month she left the bakery, but the malformation was so impressed upon her mind that she was not surprised to see it reproduced in her infant.

A very strong argument in its support [the effect of maternal impressions on the fetus] is ... the popular opinion which dates back to the time of Jacob (Genesis XXX). An almost universal sentiment, running through centuries, is rarely wholly fallacious.

John M. Keating (1889)

John M. Keating (1852–1893), whose father was professor of obstetrics at the Jefferson Medical College, graduated from the University of Pennsylvania Medical School in 1873. His life was devoted to the task of making mothers and children healthy and happy through his practice and writings. Keating's most ambitious work was his editing of the *Cyclopaedia of the Diseases of Children, Medical and Surgical,* issued in 1889 as a massive four-volume treatise, totaling more than 4,500 pages; a later supplementary fifth volume edited by William A. Edwards (1860–

1933), published in 1899, contained an additional 1,368 pages. This was the first work of its kind published in the English language. Until the *Cyclopaedia* appeared there was no American pediatric publication in which was gathered the consensus of the leading English-speaking pediatricians.

The articles were written especially for the work by American, British, and Canadian authors. The editor wrote that "his object has been not only Medicine and Surgery of Pediatrics, but also all the specialties tributary to it, as well as all collateral subjects of interest and importance."

Keating successfully united in this massive single work a collection of more than a hundred monographs that expressed the views of most of the distinguished teachers of this country and Great Britain. His goal was to make his treatise of equal importance to the busy practitioner and to the student and teacher. It should be remembered that in 1889 the vast majority of sick children were treated by general practitioners and not by the very few (probably not more than thirty to forty) true specialists in pediatrics. All of these pediatricians were located in the large cities and nearly all of them saw adult patients as well as children.

The publication of this work demonstrated to the profession that American pediatrics was an emerging and vital field. It also showed European physicians that an American editor was confident enough to try to emulate the great sixteen-volume *Handbuch der Kinderkrankheiten*, edited by the German pediatrician Carl Gerhardt and published between 1877 and 1893.

Keating, like many of his generation, was not embarrassed to show a patriotic streak:

It is a matter of regret to us in this country that many of our practitioners enter upon their careers with but a meagre acquaintance with all that pertain to pediatrics. Fortunately, however, nature has endowed the American mind with energy, enthusiasm, penetratation and natural aptitude, and as a consequence we are enabled to point to a brilliant array of honored names, of those who have fought the battle single-handed in the conflict and struggle of an active and extended practice.

Louis Starr (1894)

Louis Starr was born in Philadelphia and received his M.D. in 1871 from the University of Penn-

sylvania (Fig. 5-6). In 1884 he became clinical professor of the diseases of children at the University of Pennsylvania. He first appeared in scientific literature in 1885 as an assistant to William Pepper, who was then editing the five-volume *A System of Practical Medicine* (1885–1886). Starr's most successful publication was *Hygiene of the Nursery* (1888), one of the first books on nursery care written for parents; his most ambitious was *An American Text-Book of the Diseases of Children by American Teachers* (1894), in two volumes totaling 1,190 pages. All of the sixty-three contributors were Americans; seventeen of the forty-three founding members of the American Pediatric Society contributed chapters.

Starr's object as editor was "to present a working text-book which shall be closely limited to, while completely covering, the field of pediatrics." He was aware that the average practitioner who bought his book would most often "read as he runs" and for that reason the chapters contained practical, useful information while "avoiding so far as possible, the

Figure 5–6. Louis Starr (1849–1925).

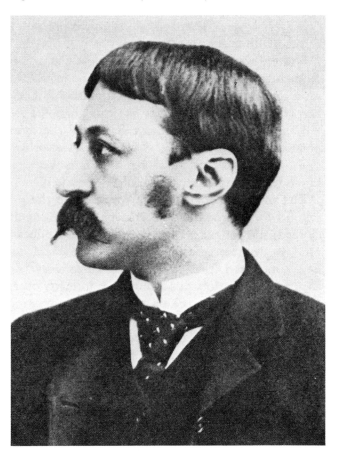

insertion of references to journals or authorities, of more interest to those engaged in research than to those in active practice."

One chapter, entitled *Sea-Air and Sea-Bathing and Convalescence,* noted that "the death rate among the resident population of a sea-coast town like Atlantic City was 12.5 per 1,000. This, according to the author, was the lowest mortality rate in an American city in the early 1890's. Sea air was thought to be particularly valuable in the treatment of children suffering from cholera infantum, asthma, rickets, Pott's disease, "rheumatic" cases, chorea, poliomyelitis, and almost all skin diseases.

Osler, then at Johns Hopkins University, wrote the chapter on tuberculosis, called then a diathetic disease. He accepted the ancient idea that there was a certain conformation of the body (diathesis) which rendered an individual more prone to tuberculosis. Hippocrates had written: "The form of body peculiar to phthisical complaints is the smooth, the whitish, that resembling the lentil, the reddish, the blue-eyed, the leuco-phlegmatic, and that with the scapulae having the appearance of wings." "In children," Osler[58] wrote, "it may be said that the build and type such as here described is certainly more prone to tuberculous affection."

Scarlet fever was described as the most widely disseminated of the exanthemata of childhood and "the most dreaded of all the diseases of children." Chilling of the surface of the body was thought to be the most likely cause of rheumatic fever and the most potent predisposing cause of rheumatic fever was said to be hereditary. Malaria and syphilis were believed to have a predisposing influence on leukemia.

The treatment for cretinism was to keep the patient in a warm room or hot atmosphere, thoroughly clothed; the patient was to be treated with pilocarpine, or the tincture of jaborandi. The bromides were considered "the surest remedy for epilepsy." In the treatment of lobar pneumonia, as in many other febrile illnesses, tincture of aconite in combination with the solution of ammonium acetate or with sweet spirits of nitre was recommended to control the temperature and "to quiet excessive action of the heart." Also, in lobar pneumonia, brandy or whiskey were to be used in liberal quantity. To "support the heart" in cases of pneumonia, digitalis was unquestioningly considered the most reliable remedy. During an attack of pneumonia the child's "general systemic tone" was to be maintained by the use of quinine in suppositories, to which asafetida was added if nervous symptoms should become pronounced.

Thomas Morgan Rotch (1895)

Rotch, in his *Pediatrics,* published in 1895, not only made a new departure by writing in the first person but also demonstrated that in his hands the method was forceful and well adapted to a textbook. Each chapter is called a lecture, and in reading it one can get the flavor of Rotch's lecture style.

In the preface he wrote:

The book begins with a consideration of the infant at birth, and follows it through its various stages of development up to puberty. After dwelling rather more at length on normal development than is usual in works on pediatrics, the abnormal conditions are discussed. Beginning with the diseases which would naturally be met with in the early periods of life, and devoting considerable space to my observations on the blood of infants and of young children, the diseases of the different organs are then considered.

With the exception of a few rare diseases, the illustrations represented actual cases theretofore unpublished by Rotch. The colored illustrations received his closest attention, and the patients were seen personally with the artist present, so as to insure accuracy.

The establishment of milk laboratories, almost entirely through Rotch's efforts, was properly viewed as one of the great advances in preventive medicine, adding "another dimension to the scientific feeding of infants." Rotch believed that the medical treatment of the various abnormal conditions arising in infants would in the future be largely dietetic rather than by means of drugs. For this reason he gave unusual prominence to infant feeding and to an explanation of the percentage method of infant feeding (132 pages).

Rotch's textbook went through five editions between 1895 and 1906 and was reissued in two volumes with major changes in 1917 by Charles Hunter Dunn (1875–1926), one of Rotch's former students.

Luther Emmett Holt (1897)

L. Emmett Holt published *The Diseases of Infancy and Childhood* in 1897. His book is considered by many an American classic and has been said to have done for pediatrics what Osler's *The Principles and Practice of Medicine* (1892) had done for internal medicine. During Holt's lifetime, his textbook ran through eleven editions and was translated into several languages including Chinese; his book was recognized at once in this country as the standard text on pediatrics. But in contrast to Osler's book, which was enlivened by a vivid writing style and frequent allusions to medical history and literature, Holt's text sacrificed everything not essential for objectivity and the logical orderly presentation of facts in all their bareness.

Edwards A. Park (1877–1969)[59] years later wrote:

"Holt" was essentially a manual for medical students, though on the shelves of every general practitioner in the country.... When struck with some rare disease or unusual manifestation, we young doctors did not get much help from "Holt." But the work was a monument, and its importance can scarcely be estimated. It lifted child illness and care out of chaos and defined and brought it all together as Pediatrics.... In concise form it furnished for the first time in any language a clear, well-balanced, complete exposition of the child in health and disease and of the principles of care.

Holt included rickets and scurvy under the rubric of "food diseases." The specific infections were placed last and more than a fifth of the book was devoted to them. The importance of diphtheria and scarlet fever at the time is evident from the more than fifty pages devoted to the former and thirty pages to the latter disease. Tuberculosis occupied thirty-six pages. The last two chapters were allotted to rheumatism and diabetes mellitus, only six pages for the former and one and a half to the latter.

Even more widely read and appreciated than Holt's textbook was his *The Care and Feeding of Children* (1895) written especially for parents. The booklet, now probably totally unknown to young practitioners, was a masterpiece of clear, incisive writing and was full of sparkling facts. The Grolier Club of America's 1946 list of the one hundred books that most influenced the life and culture of American people included Holt's *The Care and Feeding of Children* in company with such older American classics as Stowe's *Uncle Tom's Cabin*, Hawthorne's *The Scarlet Letter*, Whitman's *Leaves of Grass*, and Franklin's *Poor Richard's Almanac*.[59]

American Pediatric Journals (1850–1900)

The American Journal of Obstetrics and Diseases of Women and Children was first issued in May, 1868, and from the beginning it included articles on pediatric topics. This was the first American medical journal to include a special section for papers about children's diseases. The first of these was written by Jacobi on the pathology and treatment of the different forms of croup. The second pediatric paper, also published in the first issue, was a case report of diabetes in an infant and contained this description of how the observant mother made a brilliant clinical diagnosis: "The mother's attention was attracted to some white spots on the carpet, where a few drops of the child's urine had chanced to fall and impelled by some feeling of curiosity wet her finger, touched it to one of the spots, and tasting it, found it to be sweet. This circumstance was at once communicated to me and led to an immediate examination of the urine, which was found to be of high specific gravity and very saccharine."

The journal also contained the first study published in America of the normal temperature of infants and children by James Finlayson (1840–1906), of Manchester, England.

The Archives of Pediatrics, the first American journal entirely devoted to pediatrics, was edited from 1884 until 1893 by William P. Watson (1854–1925). It began publication in January, 1884, and continued until September, 1962, when it merged with the *American Practitioner* and the *Quarterly Review of Pediatrics* to appear under the new name of *Clinical Pediatrics*.

The first paper published in the first issue was on convulsions in children. The paper was filled with practical hints about how the young physician should evoke order from chaos when he made a house call to see a convulsing child. The secret was to keep everyone busy in preparing a warm bath, moving the patient to a larger bedroom, removing his clothing, wrapping him in a flannel blanket, and looking for mustard to put in the hot bathwater. By the time all these had been done the convulsion would probably have abated.

The *Transactions of the American Pediatric Society,* begun in 1889, was published in hardcover from 1889 to 1923, and in paperback from 1924 to the society's fiftieth anniversary in 1938. The first paper published in the *Transactions* was Jacobi's presidential address, entitled "The Relations of Pediatrics to General Medicine," in which he emphasized at considerable length the responsibility of the pediatrician to preventive medicine. As an example of this responsibility, he noted that "ninety-nine cases out of every hundred cases of rhachitis need not exist."

Pediatrics, the fourth and last nineteenth-century American pediatric journal, owned by Dillon Brown and edited initially by George Carpenter (1859–1910), of London, England, began publication in New York City in January, 1896, and continued until 1913. The first article in the first issue was a review of infant feeding by Jacobi. In it Jacobi somewhat irreverently takes Rotch to task for the "axiomatic positiveness of his assertions" about infant feeding.

As the nineteenth century ended, American pediatrics had finally been elevated from its ancillary status as a "dependent dwarf" of ordinary medical practice. The period from 1850 until 1900 witnessed not only the coining of the word *pediatrics* but also the creation of the basic discipline of that specialty, as we know it today.

Heroic therapy of sick children by bleeding, blistering, purging, and vomiting followed by dosing them with mercury, antimony, and polypharmaceutical prescriptions slowly gave way to simpler and more rational therapeutic measures.

As the twentieth century dawned, the emerging specialty of pediatrics was blessed with a handful of brilliant practitioners imbued with a zeal to foster the practice of scientific medicine and ready to jettison the dogmatism that characterized so much of the medical practice of most of the nineteenth century. Through the teaching and example of these practitioners, American pediatrics would soon obtain worldwide recognition and respect.

References

1. Abt, I. A.   A survey of pediatrics during the past 100 years. *Illinous Med. J.* 77:485, 1940.

2. Adams, S. S.   The evolution of pediatric literature in the United States. *Trans. Am. Pediatr. Soc.* 9:5, 1897.

3. Barlow, T.   On cases described as "acute rickets" which are probably a combination of scurvy and rickets, the scurvy being an essential, and the rickets a variable, element. *Med. Chir. Trans.* 66:159, 1883.

4. Bauer, L.   *Lectures on Orthopaedic Surgery.* Philadelphia: Linsay & Blakiston, 1864.

5. Bennett, J. H.   *Treatise on the Oleum Jecoris Aselli, or Cod Liver Oil.* Edinburgh: Maclachlan, Stewart, 1841.

6. Bettman, O. L.   *The Good Old Days—They Were Terrible!* New York: Random House, 1974.

7. Bolduan, C. F.   The public health of New York City: A retrospect. *Bull. N.Y. Acad. Med.* 19:423, 1943.

8. Booker, W. D.   The early history of the summer diarrhea of infants. *Trans. Am. Pediatr. Soc.* 13.7, 1901.

9. Bovaird, D.   Intubation. In W. A. Edwards (ed.), *Diseases of Children; Medical and Surgical: A Supplement to Keating's "Cyclopaedia of the Diseases of Children."* Philadelphia: Lippincott, 1901.

10. Brieger, G. H.   *Medical American in the Nineteenth Century.* Baltimore: Johns Hopkins Press, 1972.

11. Brothers, A.   Mortality in Early Life. In W. A. Edwards (ed.), *Disease of Children, Medical and Surgical: A Supplement to Keating's "Cyclopaedia of the Diseases of Children."* Philadelphia: Lippincott, 1901.

12. Brown, D.   The construction of O'Dwyer tubes with a report of three hundred and fifty cases of intubation of the larynx. *Trans. Am. Pediatr. Soc.* 2:182, 1890.

13. Caillé, A.   Tapping the vertebral canal: Local treatment for tubercular meningitis. *Trans. Am. Pediatr. Soc.* 8:76, 1896.

14. Chapin H. D.   Hereditary Syphilis. In L. Starr (ed.), *An American Text-Book of the Diseases of Children.* London: F. J. Rebman, 1895.

15. Crandall, F. M.   Scarlet Fever and Measles. In W. A. Edwards (ed.), *Diseases of Children, Medical and Surgical: A Supplement to Keating's "Cyclopaedia of the Diseases of Children."* Philadelphia: Lippincott, 1901.

16. Creighton, C.   *A History of Epidemics in Britain* (2 vols.). Cambridge: Cambridge University Press, 1891–1894.

17. Cushing, H.   *Life of Sir William Osler* (4th ed.) Oxford: Clarendon Press, 1926.

18. Dowling, H. E.   *Fighting Infection.* Cambridge, Mass.: Harvard University Press, 1977.

19. Duffy, J.   *A History of Public Health in New York City 1866–1966.* New York: Russell Sage Foundation, 1974.

20. Eliot, E.   Memorial of Job Lewis Smith. *Trans. N.Y. Acad. Med. (2nd ser.).* 13:220, 1897.

21. *Faber, H. K.* Job Lewis Smith, forgotten pioneer. *J. Pediatr.* 63:794, 1963.
22. Faber, H. K., and McIntosh, R. *History of the American Pediatric Society.* New York: McGraw-Hill, 1966.
23. Flexner, S., and Jobling, J. W. An analysis of four hundred cases of epidemic meningitis treated with the antimeningitis serum. *Trans. Am. Pediatr. Soc.* 20:17, 1908.
24. Freeman, R. G. The etiology of rickets. *Trans. Am. Pediatr. Soc.* 15:173, 1903.
25. Fruitnight, J. H. The treatment of rachitis with the lactophosphate of lime. *Trans. Am. Pediatr. Soc.* 5:168, 1893.
26. Fruitnight, J. H. Infantile scurvy, especially its differential diagnosis. *Trans. Am. Pediatr. Soc.* 6:10, 1894.
27. Gale, A. H. *Epidemic Diseases.* London: Penguin Books, 1959.
28. Garrison, F. H. History of Pediatrics: In I. A. Abt (ed.), *Pediatrics*, vol. I. Philadelphia: Saunders, 1923–1926.
29. Griffith, J. P. C. Whooping-cough. In L. Starr (ed.), *An American Text-Book of the Diseases of Children*, vol. I. London: F. J. Rebman, 1895.
30. Grulee, C. G. *Treatise on Infant Feeding* (4th ed.). Philadelphia: Saunders, 1923.
31. Haven, M. C. The etiology of rachitis. *Boston Med. Surg. J.* 114:27, 1886.
32. Hess, A. F. *Rickets, Including Osteomalacia and Tetany.* Philadelphia: Lea & Febiger, 1929.
33. Holt, L. E. *The Diseases of Infancy and Childhood.* New York, Appleton, 1897.
34. Holt, L. E. Scope and limitations of hospitals for infants. *Trans. Am. Pediatr. Soc.* 10:147, 1898.
35. Holt, L. E. Infant mortality ancient and modern. An historical sketch. *Arch. Pediatr.* 30:885, 1913.
36. Holt, L. E., and Howland, J. *The Diseases of Infancy and Childhood* (7th ed.). New York: Appleton, 1917.
37. Jackson, J. On the causes of cholera infantum. *New Engl. J. Med. Surg.* 1:113, 1812.
38. Jacobi, A. *Therapeutics of Infancy and Childhood.* Philadelphia: Lippincott, 1896.
39. Jacobi, A. The history of cerebral and spinal meningitis. *Trans. Med. Soc. State of N.Y.* 1905.
40. Jacobi, A. Diphtheria: Symptomatology and Treatment. In W. J. Robinson (ed.), *Collectanea Jacobi*, vol. 1. New York: Critic and Guide Co., 1909.
41. Jacobi, A. Preface. In W. J. Robinson (ed.), *Collectanea Jacobi*, vol. 1. New York: Critic and Guide Co., 1909.
42. Jacobi, A. The history of pediatrics in New York. *Arch. Pediatr.* 34:1, 1917.
43. Jenner, W. Lectures on rickets. *Med. Times Gaz.* (Lond.) 1:259, 333, 415, 465, 1860.
44. Jennings, C. G. The frequency and early symptoms of rickets. *Med. Age* (Detroit) 3:241, 1885.
45. Kassowitz, M. Ueber Vererbung und Uebertragung der Syphilis. *Jahrb. J. Kinderheilkd.* 21:52, 1884.
46. Kerley, C. G. A study of 555 cases of summer diarrhea among the out-patient poor. *Trans. Am. Pediatr. Soc.* 13:36, 1901.
47. Klein, E. E. Etiology of scarlet fever. *Notices Proc. Roy. Instn. G. B.* 12:150, 1887.
48. Koch, R. Weitere Mittheilungen ueber ein Heilmittel gegen Tuberkulose. *Dtsch. Med. Wochenschr.* 16:1029, 1890, 17:101, 1189, 1891.
49. LaFétra, L. E. The development of pediatrics in New York City. *Arch Pediatr.* 49:36, 1932.
50. Landsberger, M. Some pediatric milestones of the 19th century. *Am. J. Dis. Child.* 108:205, 1964.
51. Logan, G., Jr. *Practical Observations on Diseases of Children.* Charleston S.C.: A. E. Miller, 1825.
52. Lowell, A. M., Edwards, L. B., and Palmer, C. E. *Tuberculosis.* Cambridge, Mass.: Harvard University Press, 1969.
53. Meigs, C. D. On cholera infantum. *Am. Med. Recorder* (Phila.) 3:498, 1820.
54. Morse, J. L. The frequency of rickets in infancy in Boston and vicinity. *Boston Med. Surg. J.* 140:163, 1899.
55. Morse, J. L. The history of pediatrics in Massachusetts. *New Engl. J. Med.* 205:169, 1931.
56. Northrup, W. P. Scorbutus in infants. *Arch. Pediatr.* 9:1, 1892.
57. O'Dwyer, J. Intubation of the larynx. *N.Y. Med. J.* 42:145, 1885.
58. Osler, W. Tuberculosis. In L. Starr (ed.), *An American Text-Book of the Diseases of Children.* London: F. J. Rebman, 1895.
59. Park, E. A., and Mason, H. H. Luther Emmett Holt. In B. S. Veeder (ed.), *Pediatric Profiles.* St. Louis: Mosby, 1957.
60. Parry, J. S. Observations on the frequency and symptoms of rachitis with the results of the author's clinical experience. *Am. J. Med. Sci.* (n.s.) 63:17, 1872.
61. Pope, A. S. Studies on the epidemiology of scarlet fever. *Am. J. Hyg.* 6:389, 1926.
62. Portier, P., and Richet, C. R. De l'action anaphylactique de certains venins. *C. R. Soc. Biol.* (Paris) 54:170, 1902.
63. Prudden, T. M. On the etiology of diphtheria: An experimental study. *Am. J. Med. Sci.* 97:329, 1889.
64. Quincke, H. I. Die Lumbalpunction des Hydrocephalus. *Berl. Klin. Wochenschr.* 28:929, 965, 1891.

65. Ramon, G. L. L'anatoxine diphtérique: ses propri-étés, ses applications. *Ann. Inst. Pasteur* 42:959, 1928.

66. Reese, D. M. Report on infant mortality in large cities, the sources of its increase, and means of its diminution. *Trans. Am. Med. Assoc.* 10:93, 1857.

67. Reports of the Sanitary Association of the City of New York, 1859.

68. Rosen G. Acute Communicable Diseases. In W. R. Bett (ed.), *The History and Conquest of Common Diseases*. Norman: University of Oklahoma Press, 1954.

69. Rotch, T. M. *Pediatrics*. Philadelphia: Lippincott, 1895.

70. Rush, B. An inquiry into the case and cure of the cholera infantum. *Med. Inq. & Obs.* (2nd ed.). Philadelphia: J. Conrad, 1805.

71. Seibert, A. Further report on sub-membranous local treatment of pharyngeal diphtheria. *Trans. Am. Pediatr. Soc.* 3:155, 1892.

72. Shakespeare, E. O. Cholera Asiatica. In L. Starr (ed.), *An American Text-Book of the Diseases of Children*, vol. 1. London: F. J. Rebman, 1895.

73. Shattuck, L. On the vital statistics of Boston. *Am. J. Med. Sci.* (n.s.) 1:369, 1841.

74. Shryock, R. H. *Medicine in America*. Baltimore: Johns Hopkins Press, 1966.

75. Smillie, W. G. The Periods of Great Epidemics in the United States. In F. H. Top (ed.), *The History of American Epidemiology*. St. Louis: Mosby, 1952.

76. Smith, J. L. *A Treatise on the Diseases of Infancy and Childhood* (2nd ed.). Philadelphia: Henry C. Lea, 1872.

77. Smith, J. L. *A Treatise on the Diseases of Children* (7th ed.). Philadelphia: Henry C. Lea, 1890.

78. Smith, T. A comparative study of bovine tubercle bacilli and of human bacilli from a sputum. *J. Exp. Med.* 3:451, 1898.

79. Snow, I. M. An explanation of the great frequency of rickets among Neapolitan children in American cities. *Arch. Pediatr.* 12:18, 1895.

80. Starr, L. Measles. In L. Starr (ed.), *An American Text-Book of the Diseases of Children*, vol. 1. London: F. J. Rebman, 1895.

81. Sydenstricker, E. *Health and Environment*. New York: McGraw-Hill, 1933.

82. Trudeau, E. L. Animal experimentation and tuberculosis. *J.A.M.A.* 54:22, 1910.

83. Upshur, J. N. The diarrheal diseases. In W. A. Edwards (ed.), *Diseases of Children, Medical and Surgical: A Supplement to Keating's "Cyclopaedia of the Diseases of Children."* Philadelphia: Lippincott, 1901.

84. Vaughan, V. C. Toxins and antitoxins. In J. M. Keating (ed.), *Cyclopaedia of the Diseases of Children*, vol. 5. Philadelphia: Lippincott, 1889.

85. Vaughan, V. C. Diarrhoeal Diseases. In L. Starr (ed.), *An American Text-Book of the Diseases of Children*, vol. 1. London: F. J. Rebman, 1895.

86. Vieusseux, G. Mémoire sur la maladie qui a régné à Genève au printemps de 1805. *J. Méd. Chir. Pharm.* 11:163, 1805.

87. Von Pirquet, C. The relation of tuberculosis to infant mortality in prevention of infant mortality. *Am. Acad. Med. Conf.*, 1909.

88. Waxham, F. E. Measles. In J. Keating (ed.), *Cyclopaedia of the Diseases of Children, Medical and Surgical*, vol. 1. Philadelphia: Lippincott, 1889.

89. Webster, H. *A Brief History of Epidemic and Pestiential Diseases* (2 vols.). Hartford: Hudson & Goodwin, 1799.

90. Wentworth, A. H. Tapping the vertebral canal. *Boston Med. Sug. J.* 133:591, 1895.

91. Wheatley, G. M. Brief history of pediatrics in New York. *N.Y. State J. Med.* 76:1197, 1976.

92. Winslow, C-E. A. *The Life of Hermann. M. Biggs*. Philadelphia, Lea & Febiger, 1929.

93. Winters, J. E. The pathogenesis and prophylaxis of rickets. *Trans. Am. Pediatr. Soc.* 26:267, 1914.

94. Wishnow, R. M., and Steinfeld, J. L. The conquest of the major infectious diseases in the United States: A bicentennial retrospect. *Ann. Rev. Microbiol.* 30:427–450, 1976.

Infant Feeding of Paramount Concern 6

Physicians' understanding of the proper composition of diet {in the nineteenth century} was as deplorably defective as was their comprehension of public hygiene. So little solid knowledge, based on scientific observations, existed that those in authority made up their own varying rules, few of proved correctness and some with highly dangerous defects.

Harold K. Faber and Rustin McIntosh (1966)

A doleful fact of nineteenth-century pediatrics was that the first years of a child's life were by far the most treacherous. Most of the deaths were attributed to improper bottle-feeding. To learn how to overcome this formidable cause of infant mortality became the prime mission of pediatrics for the six decades between 1870 and 1930. It was not until the very end of the nineteenth century that a dent was made in the empiricism and dogmatism that had dominated the feeding of infants for almost the entire century.

As the nineteenth century ended, the infant mortality rate in New York City had fallen from a rate of 288 per 1,000 live-born infants in 1880 to 189 per 1,000 in 1900. The overall infant mortality rate for the whole country was 165 per 1,000 in 1900, with a low of 147 per 1,000 for Chicago and a high of 311 per 1,000 for Biddeford, Maine.[3] Those concerned with the welfare of infants all agreed that these figures were far too high and their reduction would primarily come about through placing bottle-feeding on a scientific basis.

Throughout almost the entire nineteenth century pessimistic opinions about the fate of bottle-fed infants prevailed; many nineteenth-century reports indicated that among infants who were not breast-fed, as many as 80 to 90 percent died. Breast-feeding, either by the infant's mother or by a wet-nurse, was thus almost a life-or-death proposition for the infant almost until the present century. For example, at the New York Infant Asylum when bottle-feeding was practiced in 1886, the deaths kept pace with the admissions; while in the New York Foundling Asylum bottle-fed infants were kept by themselves in a room known as the ward of the dying babies.[23] In the foundling home located on Randall's Island in New York City only one bottle-fed infant admitted to the hospital in a period of a year and a half had reached the age of one year.

Advocacy of Breast-Feeding

The advantages of breast-feeding were correctly extolled during the nineteenth century because of the very real dangers to the infant of artificial food. Breast-feeding had the force of Biblical injunction and almost as late as the middle of the nineteenth century women were told from the pulpit that it was their duty to nurse their own infants. But in this country, as well as in Victorian England, there were many mothers, especially those in fashion, who either could not or would not do so. The Victorian novelist Anthony Trollope (1815–1882)[11] made this point tellingly in his *Doctor Thorne* (1858), the fourth of the Barsetshire novels: "Of course Lady Arabella could not suckle the young heir herself. Ladies Arabella never can. They're gifted with the powers of being mothers, but not nursing-mothers. Nature gives them bosoms for show, but not for use." Lady Arabella, of course, hired a wet nurse as would have her American counterpart if she was wealthy and lucky enough to find the right one.

Nineteenth-Century Rules for the Selection of a Wet Nurse

In the nineteenth century there were elaborate criteria for the selection of a wet nurse. American writers, like William Potts Dewees,[10] advised:

She should neither be too young nor too old; as, before she is twenty, she has not arrived at her full development; and, after thirty-five, she is upon the decline. She should be fresh-coloured; have fine teeth, red lips, and sweet breath; her hair should not be too black nor too deep a red, nor should [she] be subject to any violent passion. Her breast should be of moderate size, with a nipple sufficiently projecting and irritable, and yielding milk upon the slightest force; her milk should neither be too thick nor too transparent and of an agreeable sweet taste. Added to these, she should have proper moral feelings, to second such qualities. Nor should these good qualities be debased by bad passions or other defect of character. She should so regulate her diet as to be entirely subservient to the advantage of the child.

Importance of the Color of the Wet Nurse's Hair

The color of the wet nurse's hair was given importance by some medical writers, at least in the first half of the century, because they believed that temperament—as a reflection of hair color—influenced the quality of her milk. Charles H. F. Routh (1822–1909),[34] a prolific nineteenth-century English writer about infant feeding practices, felt that "the milk of a brunette is generally richer in solid constituents than that of a blonde; for which reason the former are preferred as wet nurses." He called attention to the analyses of the breast milk of a blonde and a brunette wet nurse made by L'Héritier in 1842 and quoted by Simon[36] (Table 6–1). Routh added that "these are extreme cases; but the average of solid constituents lies from 120 for a blonde to 130 for a brunette."

This was the era of temperaments which were supposedly associated with certain diatheses and anthropometric observations. Routh[34] also claimed that there was "yet another reason why a brunette is to be preferred to a blonde." Blondes were said to belong "to the sanguine or scrofulous tempera-

Table 6–1. Analyses of the Breast Milk of a Blond and a Brunette Wet Nurse, (Both Age Twenty-two).

Constituents	Blonde		Brunette	
	Sample 1	Sample 2	Sample 1	Sample 2
Water	892	881.5	853.3	853
Solid constituents				
Butter	35.5	40.5	54.8	56.0
Casein	10	9.5	16.2	17.0
Sugar of milk	58.5	64.0	71.2	70.0
Salts	4.0	4.5	4.5	4.0
Total	1,000.0	1,000.0	1,000.0	1,000.0

Source: J. F. Simon. *Mother's Milk and Its Chemical and Physiological Properties.* Berlin, 1838.

ment." He claimed that "a fair skin, with brilliant colour, light blue eyes, very light or red hair, are usually present in such cases." Such individuals were thought to have weak "digestive powers" as well as "an unusual irritable manner" as a frequent accompaniment. As a consequence of this sanguine and more passionate character, "the milk of blondes is very apt to become altered under mental excitement." In extreme cases, according to Routh, "the milk of blondes has been known to produce the death of the infants."

Red-haired women were also to be avoided, according to Dewees:[10] "There may be certain moral qualities that may unfit them for the office of nurse; they are certainly of a sanguine temperament, and this temperament has attached to it great irritability of temper as one of its characteristics—hence, in a moral point of view, their unfitness as protectors of young children."

Even the highly respected, scientifically oriented English physician Frederick W. Pavy (1829–1911),[30] a leading expert on diets and nutrition in the Victorian era, believed in the importance of the color of a nurse's hair: "The difference in temperament exerts its influence in maintaining a more steady condition in the one case than in the other. For example, the sanguine temperament, with its associated susceptible organization, belonging to the *blonde*, disposes to a greater liability of sudden alterations from mental causes than the phlegmatic temperament, with its less impressionable organization, of the brunette."

It was also believed that the wet nurse's milk could transmit her moral character to the infant. Milk was thought to determine not only health but also personality.

Another widely accepted belief was that the composition of breast milk might be qualitatively changed by mental impressions. Many nineteenth-century physicians, especially in the first half of that century, reported that infants had died suddenly in the act of nursing after the mother had been violently excited. In other cases convulsions were said to have occurred. For example, Caleb Ticknor (1805–1840)[39] in his *Guide for Mothers and Nurses* (1839) wrote:

The influence of the mind upon the body is well exemplified in the case of nursing women; the milk always becoming deranged and being rendered unfit for nutrition when the mind is any way disturbed. There are frequent instances of infants being seized with convulsions after sucking an enraged nurse; and cases are not wanting where they have been destroyed by violent inflammations from the same cause. An infant of a year old, while he sucked milk from an enraged mother, on a sudden was seized with a fatal bleeding, and died; and infants at the breast in a short time pine away if the nurse be affected with grievous care.

Artificially Fed Infants

William Buchan[6] early in the century warned:

Nothing can shew the disposition which mankind have to depart from nature more than their endeavouring to bring up children without the breast. The mother's milk, or that of a healthy nurse, is unquestionably the best food for an infant. Neither art nor nature can afford a proper substitute for it. Children may seem to thrive for a few months without the breast; but when teething, the smallpox, and other diseases incident to childhood, come on, they generally perish.

And toward the century's end, Job Lewis Smith[37] was no less pessimistic about the fate of artificially fed infants than Buchan had been almost a century earlier:

In the large cities, if I may judge from our New York experience, this mode of alimentation [artificial feeding] for young infants should always be discouraged. It generally ends in death, preceded by evidences of faulty nutrition. A considerable proportion of those nourished in this manner thrive during the cool months, but on the approach of the warm season they are the first to be affected with diarrhoea and other symptoms indicating derangement of the digestive function. In my opinion, based on a pretty extended observation, more than half of the New York spoon-fed infants, who entered the summer months, died before the return of cool weather, unless saved by removal to the country.

All authors are agreed that human milk is not only the best, but one might say the only safe food for infants. The evidence adduced by Dr. [Samuel] Merriman [a nineteenth-century English physician] against dry-nursing is perfectly conclusive. He says: "It has been part of my duty to endeavour to ascertain the amount of mortality among infants from this source, and, after much careful inquiry and investigation, I am convinced that the attempt to bring up children by hand proves fatal *in London* to at least seven out of eight of these miserable sufferers; and this happens whether the child has never taken the breast at all, or, having been suckled for three to four weeks only, is then weaned. *In the country*, the mortality among dry-nursed children is not quite so great as in London, but it is abundantly greater than is generally imagined."

Early Steps in Scientific Milk Modification for Bottle-Fed Infants

Dewees,[10] like all other writers of his day, extolled the value of breast milk, and it was his opinion that "it does not happen once in a hundred times that the mother is not in every respect, competent to this end." He recommended in those rare cases where breast milk was inadequate that a "complementary feeding of cow's milk be used. The feeding should begin with two-thirds milk, one-third water, and a small quantity of loaf sugar." This formula, with only slight modification, agrees with modern pediatric practice. He was particularly critical of the "reprehensible habit" of the nurse in letting the child's food first pass through her mouth. He was also opposed to spoon-feeding and recommended the use of a bottle; he emphasized, however, that the bottle must be kept scrupulously clean and must be washed in warm water before being used again. If a bottle was given, he advised against giving too much at a time, and he preferred offering the infant small quantities at shorter intervals. After the humble beginning in infant feeding made by C. D. and J. F. Meigs, father and son,[22] of Philadelphia, in the middle of the nineteenth century, there followed many foreign investigators during the second half of the century, notably Philipp Biedert, Adalbert Czerny, Arthur Schlossmann (1867–1932), Heinrich Finkelstein (1865–1942), Max Rubner (1854–1932), Theodor Escherich (1857–1911), Otto Heubner, Wilhelm Camerer (1842–1910), and their contemporaries. The first step for all these investigators to take was a careful comparative analysis of mother's milk and cow's milk. Meigs advised the use of cow's milk if breast-feeding was not possible, adding that the chemical composition of artifical food might more nearly approximate mother's milk if water was added to cow's milk together with sugar and cream. And he wrote that "in a larger institution, the simpler the solution, the safer it will be." He believed in

long intervals between feeding and was opposed to feeding children at night after the eighth month.

It is important to note that although we now have extensive, readily accessible quantitative data on the composition of human milk and cow's milk, this was not the case less than a century ago.

Biedert[5] is usually considered to be the originator of the scientific study of artifical infant feeding. In 1878 he described "fat diarrhea," having published in 1869 one of the first scientific treatises on infant nutrition. In it he included his observations that the protein content of cow's milk was approximately twice as high as that of human milk. Biedert also studied the effect of acid on the consistency of the curd and suggested that casein curds were responsible for digestive difficulties. He maintained that the casein of cow's milk was less digestible than that of human milk; he thus suggested that instead of cow's milk, a series of graduated mixtures of cow's milk, water, and milk sugar be used. Biedert's milk formula mixture was the parent of those that followed, such as Meigs's and Rotch's mixtures.

Carefully Performed Chemical Analyses of Human and Cow's Milk

Although a start had been made on milk analyses toward the end of the eighteenth century by Boyssou and by Luissio and Rondt,[40] the first carefully performed milk analyses were carried out by the German investigator Johann Franz Simon.[36] In 1838 he published his findings in his doctoral dissertation, written in Latin, which was highly praised by Biedert and the American pediatrician Arthur V. Meigs (1850–1912). Simon's studies may well be considered the first real landmark in the exact science of infant metabolism as a basis for rational infant nutrition. His studies passed unnoticed for about thirty years.

Simon scientifically analyzed and compared the constituents of human and cow's milk. His results showed that the casein in cow's milk amounted to 7.2 percent and in human milk to 3.4 percent. He found that cow's milk contained 2.8 percent sugar. It is obvious that his figures for protein were too high, and for sugar, too low. He included all protein, including the lacto-albumin, under the term casein. He did not miss the point, however, that cow's milk contains more casein than milk. On these and other chemical studies were based the concept of the harmfulness of various constituents of cow's milk and the many attempts to imitate human milk, as exemplified by numerous milk mixtures, now obsolete, and in the various cream and top-milk mixtures.

Bottled milk, in the days before milk was homogenized, would separate within four hours after milking into a creamy supernatant fluid and a lower layer of skim milk. Varying amounts of the supernatant creamy layer, or top milk, were often used in the preparation of milk feeding formulas in order to accelerate the infant's weight gain.

The Doctors Meigs of Philadelphia and Their Contributions to Infant Feeding

An important American medical family associated with child care, more specifically with infant feeding practices, were the three Doctors Meigs—father, son and grandson.[22] The practices of these three men were to span almost a century—from 1817 to 1912.

C. D. Meigs, the grandfather, theorized that indigestion in artificially fed infants was due to the large quantity of casein in cow's milk. Later, half of this theory was substantiated when it was found that cow's milk contains more casein than breast milk. Although it has been disproved that casein is indigestible, this was one of the first attempts to explain the intestinal disturbances in infancy.

In 1850, J. F. Meigs,[26] the son, published his formulas for infant feeding in which milk, cream, and cereal decoctions were used. From this start all other methods commonly used in America have sprung. The younger Meigs made his formula from incorrect analysis of the proteins of cow's milk and diluted accordingly, adding cream and milk sugar to imitate mother's milk. It consisted of milk, cream, sugar, and limewater, so mixed as to contain 3.5 percent fat, 1.21 percent protein, 6.66 percent water, and 0.25 percent ash.

J. F. Meigs recommended that from birth to the end of the first month, and even in the second month, infant's formula should be two parts of water to one part of milk; to each pint of this mixture should be added a half-ounce of sugar of milk, or half the quantity of cane sugar. In the second month, and up to five or six months of age, the pro-

portion ought to be half and half in healthy infants. After this period it could be made two parts milk and one water until the end of the first year.

Meigs's simple formulas were unfortunately soon to be replaced by Rotch's cumbersome and complicated percentage-feeding regimen.

A. V. Meigs[24, 25] the grandson, made a number of significant contributions to American pediatrics (Fig. 6–1). Perhaps the most important was his accurate chemical analysis of human and cow's milk, which has served as a basis for modern infant feeding. His chemical studies were published in 1885 in his book *Milk Analysis and Infant Feeding*, which, although only 120 pages in length, deserves to be considered a pediatric classic. Meigs stressed that "human milk never contains more than seven-tenths to one and a half percent of casein and about seven percent sugar." Some investigators, prior to Meigs,

Figure 6–1. Arthur Vincent Meigs, A.B., M.D. (1850–1912).

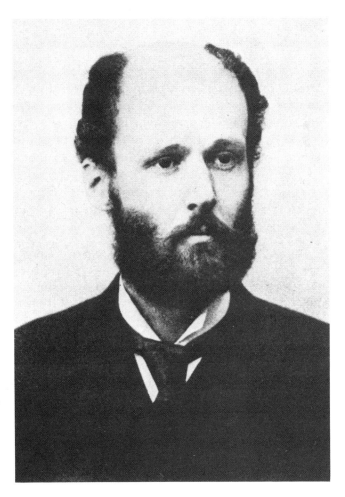

had claimed that the amount of protein in human milk was as high as 3.35 to 3.9 percent. Time has proven the correctness of Meigs's analysis; most of the systems of infant feeding developed during the later part of the nineteenth and the early part of the twentieth century have taken into consideration the low casein content of human milk.

Meigs's mixture, which he contended never needed to be altered throughout the infant's entire nursing period, was prepared as follows:

8 ounces $\begin{cases} 3 \text{ ounces of top milk [7 to 8 percent} \\ \quad \text{of fat]} \\ 3 \text{ ounces of sugar solution [15 percent]} \\ 2 \text{ ounces of limewater} \end{cases}$

Meig's mixture was thus designed to provide an infant formula made up of:

Water	87.8 percent
Fat	4.7 percent
Casein	1.1 percent
Sugar	6.2 percent
Salts	0.2 percent
Calories per ounce	21.72

The advantage of his "artifical food," Meigs wrote, was that its strength remained constant, in contrast to the usual contemporary directions for artificial feeding which recommended that the food "be increased in strength every few weeks from the time an infant is a few days old until it is old enough to take pure cow's milk." Meigs[25] found the reason for the recommendation for making frequent formula changes difficult to understand, and for him it was "a cardinal error" for these reasons:

For infants nursed by their own mothers nothing of the sort is accomplished. Although some milk analysts have tried to show that human milk changes in composition as the weeks and months go by, not one of them has ever succeeded in bringing forward sufficient reasons to establish this theory. On the contrary, it is much more reasonable to suppose that after the colostrum once disappears no further change takes place, and that the only difference between the human milk provided for an infant three weeks and one nine months old is in the quantity. My own analyses support this conclusion. It is therefore an error to increase the strength of an artificial food during the first six to nine months, and in *the frequent infringement of this law lies the explanation of many failures of bringing up infants by hand* [italics mine]. The correctness

of this view is supported by the fact that practical experience bears out the theory. In a great many cases I have pursued the plan with the most satisfactory results.

Meigs's mixture contained 21.72 kcal/oz and in light of our present knowledge was a satisfactory formula. Unknown to Meigs when he calculated his mixture was that the average requirement for growth in the first year is approximately 50 kilocalories per pound of body weight per day. Meigs suggested that "the daily amount required would gradually increase, until at the end of twenty-one days it will be found that the infant is taking two and a half ounces at a time and still about seven or eight feedings in each day, making a total of from 17.5 to 20 ounces [377 to 434 kcal/day*].When the sixth week was reached, about four ounces will be required at a time, making a total of nearly 32 ounces [700 kcal/day*]."

Meigs wondered why so many of his contemporaries were unwilling to offer the infant his artificial food but would prefer to use sweetened condensed milk, which had become popular. (Gale Borden's patent for condensed milk had been granted in 1856). The only two explanations Meigs could offer were that the profession had not yet accepted the truth of his analysis showing that "the amount of casein in human milk was only about one percent and that many still believed "milk to be a fluid of unstable composition instead of being very constant in composition, as it really is."

Meigs's formula was really a single-formula mixture that closely resembled human milk, and if he had recommended sterilization as a "matter of general application," the formula would have satisfied the nutritional and caloric needs of most infants and would have been bacteriologically safe.

Meigs advanced infant feeding significantly. Unfortunately, this greatly admired physician refused to fully accept the discoveries of bacteriology and opposed the germ theory of disease until his death in 1912.

Thomas Morgan Rotch and the Percentage Method of Infant Feeding

Rotch's percentage feeding,[33] or as it was also called, the laboratory or American method, was based, as

*Author's calculations.

was Biedert's mixture, on the idea that the protein of cow's milk is the one food element that is difficult to digest and, on the other hand, that the fat is comparatively harmless and easy to digest. It further assumed that in feeding an infant the important thing in modifying the food was to offer the infant a certain percentage of each food element, rather than to give it a certain amount of food. Rotch contended that what is good for or adapted to one infant may not be suitable for another. In his own words: "What is one infant's food may be another's poison."

John Lovett Morse,[29] one of Rotch's staunchest disciples, rightfully called attention to the dismal conditions under which infants were artificially fed toward the end of the last century. He wrote:

Most babies were fed on proprietary foods, a considerable portion of which contained no milk and were mixed with water. Very few physicians had any idea what the mixtures contained, or would have understood if they knew. They simply tried one after another, hit or miss. Those who used milk, with the exception of Meigs, Rotch, Holt, and a few others, had no definite plan. It was impossible to get clean milk. The importance of tuberculosis in cattle was unappreciated. The long tube nursing bottle was still in use. No one had ever heard of vitamins or calories.

Rotch[31, 33] taught that not only the proteins but the fats and sugars of cow's milk might also be the cause of disturbance of the infant's digestion. He was unquestionably the father and greatest proponent of the method commonly used in this country from 1890 until 1915—the percentage method. This was further elaborated by Holt and Henry E. Koplik (1858–1927). All three of these pediatricians taught that the basic factor underlying the modification of milk was that cow's milk contains more casein than human milk. Thus, cow's milk must be diluted to lower the percentage of casein, but in so doing the amount of sugar and fat is reduced below the level found in breast milk. Consequently, besides a water or cereal diluent, cream and sugar were added.

Rotch[33] had correctly pointed out that "percentage feeding" is a method of calculation rather than a method of feeding; he often wrote that "no one can satisfactorily prescribe food for an infant who does not have knowledge of the composition of that food." Rotch assumed from the analyses then available that the average composition of human milk was about 4 percent fat, 7 percent sugar, 1.5 percent protein and 0.2 percent ash. He used these figures as the basis of his calculations. Rotch further taught that ordinary cream contained about 20 percent of fat. He therefore developed the following mixture: ¼ part cream, ⅛ part milk, 1 part water, and one measure (3⅜ drams) of lactose and 1/16 part limewater for each 8 ounces of mixtures.

The whole idea was to provide a way by which the composition of the food was equal to the digestive capacity of the individual infant. Rotch saw more clearly than had Biedert that the tolerance of cow's milk varied enormously according to age. But as time went on, he grew to believe that minute variations in the composition of the food, perhaps as little as 0.1 percent variation in a single food element, could make the difference between its being digested or not. The percentage system of feeding insisted upon the very careful gradation of the size and composition of the feedings from week to week, with the result that milk was prescribed with the same accuracy and precision as dangerous drugs.

But for such accurate composition of formulas as demanded by the percentage method a well-managed milk laboratory was needed. Such a laboratory became the cornerstone of Rotch's method. Although most of his contemporaries agreed that his results were better than anything that had been accomplished previously, one wonders how much this was due to his requirement for a very pure quality of milk and how much to the percentage system. Rotch had found that no one formula was suited to all infants, and this led him to develop a system of complex formulas with varying percentages of protein, fat, and carbohydrate. To do this, according to one pediatrician, "required almost the equivalent of an advanced degree in higher mathematics, employing algebraic equations to compute the food mixture for a baby."[27]

To solve this mathematical difficulty and to put Rotch's system into practical use, the first Walker-Gordon Laboratory was established in 1891 in Boston to produce and use clean "modified" milk in preparing the formulas. Branches of this laboratory were opened in other large cities in the United States as well as one in London. Here, according to Herman F. Meyer (1900–1974):[27] "By means of slide rules and arithemetical gymnastics, these laboratories supplied the computed formulae on data submitted to them by the physician. The practitioner readily got the impression that this subject was too complicated to apply to practice, and he soon left it for the simple, patented food mixture, or for some simple milk dilution with a well-advertised carbohydrate added."

In the early days of percentage feeding the casein in cow's milk was Rotch's prime concern. But later, when it was proved that the common curds in infant's stools were often fatty, rather than containing the suspected protein, the needed modification was made in the amount of cream added to the feeding.

From the beginning, physicians had no end of trouble with percentage feeding in a large proportion of their patients; most of these absolute and relative failures, according to F. L. Wacherheim,[41] a New York pediatrician, "were wrongly attributed to an excess of casein, whereas we now know that the high fat ratios were to blame." He further described the problems with percentage feeding as follows: "These experiences led to a desire to vary the percentage plan according to the individual, so as to give different proportions of the various milk ingredients; this in turn gave rise to a large series of new tables. Holt refers to one ambitious author with 579 formulas, a vivid commentary on the riot of mathematics inherent in a consequential study of Rotch's method."

Rotch's method had been adopted almost universally by American pediatricians by the end of the 1890's, though it found little favor abroad, being considered too complicated and artificial. But by the end of the first decade of the twentieth century, percentage feeding was on the wane, largely because of the mounting criticisms of American authorities.

Henry Koplik[20] gradually came to the view that the method was overly refined and essentially artificial, taking no consideration of the normal variations in human milk, which it tried to imitate. He also viewed the laboratories as trying to improve on nature with inferior materials. He satirically commented on the "idea of trying to benefit a sick infant by offering him a food which is fundamentally unsuitable, yet figured out to amazing nicety." Abraham Jacobi,[19] as will be seen, ridiculed what he called the heresy of "the top milk gospel." He often commented at medical meetings that "you cannot feed babies with mathematics; you must feed them with brains."

By 1915 many pediatricians had begun to discard the whole rigmarole of top milk and percentages and return to simpler methods that had proved themselves at least as successful, but were laid aside because they did not achieve the impossible, namely to make cow's milk an equal substitute for human milk.

Jacobi,[18] in a veiledly sarcastic commentary, had this to say about Rotch's method:

But it must be far from me not to present Dr. Rotch's case in full. His standing and merits are such as to give him a hearing wherever and whatever he discusses.... I know of a number of babies who in health and disease have done well on the protracted use of [his] laboratory milk. Only one observation struck me in a few cases. The formation of muscles and particularly of the bones appeared to be slow, the teeth came in a number of weeks or even months too late, the cranial bones turned slightly soft in a few instances. In a few such cases I had to add animal broths of juice before the usual time; in one I tried phosphorus (elixir phosphori) which was rejected.... It is only to be deplored that for the present it is a method only for the rich; mine has the advantage of being one for the people both rich and poor.

Today the minutiae of percentage feeding seem amusing; nevertheless, the attention paid to the composition of milk and the teachings of Rotch and his colleagues unquestionably advanced materially the knowledge of infant nutrition.

Figure 6–2 illustrates an example of Rotch's calculations to prepare a percentage feeding formula. Even a short review of the intricacies of Rotch's many publications on the value of percentage feeding makes Oliver Wendell Holmes's[15] quotation seem more appropriate than ever: "A pair of substantial mammary glands has the advantage over the two hemispheres of the most learned professor's brain in the art of compounding a nutritious fluid for infants."

Abraham Jacobi and Infant Feeding

Jacobi[17] reminded his contemporaries: "Babies are the most philosophic people. They thrive or die, crow or wail without regard to the half million or more books and pamphlets which have been written about them in all countries in the course of a cen-

Formulæ for Cream and Whey.—In order to calculate the amount of whey which is needed for various combinations, the general formulæ (5), (6), and (7) can be applied by considering whey as a milk containing very low proteids (lactalbumin) and fat. Taking König's formula for whey as a standard,

Fat..............................	$0.32 = a'$
Sugar..............................	$4.79 = c'$
Proteids..............................,	$0.86 = d'$

we can then represent a′ of the general formula by 0.32, b′ by 0.86, and c′ by 4.8, and the special formula will then be

(24) $$C = \frac{Q\,(0.86 \times F - 0.32 \times P)}{9.1 \text{ or } 12.6},$$

according as twelve per cent. or sixteen per cent. cream is used.

(25) $$\text{Whey} = \frac{Q\,F - 12\,C}{0.32} \text{ or } \frac{Q\,F - 16\,C}{0.32}$$

and

(26) $$L = \frac{Q\,S - (4.8 \times \text{whey} \div 12 \text{ or } 16\,C)}{100}.$$

In such a combination sufficient diluent must be added to make up the total quantity.

The following formulæ are derivable from equations expressing the fact that the proteid or fat percentage of the mixture is equal to the sum of the proteid or fat percentages contributed by the cream and the whey.

(27) $$P = \frac{C}{Q} \times b + \frac{\text{whey}}{Q} \times b'$$

(28) $$F = \frac{C}{Q} \times a + \frac{\text{whey}}{Q} \times a'$$

whence, by deduction,

(29) $$C = \frac{Q\,(F - a')}{a - a'}.$$

One or the other of these formulæ may be used according as a definite fat or proteid percentage is desired. The constants a and a′ represent the fat percentages of the cream and of the whey respectively, and b and b′ represent the corresponding proteid percentages.

Thus, for 20 per cent. cream ($F = 20$. $P = 3.20$, $S = 3.80$) and whey ($F = 0.32$, $P = 0.86$, $S = 4.8$) the formulæ would become

(30) $$C = \frac{Q\,(P - 0.86)}{3.20 - 0.86} = (31)\ \frac{Q\,(P - 0.86)}{2.34},$$

and

(32) $$C = \frac{Q\,(F - 0.32)}{20 - 0.32} = (33)\ \frac{Q\,(F - 0.32)}{19.68}.$$

The formula for L can be derived from the general formula (7) by substitution, which gives

(34) $$L = \frac{Q\,S - (4.8 \text{ whey} + 3.8\,C)}{100}.$$

In the same way, for 16 per cent. cream the formulæ become, after substitution,

(35) $$C = \frac{Q\,(P - 0.86)}{2.74},$$

(36) $$C = \frac{Q\,(F - 0.32)}{15.68}.$$

For 12 per cent. cream,

(37) $$C = \frac{Q\,(P - 0.86)}{2.94},$$

(38) $$C = \frac{Q\,(F - 0.32)}{11.68}.$$

For 8 per cent. cream,

(39) $$C = \frac{Q\,(P - 0.86)}{[illegible]},$$

Figure 6–2. An example of Rotch's calculations to prepare a percentage feeding formula. (Reprinted from Thomas Morgan Rotch. Pediatrics *{4th ed.}. Philadelphia: Lippincott, 1903).*

tury." Jacobi's teaching in regard to infant nutrition was simple—mother's milk first and foremost, raw unpasteurized milk never, boiled cow's milk and added cereal and salt, and the use of cane sugar in place of lactose. He simply diluted the milk with barley water or oatmeal water and added cane sugar to make up for the deficit in carbohydrates. He varied the degree of dilution according to the infant's age but studiously avoided the error of laying down any hard and fast rules; the infant's general condition, especially weight, was the criterion by which the formula was prescribed.

He was an early proponent of boiling milk and often told the story of how, in the beginning of his practice, many of his patients were dying of infantile diarrhea. One morning, disheartened by his failure in treating the disease, he met two colleagues who explained to him that cow's milk was often obtained from animals that were fed distillery slops, and that the secret of cure was to boil the contaminated milk before giving it to infants. Jacobi proceeded to do this; years of subsequent experience convinced him that it was the only correct way to treat milk for infants' use. However, most physicians feared that boiling altered the milk in some unknown way. Jacobi was probably the first American pediatrician to suggest heating whole milk. He fought against the widely approved use of top milk in infant feeding because of the excess of milk fat given to the infant. He wrote:[19]

The worst cases of this kind [use of top milk] are not solely among the poor, on the contrary, many occur among the well-to-do, that is, those who can afford the expensive luxury of filling their offspring with high-priced food.

There is a medical man . . . brought up on the gospel of fat feeding, and took it without thinking, as we get our religion. Then, being a man of means, he buys for his baby certified milk, four bottles [daily], and gives him [his infant son] the upper fourth part of the four bottles. When the baby was seen, it was shriveled up, the stools were putrid, the urine ammoniacal, the eyes retracted into the orbits and big, and pitifully pleading for delivery from his father. . . . The top milk gospel is heresy.

The Calorimetric Method of Infant Feeding

Rubner and Heubner's[35] classical monograph on the metabolism and average daily caloric needs of the normal and "atrophic" infant appeared in 1898. From their studies it was possible, for the first time, to feed infants according to their caloric requirements. These studies also became the starting point for all modern investigations on infant metabolism. Heubner had been impressed by Camerer's research into the significant energy values in infant nutrition. At Heubner's suggestion, Rubner began metabolic studies on young infants and devised a respiratory apparatus by which he could determine the metabolism of three infants: a breast-fed infant, a normal one artificially fed, and a sick infant similarly fed. Later a strong, healthy breast-fed infant was similarly investigated by way of comparison.

Isaac A. Abt[2] described these investigations:

Thus it was possible for the first time to estimate the complete metabolism and energy quotient in infants in various conditions; it was also determined that only a small amount of protein was required for infant nutrition. The activity of the alimentary canal in infants suffering from digestive disturbances, the utilization of the food consumed and the variation of water elimination in rest or activity of the infant were investigated, and the carbohydrate metabolism and other problems were also studied. These observations conducted over a period of time led Heubner to a new conception of energy quotients. He learned that the food requirements of infants of various ages could be calculated, which proved to be of practical and fundamental value in infant feeding.

Among the first in America to use the caloric method was Morse,[28] who in 1904 recommended this method for the feeding of premature infants. Knowing the amount of milk the infant needed per pound of body weight was a tremendous advance and gave physicians a much more scientific and rational base from which to prepare the infant's formula than the use of the percentage or other methods based on dilution and modification of cow's milk.

Starch and Cereal Diluents in Infants' Formulas

In the early 1890's there were heated discussions about the use of starch and cereal diluents in feeding infants. Rotch[32] argued persuasively that since there was no starch in human milk, none should be added to artificial food. Chapin,[9] on the other hand, answered that as an artificial food was not human milk, it might be a good thing to add starch to the infant's formula. As late as the early nineties it was thought that the infant could not digest starch; however, by the early 1900's it was proved that the infant could convert starch into sugar at birth. Rotch countered teleologically by writing that this function was in process of development and that it was not "rational to tax a developing function." The cereal diluents were added, as a rule, not for their food value, but for their supposed action in preventing the formation of large casein curds.

The Amount and Frequency of Feeding the Infant

A great deal was written, especially in the 1890's, about the amount of milk the infant should be given at a feeding and at what intervals of time. Holt[16] was the first in this country to investigate "the quantity of food to be allowed artificially-fed infants." To determine this figure, he measured the fluid capacities of the stomachs obtained at autopsy from ninety-one infants ranging in age from birth to fourteen months.

Rotch[32] also studied the capacity of the infant's stomach, which he measured with painstaking care after death; he arrived at a number of feedings to be given in twenty-four hours by estimating the amount of breast milk taken and dividing it by the infant's gastric capacity. Holt[16] wrote, "I believe that if we take this capacity as a guide to the amount of food to be allowed to an average infant in health, we shall not go far wrong." Table 6–2 depicts Holt's feeding schedule, published in 1899, for a healthy infant during the first nine months of life.

As Morse[29] has correctly reminded us, "if anyone feels like ridiculing this table, please remember that

Table 6–2. *L. Emmett Holt's Schedule for Feeding a Healthy Infant During the First Nine Months of Life.*

Formula	Age	Feedings in 24 hrs.	Interval between daytime feedings (hrs)	Feedings 10 P.M.–7 A.M.	Quantity for one feeding (oz.)	Quantity for 24 hrs. (oz.)
I	2–14 days	10	2	2	1–2½	10–25
II	2–5 wks.	10	2	2	2–3¼	20–32
III	5–10 wks.	8	2½	1	3–4½	24–36
IV	10 wks.–4 mos.	7	3	1	4–6	28–42
V	4–9 mos.	6	3	–	5–8	30–48

Source: L. E. Holt. *The Care and Feeding of Children* (2nd ed.). New York, 1899.

the roentgen ray had just been discovered and that the caloric needs of infants and the caloric values of foods were, as far as the practical application went, unknown."

Regularity in feeding was considered important because, as Holt reminded mothers of his day, the baby should be *taught* to be regular in its habits of eating and sleeping, and regular training should be begun during the first week of life.

To Boil or Not to Boil

A burning question in this country in the 1890's was whether to boil or not to boil the milk meant for the infant. It was widely believed then that infants fed continuously on cooked milk—or on pasteurized milk—did not thrive so well as those fed on raw milk and that boiling or pasteurizing the milk predisposed to rickets and especially to scurvy. At the same time European physicians believed that infants thrived just as well, or perhaps better, on boiled than on raw milk. Jacobi always recommended boiled milk. As usual, his reason was explained in a manner that left little room for rebuttal. "Now, what is it that boiling can and will do? Besides expelling air, it destroys the germs of typhoid fever, Asiatic cholera, diphtheria and tuberculosis, also the many bacteria which cause the change of milk-sugar into lactic acid and the rapid acidulation of milk with its bad effects on the secretion of the intestinal tract." However, A. V. Meigs[25] expressed in 1896 the more commonly held belief that boiling the infant's milk was not to be recommended as a general rule:

The sterilization of milk [this term as well as pasteurization were often used loosely] has been vaunted very much in recent years. . . . But latterly there seems to be a tendency to the general agreement that so high a temperature produces changes which render the milk less desirable as food for young infants, if it is not put in a condition to be positively injurious. . . .

As time goes on there is more and more heard of the damage done by the heating of milk, and many now oppose the system altogether. For my part I have never been an advocate of its use under ordinary circumstances.

Others, notably Rotch, Henry L. Coit (1854–1917), and Koplik approached the problem differently by trying to improve the quality of milk.

Spearheaded by Rotch, the Walker-Gordon farms, upon which the success of the first milk laboratory depended, served as an example for other dairy farms. Coit, as will be seen, originated the plan to produce certified milk in 1889 which was first put into operation in New Jersey in 1893.

Sanitary Milk Supply

Despite the contributions of Rotch and others to infant feeding, none could match in importance the campaign for a sanitary milk supply. Two different methods were advocated to keep milk free of disease-producing bacteria, certification and pasteurization. As early as 1830 Robert Hartley[14] (1796–1851) set in motion a drive to improve the milk supply. A pure-milk campaign was started soon thereafter as a by-product of the temperance movement, but it was not until the nineteenth century was nearly over that the campaign culminated in success. Linnaeus E. LaFétra (1868–1965)[21] described New York City's milk supply in the mid-1860's as follows:

More than half of the milk used in the city came from cows fed only on distiller's mash. At Ninth Avenue and 18th Street, adjoining a distillery, were sheds containing 2,000 cows. The animals were kept in incredible filth; they had no exercise, no fresh air, no fresh food and no hay.

The stables were rented at five dollars per year per cow and mash supplied at nine cents a barrel. City tramps were the milkers, being paid for their labor by night shelter in the stables. The cows were diseased and the milk filthy.

Distillery cows produced what was known as "swill-milk" (p. 74). This particular liquid, which was said to make infants tipsy, caused a scandal in the New York of 1870 when it was learned that some of the cows cooped up for years in filthy stables were so enfeebled from tuberculosis that until they died they had to be raised on cranes to be milked (Fig. 6–3).

As the nineteenth century was ending, all physicians recognized that dirty milk disastrously affected the health of the child, but there was little unanimity about a solution to the problem.

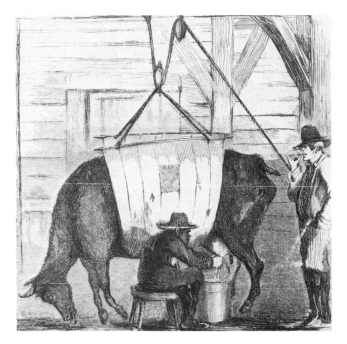

Figure 6–3. A diseased cow, unable to stand, is pulled up to be milked. (Harper's Weekly, January 22, 1870.)

Even in the early twentieth century, dirty milk was usually found in most large American cities. Abt[1] vividly described the odorous tin cans from which it was sold, "with flies festooning the open containers and customers carrying the milk home in open pitchers or pails in the hottest months." Then once at home, Abt wrote, "the milk container was set out in a hot room on a table because there were no ice boxes."

It was common knowledge that milk was diluted and the dealers were neither subtle nor timid about it; all they required was a water pump to boost two quarts of milk to a gallon. Nor was that the end of the mischief; to improve the color of milk from diseased cattle they often added molasses, chalk, or plaster of Paris. No wonder that in 1889 New York's public health commissioner reported seeing in certain districts a "decidedly suspicious-looking fluid bearing the name of milk."[4]

In the latter part of the nineteenth century milk was delivered to city dwellers by a horse-drawn wagon bearing two big milk cans. If the supplier catered to the "upper class," there were spigots on the cans from which the housemaids filled the pitcher or bucket. On streets further down the economic scale, the lid was slid off the top of the can and the milk was ladled out at a few pennies a pail. The milk handling at the farm was often worse than the delivery service.

When in 1902 the New York City Health Commission tested 3,970 milk samples, it was found that 2,095, or 52.77 percent, were adulterated. In 1902, the Rockefeller Institute reported that half of all New York milk was diluted. Dairymen, it was said, "cheat as meanly as faro dealers."[4]

Bacteriologic Studies of Milk

The association of infant feeding with research in bacteriology has always been a close one, beginning with the pioneer work of Escherich on the relationship of the colon bacillus to disease (1886). The most dramatic contribution, according to Grover F. Powers (1887–1968),[31] was doubtless the demonstration by investigators at the Thomas Wilson Sanitarium in Baltimore in 1902 that ileocolitis, or bloody diarrhea, in infants may really be dysentery caused by an organism of the groups of bacilli described in part by Kiyoshi Shiga (1870–1957) in 1898 and by Simon Flexner in 1900. The science of bacteriology should be credited more than any other single development in reducing the morbidity and mortality of artificially fed infants.

Infant feeding is under its heaviest debt to bacteriology for the use of pasteurization (first begun on a commercial scale in Denmark in 1890). This method originated with Pasteur's announcement in 1864 that keeping wine at a high temperature killed the bacteria that caused the wine to sour. In 1886, Franz von Soxhlet (1848–1926),[38] a German chemist, recommended that this procedure be used for milk; the method came to be known as pasteurization. It is of interest that pasteurization was first used in the dairy industry about 1890 more as a means of increasing the "life" of the milk than to kill the bacteria likely to cause harm to the consumer. For example, milk arriving in town in the late afternoon after a long railway journey, and not refrigerated en route, would probably turn sour before it could be distributed the next morning. Pasteurization was found to retard souring by killing most of the bacteria which produce acid. It was a few years later, about 1896, before it was appreciated that pasteurization also provided a valuable protection against milk-borne disease. However, the movement for pasteurized milk gained acceptance slowly. It was not until 1908 that Chicago became the first city in the world to require pasteurization; in the next few years many others followed.

Henry L. Coit and the Fight for Clean Milk

A vigorous fight for clean, wholesome milk, to be known as certified milk, was led by Henry L. Coit[42] (Fig. 6–4). His interest in clean milk and infant feeding began in 1887, as a result of watching his firstborn son as he lay dying of diphtheria while the desperate father sought pure milk for him. He poignantly described this experience:

With an eager mind I pored over the scanty scientific

Figure 6–4. Henry Lever Coit, Ph.G., M.D. (1854–1917).

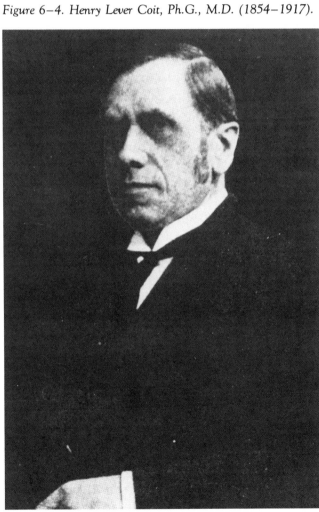

literature on infant dietetics [and] thus equipped I spent two years at the feet of this child. . . . The vicissitudes through which I passed on the question of pure materials with which to nourish this child, will never be told. It is sufficient to state that, in order to obtain sound milk for his needs, I was driven from one source of impoverished and contaminated milk to another until, in desperation, I sought a small suburban dairyman who . . . delivered the milk of four cows. An honest and industrious man, but without a knowledge of hygiene, he became unwittingly a dangerous element in my family life.

"A baby consumes about 500 quarts of milk during the first year," wrote Coit,[8] "and a very slight variation in the chemical contents of milk may cause fatal disturbances. A direct relation is at once established between the character of the food supply and infant mortality." Coit's plan for clean milk, according to Manfred J. Waserman,[42] included three general requirements:

First, that physicians give support to a medical commission that would insure the production of a pure milk produced under prescribed regulations; *second*, that an approved and trustworthy dairyman, possessing honor, financial ability, and dairy facilities, collect and handle the product in conformity with the commission's requirements; and *third*, that the commission, without pecuniary compensation, establish clinical standards of purity for the milk, be responsible for the inspection of the dairy or dairies under their patronage, and provide for examinations of the dairy stock and be responsible for the chemical and bacteriological testing of the product. The expense of all examinations would be defrayed by the dairyman. The milk produced in this manner would be know as *certified* milk, sealed in separate quart containers, and bear the name of the producer and the date of milking.

The milk was "designed especially for clinical purposes," and while Coit stated that this product should be used by the physician to "secure results in his professional work among the sick," he also stressed that the plan could be a "remedy for the difficulties which surround the milk supply in large cities."

Certified milk attempted to incorporate three important features: "uniform nutritive values, reliable keeping qualities and freedom from pathogenic bacteria." Among the standards adopted by the American Association of Medical Milk Commissions was that "certified milk shall contain less than 10,000 bacteria per cubic centimeter when delivered" and that "the fat standard shall be 4% with a permissible range of variation of from 3.5% to 4.5%. . . .the protein standard shall be 3.5% with a permissible range of variation from 3% to 4%."

In 1892, Mr. Francisco, owner of the Fairfield Dairy in Caldwell, New Jersey, produced the first bottle of certified milk and the first commercial milk to be dispensed in individual bottles. Mr. Francisco's first bottle, tied with a blue ribbon, was personally delivered to Mrs. Coit, whose encouragement and loyalty had been an important factor in the program. It was Emma Coit, the two-year-old daughter, who became the ultimate consumer and symbolically the goal of the entire program. The Fairfield Dairy in the late 1890's sold a quart of certified milk for twelve cents, which was twice the cost of a quart of ordinary milk at that time. Although certified milk was vigorously promoted in some cities, its production was too difficult to monitor to be feasible on a large scale.

Nathan Straus and Milk Stations for the Poor

In 1900 newspapers praised Nathan Straus (1848–1931), the part owner of Macy's department store, for establishing in the spring of 1893 a number of pure milk depots in New York City and for providing a pasteurization plant in the foundling hospital located on Randall's Island, where the infant death rate dropped from 51 to 18 percent within the first year after the milk plant was established.[12] This philanthropic effort had been prompted by Dr. Coit.

Actually, Koplik had established the first American milk depot in 1889 in the Good Samaritan Dispensary, which was located in the Lower East Side of Manhattan in one of the most crowded slum districts of the city. From six to eight bottles of milk were dispensed per infant, depending on the doctor's orders. Six bottles sold for eight cents; the deposit on the bottle was three cents and on the rubber stopper one cent. About two hundred bottles were dispensed daily and on Saturday the number ran as high as two thousand.

Another Straus Milk Charity pasteurization plant was established on the advice of the pediatricians of New York City on a public pier at the foot of East Third Street, close to a large and poor tenement house population (Fig. 6–5). But the demand for this milk was so great that the original plant on the pier was too small to meet the demand, and a larger building was then acquired.

The milk was pasteurized at the plant and was dispensed with the direction that it be kept cool and used within twenty-four hours. At first, two milk preparations were furnished: pure milk, pasteurized in eight-ounce bottles, and milk especially prepared for feeding small infants, a one-half dilution with water, lactose and limewater to make up a formula containing 2 percent fat, 2 percent protein and 7 percent sugar. Later, on Jacobi's advice, there was added a third preparation of a one-half dilution of milk with barley water sweetened with cane sugar, according to the following formula:

table salt	¼ oz
white cane sugar	10 oz
milk	1 gal
barley water	1 gal

This was dispensed in six-ounce bottles that were sold for one cent each. The eight-ounce bottles of pure milk were sold at one and a half cents each.

During the first summer (1893), thirty-four thousand bottles were sold, during 1894 more than three hundred thousand, and during both 1895 and 1896, more than six hundred thousand. During the first five summers this charity was in existence, more than two million bottles were distributed. These bottles were specially designed with sloping necks so as to be easy to clean and spheroidal bottoms so that they could not stand upright. This was done so that the bottles could not be left standing unstoppered, thus allowing contamination.

Did Straus's effort affect the infant mortality? Freeman[12] tabulated the deaths from diarrheal diseases in infants for the three years just prior to the opening of the milk stations and for the first three years afterward. His study, though it was not well designed, found that the number of deaths from diarrheal diseases fell from 6,122 to 5,262 during these two periods.

Proprietary (Artificial) Infant Foods

The studies of the chemist Justus von Liebig (1803–1873), a pupil of Francois Magendie (1783–1855),

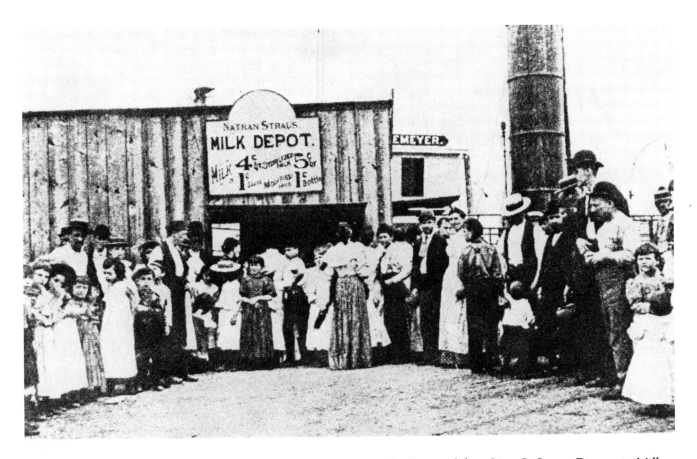

Figure 6–5. Nathan Straus Infant Milk Station, New York City, 1893. (Reprinted from Lina G. Straus. Disease in Milk *{2nd ed.}. New York: Dutton, 1917.)*

on the chemistry of food had both a direct and indirect influence on the artificial feeding of children. Indirect, because of Liebig's biochemical classification of the organic foodstuffs and the processes of nutrition, and direct because he himself devised and marketed a patented infant's food. The beginning of the proprietary food industry might be dated from 1867, when Liebig marketed his "perfect" infant food.[9]

Liebig's Mixture

The formula Liebig devised was a mixture of wheat flour, cow's milk and malt flour, cooked with a little potassium bicarbonate, which he added to reduce the acidity of the wheat and malt flours. Liebig's food was the first to take into account the infant's supposed physiological needs (caloric feeding was developed about thirty years later). Actually, as so often happens in medicine, Liebig's idea was not entirely new, for in 1862 an English chemist had taken out a patent for preparing infants' food from cooked

flour to which sugar and potassium bicarbonate were added. It was sold as a powder and was entirely farinaceous. Such foods Liebig correctly condemned as unsuitable for infants and for this reason he included milk in his own formula. At first Liebig's food was sold as a liquid, but as it did not keep well in this form, it subsequently was sold in powder form. Two years after Liebig first introduced his infant food on the market it was widely advertised in America as "the most perfect substitute for *mother's milk.*"

This was the beginning of an almost endless variety of infant foods which appeared during the last quarter of the nineteenth century. Often totally unwarranted claims were made for them. They consisted either of dried milk, in combination with a cereal or alone, and with or without the addition of a malt preparation of some kind. Again, many of the infant foods contained nothing but a dry, carefully prepared cereal.

The proprietary foods sold in the United States

could roughly be divided into three groups. The first group contained dried cow's milk, combined with some cereal and sugar. Examples were Nestlé's Food, which contained much unchanged starch, and Horlick's malted milk, in which the starch was largely converted into soluble carbohydrates such as maltose and dextrin. These foods were intended as an exclusive diet for infants and were violently criticized by the leading pediatricians of the day. The second group contained some form of malted carbohydrate. The starch was completely changed to dextrin and maltose. The most widely used of this group was Mellin's Food, which was a desiccated malt extract. The third group of infant foods consisted of those composed of a pure cereal to be used with fresh cow's milk; the best-known brand names were Eskay's Food, Imperial Granum, and Robinson's Patent Barley (Fig. 6–6). The great harm of these foods was that they were often used as the infant's only article of diet. Since most of them contained little more than concentrated carbohydrates, the results were usually disastrous.

Introduction to Solid Foods

In contrast to present-day practice, in which solid foods such as cereals, strained fruits, vegetables, soups, and meats are usually offered to infants during the first three months of life, infants in the latter part of the nineteenth century customarily received nothing but milk until their tenth month. Holt's[16] 1899 feeding regimen (below) was similar to those published by his contemporaries. He recommended:

Feeding During the First Year

a. Nothing but milk until the infant was 8 or 9 months old.

b. Beginning at ten months beef juice beginning with one tablespoonful and increasing to four to six tablespoonfuls daily by twelve months of age.

c. Also at ten months thin gruel made from the grains of oats, wheat or barley, from farina or arrowroot; one to three tablespoonsful may be added to each feeding.

Feeding During the Second Year

From the twelfth to the sixteenth month:

a. First meal:

A bottle made up of milk	—5 oz.
cream	—1 oz.
water	—2 oz.
thick gruel	—2 oz.

(wheat, oatmeal, or barley), a pinch of salt and a little sugar

10 oz.

b. Second meal: same as above

c. Third meal: Beef juice   2–4 oz., three times/ week

Figure 6–6. Advertisement for baby foods from Sears, Roebuck catalogue, spring, 1897.

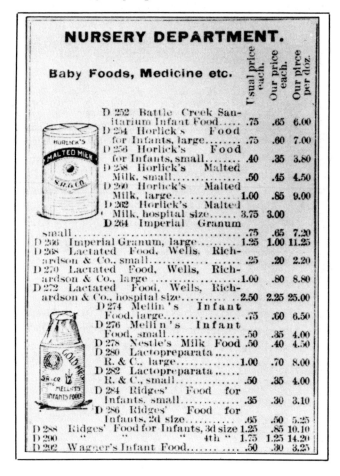

Eggs (poached or soft boiled)	2/week
Chicken or mutton broth	4–6 oz./week
Bottle as above	5 oz.
Fruit juices	1–2 oz./daily
Orange juice or peach juice or apricot juice	

As late as the latter part of the 1920's infants were usually not offered solid food until they were nearly a year of age. Even in the period before Sylvester Graham and his followers advocated vegetarianism, there was a widespread fear of giving too much animal food to children. Dewees[10] had written that "children should never make animal substances a principal part of their food, until the age of puberty." As the nineteenth century ended, many foods continued to be interdicted for children under four years of age, among them bacon, liver, tomatoes, beets, bananas, and all canned, dried, and preserved fruits.

Jacobi[18] advised: "Before children are two years of age no vegetables in any quantity should be given to them. Small quantities may be given later on; they will be acceptable and be readily digested."

Rotch was as emphatic as Jacobi about the age at which to offer solid foods to the child. He permitted baked potato at seventeen or more months of age and vegetables at thirty months, but even then only easily digested ones, such as squash, young peas, and young beans. Rotch, as well as Holt and Jacobi, did not recommend adding fresh fruits to the child's diet until the third year of life. For some reason, all writers were particularly fearful of bananas.

The age-old belief that fruits and vegetables were bad for infants and young children lingered on until the end of the century. What finally discredited it was the discovery that "summer diarrheas," which had almost always been attributed to the "corrupting influence" of fruits and some vegetables, were in fact largely diseases of bacterial and viral origin.

Nineteenth-Century Views on Weaning

During the entire century there were no major changes in weaning practices, save for a slight de-crease toward the very end of the century in the age to begin weaning. Job Lewis Smith[37] advised:

Weaning ought to take place, as a rule, between the ages of ten or twelve months. It is well, if the mother's health is good, and her milk sufficient, to defer weaning till the canine teeth appear. The infant then, possessing sixteen teeth, is able to masticate the softer kinds of solid foods . . . nurslings in the city should not be weaned in warm weather, nor within a month immediately preceding it. If the mother's health fail, or her milk becomes deficient, in the summer months, so that she cannot continue suckling, the infant should be sent immediately to the country, or a wet-nurse be employed. Many lives are sacrificed in consquence of ignorance of the danger of weaning under the circumstances mentioned. Severe diarrhoea, inflammatory or non-inflammatory, is apt to result.

J. P.Crozer Griffith[13] in his *Care of the Baby* (1895) written for nurses and parents (as was Holt's *Care and Feeding of Children*), advised: "Ordinarily weaning should take place at about the age of ten to eleven months. . . . Another very important matter is the season of the year. It is very bad policy to wean a child at the beginning of hot summer weather if it can be avoided in any way."

Koplik's[20] explanation for the inadvisability of weaning an infant at the onset of summer was that "during the summer a bottle-fed infant is very likely to be upset should anything happen to the milk." Infants so upset often developed the "summer complaint," or acute gastroenteritis, which took an astonishing toll of lives. Holt[16] in 1897 showed that the mortality from summer diarrhea in New York showed a sharp upswing each June, reached a peak in July, and slowly declined to "normal" levels by October, with a well-defined relationship to the mean temperature.

The nineteenth century saw pediatrics emerge as a discipline *sui generis*, and for its few practitioners infant feeding was of paramount concern. Not until the latter part of the century was a dent made in the crude empiricism and blind dogmatism that dominated the feeding of infants for almost the entire century. As the century ended, the calorimetric method of infant feeding was just evolving. This, plus the science of bacteriology, set the stage for the "modern scientific period of infant nutrition and for the clean-milk campaign.

References

1. Abt, I. A. *Baby Doctor.* New York: McGraw-Hill, 1944.
2. Abt, I. A. History of Pediatrics. In I. McQuarrie (ed.), *Brennemann's Practice of Pediatrics,* vol. I. Hagerstown, Md.: Prior, 1948.
3. Baker, S. J. *Child Hygiene.* New York: Harper, 1925.
4. Bettman, O. L. *The Good Old Days—They Were Terrible!* New York: Random House, 1974.
5. Biedert, P. *Untersuchungen ueber die Chemischen Unterschiede der Menschen- und kuhmilch* (disseration). Giessen: W. Keller, 1869.
6. Buchan, W. *Domestic Medicine.* Philadelphia: Richard Folwell, 1801.
7. Camerer, W. *Der Stoffwechsel des Kindes.* Tübingen: H.Laupp, 1894.
8. Coit, H. L. Certified milk. *Arch. Pediatr.* 14:824, 1897.
9. Cone, T. E., Jr. *200 Years of Feeding Infants in America,* Columbus, Ohio: Ross Laboratories, 1976.
10. Dewees, W. P. *Treatise on the Physical and Medical Treatment of Children* (10th ed.) Philadelphia: Blanchard and Lea, 1853.
11. Evans, P. R. Fashions in Infant Feeding. In J. A. Askin, R. E. Cooke, and J. A. Haller, Jr. (eds.), *A Symposium on the Child.* Baltimore: Johns Hopkins Press, 1967.
12. Freeman, R. G. The Straus milk charity of New York City. *Arch. Pediatr.* 14:838, 1897.
13. Griffith, J. P. C. *The Care of the Baby.* Philadelphia: Saunders, 1895.
14. Hartley, R. *An Historical, Scientific and Practical Essay on Milk.* New York: Leavitt, 1842.
15. Holmes, O. W. Scholastic and Bedside Teaching. In *Medical Essays.* Boston: Houghton Mifflin, 1911.
16. Holt, L. E. *The Care and Feeding of Children* (2nd ed). New York: Appleton, 1899.
17. Jacobi, A. *Infant Diet.* New York: Putnam, 1885.
18. Jacobi, A. *Therapeutics of Infancy and Childhood.* Philadelphia: Lippincott, 1896.
19. Jacobi, A. The Gospel of Top Cream. In W.J. Robinson (ed.), *Collectanea Jacobi,* vol. 3. New York: Critic and Guide Co., 1909.
20. Koplik, H. E. *Diseases of Infancy and Childhood.* Philadelphia: Lea & Febiger, 1902.
21. LaFétra, L. E. The development of pediatrics in New York City. *Arch. Pediatr.* 49:36, 1932.
22. Levinson, A. The three Meigs and their contribution to pediatrics. *Ann. Med. Hist.* 10:138, 1928.
23. McNutt, S. A. The Babies' Hospital—A summer's work. *Med. Rec. (N.Y.)* 35:234, 1889.
24. Meigs, A. V. *Milk Analysis and Infant Feeding.* Philadelphia: Blakiston, 1885.
25. Meigs, A. V. *Feeding in Early Infancy.* Philadelphia: Saunders, 1896.
26. Meigs, C. D. *Observations on Certain of the Diseases of Young Children.* Philadelphia: Lea and Blanchard, 1850.
27. Meyer, H. F. *Essentials of Infant Feeding for Physicians.* Springfield, Ill.: Thomas, 1952.
28. Morse, J. L. A study of the caloric needs of premature infants. *Am. J. Med. Sci.* 127:463, 1904.
29. Morse, J. L. Recollections and reflections on forty-five years of artificial infant feeding. *J. Pediatr.* 7:303, 1935.
30. Pavy, F. W. *A Treatise on Food and Dietetics* (2nd ed.). London: Churchill, 1875.
31. Powers, G. F. Infant feeding: Historical background and modern practice. *J.A.M.A.* 105:753, 1935.
32. Rotch, T. M. Infant Feeding—Weaning. In J. M. Keating (ed.), *Cyclopaedia of the Diseases of Children, Medical and Surgical,* vol. 1. Philadelphia: Lippincott, 1889.
33. Rotch, T. M. An historical sketch of the development of percentage feeding. *N.Y. Med. J.* 85:532, 1907.
34. Routh, C. H. F. *Infant Feeding and Its Influence on Life* (3rd ed.). New York: W. Wood, 1879.
35. Rubner, M., and Heubner, O. Die Natürliche Ernährung eines Säuglings. *J. Biol.* 36:1, 1898.
36. Simon, J. F. *Mother's Milk and Its Chemical and Physiological Properties* (Latin dissertation). Berlin, 1838.
37. Smith, J. L. *A Treatise on the Diseases of Infancy and Childhood* (2nd ed.). Philadelphia: Henry C. Lea, 1872.
38. Soxhlet, F. Ueber Kindermilch und Säuglings Ernährung. *Münch. Med. Wochenschr.* 33:253, 276, 1886.
39. Ticknor, C. *A Guide for Mothers and Nurses in the Management of Young Children.* New York: Taylor & Dodd, 1839.
40. Underwood, M. *A Treatise on the Diseases of Children* (5th ed.). London: J. Callow, 1805.
41. Wachenheim, F. L. *Infant Feeding.* Philadelphia: Lea & Febiger, 1915.
42. Waserman, M. J. Henry L. Coit and the certified milk movement in the development of modern pediatrics. *Bull. Hist. Med.* 46:359, 1972.

The Twentieth Century

Pediatrics Comes of Age

7

{Pediatrics} is the science of the young. The young are the future makers and owners of the world. The physical, intellectual, and moral condition will decide whether the globe will become more Cossack or more Republican, more criminal or more righteous. For their education and training and capabilities, the ... {pediatrician} as the representative of medical science and art should become responsible. Medicine is concerned with the new individual before he is born, while he is being born, and after....

It is not enough, however, to work at the individual bedside and in the hospital. In the near or dim future, the pediatrician is to sit in and control school boards, health departments, and legislatures. He is the legitimate advisor to the judge and the jury, and a seat for the physician in the councils of the republic is what the people have a right to demand.

Abraham Jacobi (1904)

The most important pediatric milestone during the first quarter of this century was the gradual acceptance of pediatrics as a specialty. The important realization that children and particularly infants were not merely manikins, that they differed profoundly from adults in terms of physiology, biochemistry, pathology, and bacteriology was not fully appreciated until a few physicians toward the end of the last and the beginning of this century began to devote their whole time to the study of the diseases of children.

In 1900 there probably were not over fifty medical practitioners in the whole country who took a particular interest in this age group and not half a dozen men practiced pediatrics exclusively.[114] Possibly one doctor out of every twenty-five hundred in the United States could have been classified as a pediatrician. Today there are over twenty thousand, or about one in every twenty of registered physicians. Laboratories for clinical, pathological, or chemical investigation of pediatric problems were nonexistent, save for those few devoted to the bacteriological study of diphtheria. Diphtheria antitoxin had been introduced in 1897, but it was not in general use and its value was still regarded by many as a subject for discussion.[60]

The child welfare movement, the milk station or well-baby station, and prenatal clinics had not yet been organized. There was not a state or municipality with a special department of child hygiene or child welfare. Health supervision of schoolchildren —if it existed at all—consisted of a cursory examination to detect contagious disease. Physicians confined their efforts to the child when sick rather than the child when well. Health departments went entirely on the principle that there was no point in doing much until something had happened.[7] There was no state or municipal milk control. Full-scale commercial pasteurization of milk was still years away. Parenteral fluid and electrolyte therapy were hardly thought of, and even if they had been, appropriate needles, syringes, and tubing were not available. As late as 1915 a leader of American academic pediatrics wrote: "The method of obtaining blood from the veins of the scalp, from the jugular or other veins, is very difficult and open to frequent failures."[55]

During this period the pediatrician was often known as the "baby feeder." His activities in preventive pediatrics, if any, were linked with milk and infant health stations. His other principal medical duty was to do battle with the "summer complaint" and his weapons were, as Grover F. Powers[95] so aptly put it, "tea, barley water, protein milk, floating hospitals and seaside or country sanatoria."

Summer diarrhea of infants remained a prevalent and serious disease without an effective method of treatment. In New York City, for example, during the first decade and a half of this century, fifteen hundred babies would be killed by it each week all through the hot weather.[7] Numerous studies in the period between 1900 and 1920 showed that of the babies who died from diarrheal disease, and especially from summer diarrhea, 80 to 90 percent had been exclusively bottle-fed.[6]

Therapy, even in the hands of one so experienced as Abraham Jacobi,[70a] remained empirical and even drastic. For example, he stated that he "rarely treated an adult or child pneumonia without digitalis." He warned the practitioner that in pneumonia, "the heart loses strength from day to day. . . . Digitalis alone may not be sufficient. Spartein sulphate should accompany it in good doses . . . big doses save your babies." In urgent cases of pneumonia, even in infants, he recommended as much as 10 grains of camphor a day and if the infant continued to fail, Jacobi recommended that the camphor be given subcutaneously "in 4 parts of sweet almond oil." All of

these things, "namely digitalis, spartein sulphate, camphor, sodio-caffeine benzoate, strychnia and alcohol," he claimed, did "no harm."

Aerotherapy, or fresh air therapy, was given almost mystical preventive and healing properties. It was believed that the course of many pediatric diseases could be favorably influenced by judicious airing, while disastrous results could ensue from its improper use.[39] Climatotherapy and heliotherapy became almost specialties in their own right, because it was both an art and a science to select the proper climate and the precise amount of sunlight in the treatment of childhood diseases such as pulmonary and bone tuberculosis, skin diseases, the anemias of childhood, and particularly rickets.

It was this belief in the beneficial effect that cool, fresh sea air would have on sick infants which led to the founding of one of our most important children's hospitals—the Boston Floating Hospital.[10] This hospital had its origin on July 25, 1894, when the rented barge *Clifford* was towed away from Pickert's Wharf in East Boston, carrying several hundred people for a day's outing—mothers, infants, crew, and medical staff. Only mothers with sick children were given tickets for the day's cruise around Boston Harbor, as it was felt that sick infants would benefit most from the salt air and harbor breezes. Until 1931, when the new Boston Floating Hospital opened its doors on dry land, the hospital remained true to its name, caring for thousands of sick infants over the years as it sailed around Boston Harbor. During its floating years the hospital made highly significant contributions to our basic knowledge of infant feeding and disease, particularly of infectious summer diarrheas and dysentery.[10]

Maternal impressions as a possible cause of malformations were still not completely discarded by some of our most respected pediatricians. For example, Benjamin K. Rachford (1857–1929)[96] in 1901 described the effects on the offspring of an appendectomy performed on the mother at the third month of pregnancy: "When the infant was 1 year old, marks resembling "stitch-scars" began to appear on the infant's abdomen. These markings became more pronounced, so that at the present time the appearance is such as would be produced by an operation for appendicitis, except there is no scar marking the line of incision."

The Milk Problem

The effect of milk on the health of children, once the relationship between bad milk and the health of children had been defined, led to two general approaches toward solving the problem of keeping milk free of disease-producing bacteria, namely, pasteurization or certification. Certified milk was nonpasteurized milk that had been produced only in carefully supervised dairies which met rigid standards set by the American Association of Medical Milk Commissions. Among these standards was that "certified milk shall contain less than 10,000 bacteria per cubic centimeter when delivered."

Prior to pasteurization, the great bulk of milk consumed by the urban poor was "grocery" or "loose" milk. Unpasteurized, originating from all sorts and conditions of dairies, and sold in dubious containers, milk was undoubtedly one of the most prolific sources of infants' and children's diseases. Milk arrived in New York City, for example, from six different states, all with different sanitary regulations and standards of enforcement, and was never less than twenty-four hours old when it entered the grocery store, to be dipped into for bulk sale. Under these circumstances, telling a tenement mother to give her child so much milk a day was like telling her to give him diluted germ culture daily.[7]

By 1910 it had become obvious that pasteurization of milk greatly reduced the "summer complaint" that annually killed an untold number of infants. In 1914 the discovery of tuberculosis in cows on a certified farm proved even more firmly that pasteurization was the only way to ensure safe milk.[6] The publication of a special bulletin, *Milk and Its Relation to the Public Health,* by the U.S. Public Health Service in 1908 was largely responsible for the general enforcement of special measures to safeguard the milk supply and to make it fit for infants and children.[7] Chemistry and the evolving science of bacteriology were essential to the solving of the milk problem. Both fields developed into modern sciences in the first quarter of the century.

The Infant and Child Welfare Movement

The concept that the health of mothers and children was a public responsibility, and as such deserved official status in public health agencies, grew slowly. It is only within the past century that the race as a whole has been seriously concerned with the care and protection of the child.[118] There is little doubt that more has been written about the child in this century than in all the preceding centuries.

In 1900 efforts directed toward the welfare of infants and children in this country were largely sporadic and disjointed. Most of the early measures designed to improve the health of mothers and children were entirely due to the pioneer work of voluntary organizations. The beginning of child welfare legislation in the United States was the act passed by the New York State Legislature in 1876 granting to the Society for the Prevention of Cruelty to Children a charter giving it wide power with regard to the protection of child life. The inception of this legislation—as has been mentioned in Chapter 5—was based upon the well-known case of little Mary Ellen, a child who was found, neglected and abused, in filthy surroundings. When it was known that a society for prevention of cruelty to animals already existed and could have cared for an animal who was found in the same unfortunate condition, it was determined that children should have at least equal protection. From this simple beginning have arisen all of our child welfare laws.[6]

The idea that the protection of motherhood was inseparably bound up with the protection of infancy was to become the keynote of modern infant welfare work. A few visionary thinkers came to realize that the most rational way to prevent prematurity, the deadly diarrheal diseases of infancy, and injurious environmental influences, which were largely responsible for poor health and death among babies, would best be accomplished through the education of the mothers.

In 1908 the Division (later Bureau) of Child Hygiene was established in the New York City Health Department, the first of its kind in the world. Its mission was to control all public health matters affecting children from birth to puberty. Among these were the regulation and standardization of obstetrical procedures, the establishment of prenatal or maternity centers, the reduction of infant mortality, the supervision of preschool children, school medical inspection, and the establishment of legal standards controlling the employment of children. Previous to 1908 there were limited types of child hygiene efforts in existence in a few of our cities but these were mainly directed toward prevention of the spread of contagious diseases among school children.[6]

S. Josephine Baker (1873–1945)[7] (Fig. 7–1), the first head of this bureau, has described the problems of a pioneer in this field in her book *Fighting for Life*. She soon found that there was no endeavor in infant welfare work that met with such instant success and was capable of such great development as the infant health center. She increased the number of infant milk stations; increased the number of trained visiting public health nurses, already under the direction of Lillian D. Wald (1867–1940) at the Henry Street Settlement for Nurses, available to make home visits to every infant out of reach of the health stations; and established the Little Mothers' League, numbering over twenty thousand schoolgirls from twelve to fourteen years of age. These girls were taught practical methods of infant hygiene and feeding and were able to help in raising infants of mothers who were forced to work. The primary purpose of the Little Mothers' League was to reduce infant sickness and death rates. The second purpose was the education of adolescent girls for potential motherhood. The league's third purpose was to have the girls carry to their own families the knowledge of enlightened child hygiene practices they had gained.

When the New York City Division of Infant Hygiene was established, there were no previous guidelines to follow. There had been only a few sporadic efforts of private organizations to solve certain problems, such as the establishment of milk stations in Cleveland, New York, Boston, Philadelphia, and Rochester, where modified milk for infant feeding was dispensed by private philanthropy to a handful of mothers, and of school medical inspection, of the most elementary type, in a few cities.[6]

The development of infant health stations began about a century ago. Starting initially as centers to dispense pure milk, modified according to set formulas supposed to be adapted to the average child at certain ages, but without any medical supervision or instruction of the mothers, these milk stations were found to be of limited value. The purest of milk improperly kept could do an immense amount of harm. In the beginning, these stations also played an unintended role in stimulating the use of artificial feeding by giving mothers a false sense of security in regard to the safety of bottle-feeding. Further, they taught the mother nothing. Moving to a place where such a milk station was not available, she was as badly off as before, if not worse off.[118]

By 1910 there were forty-two organizations maintaining some type of baby health station located in thirty different cities. There was a general tendency in time to change the name of these centers from a designation featuring milk, such as infant milk stations or depots, to one that stressed the concept of health, such as infant health stations, baby clinics, and the like. In the early milk stations physicians and nurses were rarely in attendance, though on occasion physicians were employed to care for sick children. Between 1905 and 1910 these stations in-

Figure 7–1. S. Josephine Baker (1875–1945).

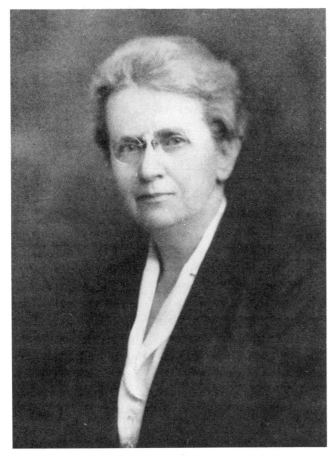

creasingly began to stress the idea of prevention of illness in infancy along with milk distribution. Almost all of these stations prior to 1911 were maintained by private subscriptions and were carried on under the auspices of private organizations. In New York City the first strictly municipal stations were organized in 1911 under the jurisdiction of the Department of Health, with the full cost of the work borne by the municipality.[6] It will be recalled that the first infant milk station in the United States was established by Nathan Straus in New York City in 1893 (p. 114).

The value of infant welfare stations in reducing infant mortality was conclusively shown by a study performed in 1911 by the New York City Milk Committee. This organization, created in 1906, was a powerful factor in stimulating better milk supply, infant welfare work, and better statistics on infant mortality. A vigorous campaign for the reduction of infant mortality was carried out through the establishment of thirty-one milk stations in the most congested districts of the city. The association also cooperated with the health department and a number of other organizations to demonstrate to the city officials that money spent for this purpose was well spent. Between June 1 and November 1, 1911, a total of 5,379 infants under a year of age came under the care of the milk stations. The mortality rate per thousand enrolled infants, however short their period of attendance and whether they died under the supervision of the stations or not, was 26.9.[4] The general infant mortality rate among unenrolled infants in these same districts for the twelve months preceding November 1, 1911, was 53.2, or 98 percent higher than for the enrolled infants. While there is the possibility of considerable error in interpreting these figures, the difference was so striking that the general result was quite convincing to the health and municipal authorities. Moreover, the Milk Committee's report showed that over a quarter of the infants under the care of the milk stations were sick on enrollment.[4]

By 1910 milk stations had been established in thirty cities with a population of over fifty thousand and several hundred in smaller communities.[6] At the outset most of these stations were open only during the summer months in an attempt to reduce the greatest cause of infant mortality, which was summer diarrhea. But it soon became evident that to accomplish permanent results the stations had to remain open all year.

The Department of Health of New York City gave as its fundamental precept: "Public Health is purchasable; within normal limitations a community can determine its own death-rate."[7] At the same time, a wellspring of interest arose in "baby-saving" as a public responsibility. It was this awakening of the public mind that caused newspapers, beginning about 1910, to print infant mortality statistics for the first time as "news" and many magazines to publish articles about baby-saving campaigns.

France and the Infant Welfare Movement

The infant welfare movement was strongly influenced by France. French physicians were the first to establish infant welfare organizations in the hope of reducing their country's inordinately high infant mortality. During the second half of the nineteenth century they had viewed with apprehension the fact that despite a high infant mortality rate the French birth rate was the lowest in Europe.[60] How to save French infants became a public question of the first importance. With a smaller loss by emigration than either Germany or England, the population of France, in the twenty years from 1891 to 1910, had increased less than a million, while during the same period Germany had grown by over fourteen million and England by over seven million.[60]

The first effort was the founding of the Société Protectrice de l'Enfance in 1865 whose chief aims were to encourage breast-feeding, to supervise the health of infants sent out to be wet-nursed, and to instruct mothers of all social classes in the care of their children. As a result of ten years' work this society was responsible for a great reduction in the infant mortality in the district in which it operated. This organization was followed in 1876 by the Society for Nursing Mothers (Société d'Allaitement Maternelle) whose aim was to encourage breast-feeding by providing health care for both the expectant and nursing mother. Visitors were sent into the home to assist mothers during the prenatal period and after confinement; facilities were also provided for expectant mothers to consult a physician from time to time during her pregnancy. Confinement homes were established and maternity grants allowed. Regular monthly observations of the infants by physicians and home visitors were provided. During a sixteen-year period the society cared for about ten thousand mothers in preconfinement homes with such excellent results that no mother received into maternity hospitals from these homes died in childbirth. There was also a perceptible improvement in the children born; they were said to be above average weight and were much more vigorous than the children of women not receiving such care. Another benefit resulting from prenatal care was a marked reduction in the neonatal mortality rate.[60]

In 1892 the first fully developed Consultation de Nourissons was opened in Paris by Pierre Constant Budin (1846–1907), a professor of obstetrics, in connection with a maternity hospital (La Charité). Its main object was the supervision and hygienic care of infants born at the hospital with great stress being placed on breast-feeding. Regular medical supervision, including measurement of height and weight, was kept up for a period of two years. The mothers were instructed in infant hygiene and feeding and advised about the treatment of minor ailments. Breast-feeding was encouraged and assisted; when it was not possible, sterilized milk in separate feeding bottles was supplied. The great advantage secured by this plan was continuous educated supervision of the mother, and through the mother, the care of the infant from its birth. Under this kind of supervision, infant mortality was reduced in less than five years from 178 to 46 per 1,000 live births.[60]

In 1894 the first Goutte de Lait was established by Leon Dufour, a doctor in the small Norman town of Fechamp. Its purpose was proper artificial feeding under medical supervision. Dufour was the first to give the name Goutte de Lait to these milk stations. He was successful in reducing infant mortality from diarrheal diseases to 2.8 percent. The mortality from these affections in Rouen, Bolbec, and Le Havre had been as high as 76.6 percent and 51.2 percent.[15] While in the Consultation de Nourissons the majority of the infants were breast-fed, the opposite was true in the Goutte de Lait. There, almost all of the infants were bottle-fed. In time these two organizations, the Consultation and the Goutte de Lait, were merged into one. They may truly be considered as marking the beginning of the modern movement for the reduction of infant mortality.

Establishment of the U.S. Children's Bureau

The National Child Labor Committee, begun in 1904 by four women advocates of reform and promotion of child health, was an influential and vigorous forum in stimulating a drive for the establishment of a national children's bureau. The women were Florence Kelley (1859–1932), a factory inspector in Illinois and founder of the National Consumer's League; Grace Abbott (1878–1939), head of the Immigrants' Protection League; Julia Lathrop (1858–1932), who was to become the first chief of the Children's Bureau; and Lillian Wald, director and founder of the Henry Street Settlement in New York. This committee pointed to the dearth of national statistics about the health of American children and urged the federal government to investigate the welfare of children and to gather data about infant mortality.[6] The committee also pointed out that the federal government knew much more about fish and wildlife, and even the boll weevil, than it did about the numbers of children who were born or died, because no government agency kept such statistics. Forceful impetus for the Committee's efforts came from the first White House Conference on Children and Youth, called by President Theodore Roosevelt in 1909. The theme of this conference was the dependent child. It resulted in fifteen recommendations, the most important of which called for the formation of a Children's Bureau as the first national activity directed toward child welfare.

After six years of debate, much of it acrimonious, legislation was finally passed in 1912 creating the Children's Bureau within the Department of Labor. In 1913 the bureau was allowed an appropriation of only twenty-five thousand dollars to carry out its work and was charged with the obligation to investigate and report on all matters affecting children and child life.[118]

Once the Children's Bureau was established, it set out as its top priority the promotion of birth registration as a means of attacking infant mortality, and by 1915 thirty-two states had enacted laws and procedures ensuring reasonably accurate records. The Census Bureau had been authorized in 1902 to issue statistics on births and deaths, but the accuracy of these data depended on local compliance, and many states had no birth-registration laws.[18] It would not be until the late 1920's that the Birth-Registration Area was complete.[6]

A second objective of the Children's Bureau was to investigate in detail for the first time the infant mortality rates in certain industrial towns. A 1913 study of Johnstown, Pennsylvania, involved interviewing the mother of every child born in 1911, whether the child was living or dead.[31] The infant mortality rate was found to be lower for babies delivered by physicians than for those delivered by midwives. The highest infant mortality rate was noted in mothers over forty years of age and the lowest in mothers from twenty to twenty-four years of age. As had been expected, but not previously documented statistically, children of newer immigrants, of illiterates, and of those who could not speak English had the highest infant mortality; these were generally the poorest families housed in the most unsanitary and unhealthful parts of the city.

The infant mortality varied inversely with the father's annual earnings from 197.3 per 1,000 for fathers with an annual income under $521.00 to 102.2 per 1,000 for those with an annual income of $1,200 and over, and there was a definite correlation between infant and maternal mortality. Low income was the underlying factor in high infant mortality.[31] From this study and others like it the Children's Bureau concluded that prenatal care would be the most direct way to improve the health of mothers and infants. Laws forbidding the employment of women for a stated period before and after childbirth had been enacted in only five of our states by 1919—in Massachusetts in 1911, in New York in 1912, in Connecticut and Vermont in 1913, and in Missouri in 1919.[6] The periods varied during which gainful employment was forbidden, ranging from two to four weeks before, and from four to six weeks after confinement. In none of these laws was there any provision for payment of wages or maternity benefits during this period of enforced idleness.

The bureau, in conjunction with the emerging feminist movement and a few socially directed physicians, began a campaign for federal legislation to provide funds for states to educate women about prenatal and postnatal care. The proponents could now use deaths of men in battle in World War I as a standard of comparison by pointing out that childbirth was a battleground every bit as dangerous as had been the trenches in France. Josephine Baker,[5] although stretching her statistics a bit, offered this telling comparison: "During the nineteen months we were at war [World War I], for every soldier who died as a result of wounds, one mother in the United States went down into the valley of the shadow and did not return." By 1921 the efforts of these socially minded proponents led to the passage of the Sheppard-Towner Act, or "the Act for the Promotion of the Welfare of Maternity and Infancy." This was one of the earliest health acts of the federal government and was meant to benefit poor women and their children; it also provoked the first public assertions that health care should be the right of every citizen regardless of background. This act provided grants to states to develop health services for mothers and children and soon led to the establishment in almost every state of a division of maternal and child health. It is of interest that every state accepted these grants except Massachusetts, where the organized medical lobby in opposition to the act was strongest.[123]

The Sheppard-Towner Act was attacked and vigorously denounced in Congress as "socialistic" and was accused of being "drawn chiefly from the radical, socialistic, Bolshevistic philosophy of Germany and Russia." The American Medical Association denounced it as an "imported socialistic scheme." By the end of the 1920's opponents of grants-in-aid for maternity and infant care prevailed, at least for the time being, and the Sheppard-Towner Act lapsed in 1929. Federal involvement in maternity care came to an end until 1935, when the Social Security Act revived it.

Pediatrics and the Child Welfare Movement

At the first meeting of the American Pediatric Society, held in September, 1889, in the library of the Surgeon General's office in Washington, D.C., Jacobi, in his presidential address, "The Relations of Pediatrics to General Medicine," outlined a broader field for pediatrics than just the advancement of physiology, pathology, and therapeutics of infancy and childhood, the society's goal as outlined in its constitution. Jacobi was by temperament socially minded and prophetically pointed out the preventive medical benefits of organized medical inspection and health supervision of schoolchildren long before they became *faits accomplis*. Jacobi also stressed the importance of the society's participating in the solution of public health problems of the day so as to raise "the standard of physical and mental health to possible perfection thereby contributing to the welfare and happiness of the people." Samuel McC. Hamill (1864–1948) termed this address "Jacobi's first epistle to the pediatrists."

Walter S. Christopher (1859–1905), in his presidential address at the 1902 meeting of the American Pediatric Society, stated that "pediatrics is preventive medicine of the highest order." This, with the exception of Jacobi's address, was the first reference to preventive medicine, health, or hygiene in any paper presented up to that time to that society.[35]

Two years later August Caillé[18] spoke about the broader field of child welfare as distinguished from clinical pediatrics. His main topic was the need for improvement of conditions in the public schools as they affected the health of children; this was to be achieved by daily inspections of children for infectious diseases and parasites, by properly designed desks, by encouragement of proper posture, and by the detection of defects in the children's vision and hearing. He saw the society as a potent influence to shape and promote the public understanding of the nature of child health and education. "Pediatric societies," he said, "should be the guardians of our children in all sanitary questions."

Pediatrics and Social Reform

At the 1909 meeting of the American Pediatric Society the members who attended were challenged by Thomas Morgan Rotch[100] in his leadoff address, "The Position and Work of the American Pediatric Society Toward Public Questions," to direct the society to assume an active role in social and public welfare work, such as child labor legislation, and in the assessment of fitness of schoolchildren for their tasks, either in school or at work. Rotch vigorously defended this course by declaring that "prophylaxis is the greatest principle of medical work of the future." Many in discussing the paper agreed with him, but not L. Emmett Holt, who felt that he would "feel sorry to see a large part of the work of this Society devoted to subjects of this kind, which, though of sociologic interest, are not so much along

the line of work of most of us as other matters more strongly medical: I believe we can do our best work along lines of research." Isaac Abt agreed with Holt in not wishing to see the society enter the sociologic area. "It seems to me," he noted, that "it is our mission to stimulate and encourage scientific work to the very highest degree. It should be the farthest from our purpose to become entangled in political or legislative questions." John Lovett Morse concurred with Holt and Abt. Linnaeus LaFétra, on the other hand, sided with Rotch because he believed the American Pediatric Society should take the lead in developing programs to protect the child. He mentioned child labor, ophthalmia neonatorum, epidemic vulvovaginitis, and school health supervision.

Rotch, in closing the lively discussion, insisted that to him his paper pertained as much to medicine as any scientific paper anyone could have presented and argued that if the society as a whole did not lend its influence to broad questions of this kind connected with pediatrics, these questions would then be discussed and acted upon elsewhere.

By 1923 Holt had radically changed his views since he had discussed Rotch's paper fourteen years before. In his 1923 presidential address, "American Pediatrics: A Retrospect and a Forecast," Holt[62] wrote: "We must be teachers and leaders in all subjects related to the growth and health of children. This field we have neglected in the past; we have left the subject of popular health education too much to the nurse, the social worker and the nutrition worker, and some of these groups, largely owing to our neglect, have gotten somewhat out of hand."

By 1930 when President Herbert Hoover called the third White House Conference on Children and Youth, devoted to the growth and development of children, pediatricians made up almost all of the participants. Involvement in problems of public health and social reform had now been accepted by most pediatricians as an important and necessary part of their professional lives.

The value of child hygiene activities in this country was recognized by private organizations and interested individuals long before it became a subject of governmental concern. Similar experience has been the rule in nearly all of our great matters of public welfare. Governments are slow to act and nearly every great welfare movement has received its first impetus from private initiative. A case in point was the American Association for Study and Prevention of Infant Mortality, which was organized in New Haven, Connecticut, on November 12, 1909. This was the first nationwide association to stimulate interest in the study and prevention of infant mortality; it had a profound influence in bringing about registration of all infant births and deaths in this country, records of which until then had not been kept. Until 1900, the Census Bureau was not even a permanent organization. The population was enumerated and classified each ten years, and that was all.

The object of the American Association for Study and Prevention of Infant Mortality was to direct public attention to the problem of infant mortality and bring together the experiences of various agencies—governmental, philanthropic, social, and medical—concerned with infant mortality.

As time went on, the objectives originally sought by this society were widened into many more and greater goals for child welfare. In 1919, the association changed its name to the American Child Hygiene Association, a name which by that time was far more descriptive of its aims and objectives, and in 1923 merged with the Child Hygiene Organization of America, formed in 1918 to study the health of the schoolchild, to become the American Child Health Association. Its record was one of great accomplishments for child welfare. In 1935, it voted to

dissolve. Its school health interests were passed on to the National Education Association and all other interests to the American Public Health Association. Private organizations such as the Commonwealth Fund and the Russell Sage Foundation were also active in child health work.

Reduction in Mortality Figures

The mortality figures for children under five years of age for New York City (boroughs of Manhattan and the Bronx) for two years, 1921 and 1922, showed some interesting comparisons with those of 1896–1897, a quarter of a century earlier. While the population under five years of age had increased from 225,000 to 297,000, or 32 percent, the actual number of deaths under five had decreased from 32,202 to 28,519 and the death rate had fallen from 14.3 to 9.6 percent.

Table 7–1 lists the ten most common causes of death for these two periods in children under five years of age. The most striking change in those twenty-five years was that the actual deaths from diarrheal diseases in children under five had dropped from 7,224 to 1,942. By 1921–1922, diarrheal diseases, which had occupied first place in mortality figures for this period of life as long as our records had been available, had now fallen to third place,

Table 7–1. The Ten Most Common Causes of Death in Children under Five Years of Age in the Boroughs of Manhattan and the Bronx, 1896–1897 and 1921–1922.

Rank	1896–1897 Cause	Deaths	1921–1922 Cause	Deaths
1.	Diarrheal diseases	7,224	Malformations and diseases of early infancy	4,972
2.	Malformations and diseases of early infancy	5,841	Pneumonias	3,413
3.	Pneumonias	5,169	Diarrheal diseases	1,942
4.	Diphtheria and croup	2,703	Measles	694
5.	Acute bronchitis	1,892	Diphtheria and croup	677
6.	Measles	1,042	Whooping cough	337
7.	Convulsions	1,010	Tuberculous meningitis	294
8.	Tuberculous meningitis	919	Scarlet fever	240
9.	Whooping cough	719	Acute bronchitis	171
10.	Scarlet fever	655	Convulsions	24
	Totals	32,202		28,519
	Estimated population under five years of age	225,000		297,000
	Death rate under five years of age (%)	14		9.6

Source: L. Emmett Holt. Trans. Am. Pediatr. Soc. 35:9, 1923. Reprinted by permission.

and malformations and diseases of early infancy headed the list as causes of death in children under five years of age, with pneumonia in second place.

The Emergence of Biochemical Research in Pediatrics

Biochemical investigation in pediatrics began during the first two decades of this century with the establishment of two research laboratories: the first, in 1910, by Holt at the Babies Hospital in New York, with the aid of the Rockefeller Institute for Medical Research, and the second, in 1912, by John Howland (1873–1926) at the Harriet Lane Home in Baltimore. Both men brought the beginnings of academic medicine to pediatrics because of their belief that scientific progress in pediatrics had to be built on integration with the basic sciences. This new emphasis on laboratory investigation led to major discoveries in the fields of immunology, serology, and biochemistry.

L. Emmett Holt

Beginning in 1911 the first of a series of biochemical studies appeared from Holt's laboratory. The problems which interested Holt and his colleagues were biochemical, but since he lacked special training in biochemistry, he appointed to his staff two highly experienced chemists, Angelia Courtney and Helen Fales. A score of studies, published jointly from the Rockefeller Institute and Babies Hospital, bearing the names of Holt, Courtney, and Fales, or of Holt and Fales, were the result. These papers dealt with problems encountered in infant feeding, such as the composition of casein curds, chemical analyses of human milk, the excretion of sodium chloride solution injected subcutaneously in severe diarrhea or protracted vomiting, the absorption under varying conditions of calcium and fat, the electrolyte losses in diarrheal versus normal stools, and the effects of high protein intake in the infant's diet.

John Howland

Howland, one of Holt's former associates, came to Baltimore from St. Louis in 1912 to succeed Clemens von Pirquet (1874–1926) as full-time head of

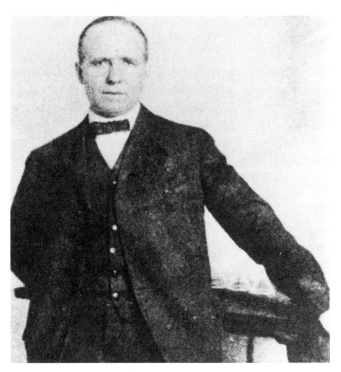

Figure 7–2. John Howland (1873–1926).

the Pediatric Department of the Johns Hopkins Medical School. Von Pirquet, an Austrian, had been appointed professor of pediatrics in 1908 when he was thirty-four years of age. He occupied the chair of pediatrics from 1909 to 1910. No building existed for pediatric patients at that time, and the Harriet Lane Home was not ready to receive patients until 1912.[91] At the end of the year 1910 von Pirquet asked for a leave of absence and went to Breslau, Germany, where he had been called to the chair of pediatrics vacated by Czerny, with the understanding that if he found the position not to his liking, he would return to Baltimore at the end of the year. While at Breslau, von Pirquet was appointed director of the Imperial Pediatric Clinic of the University of Vienna—the foremost pediatric clinic in the world at the time. Although he had accepted the chair of pediatrics at Vienna, he still expressed his willingness to return to Johns Hopkins. He wrote that he had no interest in medical practice and that he would accept the professorship at a salary of ten thousand dollars a year, but the board of trustees would offer him no more than eight thousand. According to Edwards A. Park,[91] this was the reason von Pirquet did not return to Baltimore.

During the decade and a half following Howland's arrival in Baltimore, pediatric biochemistry was solidly established as a vital component of pediatrics. Actually, the transition from unsupported individual effort to the combined attack of well-equipped laboratories as we know them today can be attributed to Howland. He, even more than Holt, has been acclaimed as the founder of academic pediatrics in this country and a pioneer in the full-time movement. Much of the basic work in pediatrics during this period was performed by Howland and the extraordinarily talented young men associated with him in the Harriet Lane Home. He more than anyone else perceived the importance of chemistry for the investigation of disease in children. His studies on acidosis, rickets, and tetany were to become landmarks in the history of pediatrics.

Within a few years Howland's staff consisted of a number of exceptional men, each of whom contributed enormously to pediatrics. Edwards A. Park (Fig. 7–7) joined him as chief of the outpatient department and Kenneth Blackfan (1883–1941) was appointed chief resident on the inpatient service. Grover Powers joined the group in 1913, William McKim Marriott (1885–1936) (Fig. 7–4) in 1914, and James L. Gamble (1883–1959) in 1915. Marriott left in 1917 to become professor of pediatrics at Washington University, and Benjamin Kramer (1882–1972) (Fig. 7–6) replaced him.[53]

A landmark paper in the history of American pediatrics was Howland and Marriott's[64] study of severe diarrhea in infancy, in which they proved that infants with this disease were in a state of acidosis and furthermore that the acidosis was not due to organic acids. This paper, presented at the 1915 meeting of the American Pediatric Society, gave an explanation differing from the existing one suggested by Heinrich Finkelstein, of the Kaiser and Kaiserin Friedrich Children's Hospital of Berlin, for the symptoms of what was then commonly termed "alimentary intoxication," namely, marked dyspnea without signs of respiratory obstruction, restlessness, stupor, and even coma. Finkelstein had attributed these symptoms observed in some infants suffering from severe diarrhea to the toxic effects of intermediary products of metabolism. Howland and Marriott, however, proved that these symptoms were due to loss of base, thus producing a state of acidosis in the infant. To prove this they demon-

strated an increase of urinary ammonia, a marked reduction in carbon dioxide tension in the alveolar air, an increase in the hydrogen-ion concentration of the blood, and a significant increase in the amount of sodium bicarbonate required to alkalinize the urine, which was highly acid.[65] They found they could correct the acidosis in part or wholly by administration of sodium bicarbonate, preferably intravenously, or if this was not possible, subcutaneously.[64] However, Howland and Marriott admitted that the "acidosis may be entirely overcome, and yet death ensue as a result of it," because "it probably initiates many abnormal processes that we do not understand and that we have no way of overcoming." Their conclusion was that it was not the intermediary products of metabolism that were involved; "indeed, all proof of their presence is lacking. The condition depends on acidosis such as is found in cholera and a variety of other different diseases. This condition should not be, therefore, termed a food intoxication," for it is not "due to the presence of abnormal substances— it is the absence of substances that are very normal and very necessary to life."

A few years later, Marriott[83,84] enlarged and strengthened his explanation of these symptoms by demonstrating the critically important role played by anhydremia in infants with severe diarrhea. Marriott thus supplied the concept missing from previous studies of fluid replacement therapy, which had failed to recognize the importance of the physiologic dimension of volume.

Oscar Schloss

At about the same time, Oscar Schloss (1882–1952)[105] (Fig. 7–3), of New York, had also discovered the presence of acidosis in infants and children with so-called "alimentary intoxication." Learning that Howland and Marriott had made independent studies with similar results, Schloss generously withheld his publication until theirs had appeared, in order to give them the priority which he felt they deserved.[47] This was an act of courtesy that was perhaps more common among physicians a generation or so ago than would be the case today.

Schloss made a number of outstanding contributions to our understanding of the physiological imbalance in infants with diarrhea. He described the importance of acidosis in infants with diarrheal dis-

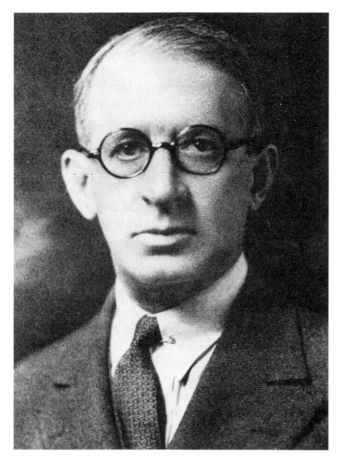

Figure 7–3. Oscar M. Schloss (1882–1952).

tant paper which described the importance of impaired renal function in explaining the development of structural defects in the body fluids. The understanding of events in dehydration offered by these studies clearly demonstrated the urgency for replacement of fluid losses. He prophetically noted that "pediatric literature contains many references to protein, sugar, and fat but contains very little about water."[103]

Marriott's Studies on Acid-Base Balance and Water Loss

In 1919 Marriott[83] presented his paper "The Pathogenesis of Certain Nutritional Disorders." Faber and McIntosh[35] have written that with this "revolutionary paper," Marriott, at one stroke, finally "destroyed a long-established misconception and initiated new and effective therapy in the depleting nutritional disorders of infants and children." The misconception, already mentioned, was Finkelstein's

Figure 7–4. William McKim Marriott (1885–1936).

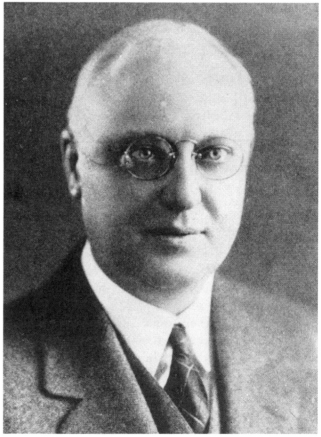

orders in 1917,[105] and in 1919 his paper with Helen Harrington (b. 1890)[104] compared the carbon dioxide tension of the alveolar air and the hydrogen-ion concentration of the urine with the bicarbonate of the blood plasma, using the newly developed method of Donald D. Van Slyke (1883–1971) and those of Howland and Marriott and others. The purpose of the latter paper was to apply these methods as a guide to regulating the dosage of sodium bicarbonate in the treatment of acidosis. Schloss[105] also noted: "In our experience the most satisfactory method of administration is by intravenous injection." This is one of the first times that the intravenous route was suggested in American pediatric literature. Schloss's studies were major contributions to pediatrics, and they enhanced and confirmed the importance of Howland and Marriott's earlier paper on the same subject.

Schloss[103] in 1918 published an extremely impor-

alimentär intoxikation or "alimentary intoxication." Contrary to Finkelstein's explanation, Marriott[84] explained the whole clinical picture as the consequence of acidosis accompanied with water loss and the resulting anhydremia. He developed his theory in the following logical and sequential steps: (a) The blood of these patients is invariably concentrated; (b) the diminished blood volume leads to diminished tissue oxidation, resulting in the accumulation of acid end products; (c) oliguria which follows causes retention of metabolic end products, including acids, leading to "a double explanation of the acidosis and the accompanying symptoms of air hunger and coma"; (d) the blood concentration causes arteriolar constriction and the accumulation of corpuscles in the "rather stagnant capillary blood; this explains the peculiar grayish color of the skin of the infants suffering from this condition;" and (e) the greatly diminished blood volume explains the hypotension. Marriott then proved conclusively that when it was possible to administer sufficient water to cause a return of the blood concentration to normal, all the symptoms abated.

He found that the "most effective method of administering fluid, when but little is retained by the alimentary canal, is by intraperitoneal injections of saline at frequent intervals, and intravenous injections of hypertonic glucose or glucose-acacia solutions." Marriott also recognized that anhydremia could result from causes other than diarrhea, such as persistent vomiting or septic conditions, and could occur in the course of pneumonia and scarlet fever, but he added that no matter what the cause, "the symptoms are the same."

Marriott's demonstration of the large reduction[84] in blood volume in dehydrated infants confirmed the urgent need to replace the infant's fluid and electrolyte losses. His studies reawakened interest in the long-forgotten publication of the first observations pointing to the existence of an acid-base disturbance with loss of body water from the blood, which were contained in a letter of about a hundred and sixty words by William B. O'Shaughnessy (1809–1889),[86] dated December 29, 1831, to the editor of the *Lancet*. O'Shaughnessy's letter described the condition of patients suffering from asiatic cholera, which at the time was epidemic in England. His letter contained an extraordinary amount of information. He identified "carbonate of soda" as the alkali and mea-

sured its loss in the stools. He also observed the loss of "neutral saline ingredients" in the water content of the serum, and gave a quantitative measurement of the degree of desiccation that was suffered in the loss of water that went with the salt and carbonate.[119]

There was almost immediate clinical application of O'Shaughnessy's observations about therapy by Thomas Latta (?1798–1833),[80] of Leith, Scotland, who successfully treated a patient with cholera on the basis of O'Shaughnessy's observations by injecting intravenously ten liters of a solution containing sodium chloride and sodium bicarbonate in the first ten hours of the disease. To Latta belongs the credit of having been the first to employ intravenous injection of a solution of sodium salts to replace losses incurred in severe diarrhea. The solution which Latta used contained about 0.4 percent sodium chloride and 0.3 percent sodium bicarbonate, so that it was an approximately isotonic solution.[44a]

With the passing of the cholera epidemic, O'Shaughnessy's and Latta's reports were forgotten until 1892, when Arnoldo Cantani, during an epidemic of cholera in Naples, once again called attention to the fluid and salt loss and to the value of parenteral fluid therapy (page 114). Indeed, it was not until Marriott directly measured the large reduction of the volume of blood in dehydrated infants that circulatory failure was recognized as the immediately dangerous event in infant diarrhea, and it soon became clear that volume was the critical dimension of effective replacement therapy. Marriott[84] showed that "the whole clinical picture could be explained as the result of loss of water and the resulting anhydremia."

Marriott spent only three years with Howland from 1914 to 1917 when he left Baltimore to become professor of pediatrics at Washington University in St. Louis, where he continued to produce many important contributions to pediatrics, among them his classic studies in the field of infant feeding. These are discussed in Chapter 10.

James L. Gamble

James Gamble joined Howland's staff in January of 1915 after having spent the previous five years in Boston developing his knowledge of the quantitative techniques used by the biochemist and physiologist in the study of disease. He worked in Otto Folin's (1867–1934) laboratory, where simple chemical procedures applicable to the study of metabolic processes in man were being developed, and then with Fritz B. Talbot (1878–1964) at the Massachusetts General Hospital, where his first undertaking was to study the effect of various protein intakes in infants upon the partition of nitrogen end products in the urine, as Folin had done in the adult.

Gamble later came under the tutelage of Lawrence J. Henderson (1878–1942), from whom he received additional training in biochemistry. Henderson, particularly, stimulated his interest in the problems of electrolyte physiology. Largely inspired by Henderson, Gamble decided to dedicate his professional life "to the study of diseases by means of chemistry." He modestly attributed his success to the coincidence "that the abrupt and rapid development in this country of quantitative methods of studying disease in the clinic came just as I was finishing my interne years."[44]

At first Howland assigned Gamble to the outpatient department for half of his time with the freedom to carry on his research in the other half. Six months after his arrival in Baltimore, Gamble decided to give up a career in clinical medicine. Thus, the influence of L. J. Henderson continued to play a guiding role in his life.

Howland's interest in the treatment of epilepsy by the ketosis of starvation stimulated Gamble[45] to work on this problem with two Canadian members of Howland's staff—S. Graham Ross (b. 1888) and Frederick F. Tisdall (1893–1949). Gamble was alert to the possibilities which this therapeutic regimen offered for the exploration of the responses and defenses of the body in acidosis. The design of the study, which began in 1919 and was finally published in 1922, was simple. Since there was no food intake or feces, the balance studies could be carried out by measurements of the daily urine collections and the blood plasma. The experiments, however, were laborious and required nearly two years to complete, and the analytical determinations were said to be tedious beyond belief.

Robert Loeb (1895–1973)[81] described the importance of Gamble's study as follows:

These experiments constituted a pioneer approach to the interpretation of quantitative description in terms of

the mechanisms involved. Meaning received the primary emphasis. . . . The general design of the experiments devised by Gamble continues to be the pattern for most studies dealing with electrolyte and water metabolism today. Even the expression of data by simple graphic means, now known as Gambelian diagrams or Gamblegrams, has been generally adopted and is a blessing for students, teachers and investigators alike.

Gamble's last paper on work done at Baltimore was presented at the 1923 meeting of the American Pediatric Society. In this study on the manner of the therapeutic action in tetany of substances producing hydrochloric acid, illustrated for the first time with the now well-known Gamblegrams, he showed how calcium chloride, ammonium chloride, and hydrochloric acid alike produced a lowering of plasma bicarbonate with a simultaneous increase in chloride and a reduction of pH, increasing the ionization of calcium and so inducing relief of tetany.[35]

In 1922, at the invitation of Schloss, who had recently been appointed professor of pediatrics at the

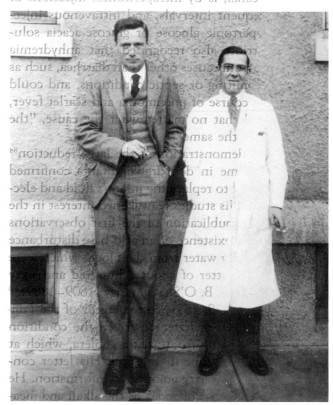

Figure 7–5. James L. Gamble (1883–1959) and Kenneth D. Blackfan (1883–1941) at the Children's Hospital, Boston, c. 1924–1925.

Harvard Medical School, Gamble left Baltimore and returned to Boston, the scene of his early training. But within the year Schloss decided to return to New York; he was succeeded in 1923 by Blackfan. Gamble and Blackfan were to spend the rest of their professional lives at the Boston Children's Hospital (Fig. 7–5). Gamble held the post of Director of the Metabolic Research Laboratory at the Children's Hospital.

Perhaps the greatest service performed by Gamble, according to Talbot,[116] was his ability to devise methods of translating biological equilibrium into terms which the average clinician could understand. He clarified the role of bicarbonate of soda in acidosis and alkalosis, demonstrated the changes in the electrolyte structure of the blood plasma in many clinical conditions, and brought out the important fact that when sodium chloride is introduced into the body, both sodium, the base, and chloride, the acid, can act independently.

Benjamin Kramer

Benjamin Kramer succeeded Marriott as a biochemist on Howland's staff. Shortly after Kramer came to Hopkins in 1918, he developed micromethods for analysis of inorganic ions in serum, particularly calcium and magnesium, which opened up new fields in the metabolic studies of children. Without these micromethods the studies on rickets would not have been possible. Park,[91] who believed that "Kramer was a far abler chemist than Marriott," wrote that "Gamble once stated that Ross, Tisdall, and he could never have performed their classic studies on the metabolism of starvation had it not been for the necessary micro-methods by Kramer." One of the immediate results from Kramer's technique was the discovery that rickets was characterized by a low plasma phosphorus.

Kramer left the Harriet Lane Home in 1923 to accept the positions of chief of pediatrics at the Brooklyn Jewish Hospital and of professor of pediatrics at the Long Island College of Medicine, which is now part of the State University of New York. He continued his interest in the application of chemistry to the diagnosis and study of disease, especially disorders of mineralization. Kramer later published many studies on the mechanism of calcification and of the

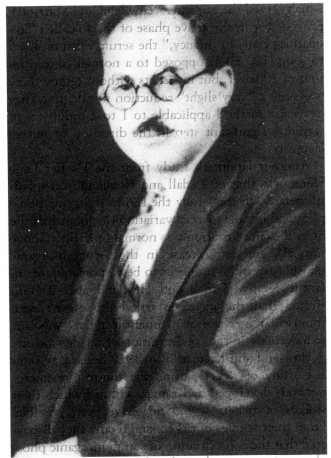

Figure 7–6. Benjamin Kramer (1882–1972).

biochemical behavior of lead in relation to calcium and phosphorus metabolism and vitamin D action.[53]

Rickets

The key to the problem of rickets was to learn what prevented the deposition of calcium salts into the bone and bone-forming cartilage. This was to be the second great triumph of the Harriet Lane staff. Howland and Marriott began their study on this problem in 1914; the first requisite was to be able to determine the concentration of the elements which made up the major part of the inorganic salts of bone, namely calcium and phosphorus in the fluid from which the bones received them. There were no techniques then available to detect these substances in the small amounts of blood that could be safely obtained from infants. This forced Marriott and Howland to develop methods, later greatly improved, which served the purpose.[53] Howland and Marriott[67] proved that in the active phase of the so-called "idiopathic tetany of infancy," the serum calcium was 5 to 7 mg/100 ml as opposed to a normal concentration of 10 to 11, but in rickets without tetany there was only a "very slight" reduction in calcium. They devised a method applicable to 1 to 2 milliliters of serum, a significant step in the direction of microchemistry.

Another landmark study from the Harriet Lane Home was that of Tisdall and Howland[75] on infantile tetany. In this study the serum inorganic phosphorus showed a marked variation (in about half the cases the concentration was normal or slightly above normal), and an increase in the serum inorganic phosphorus did not appear to be responsible for infantile tetany. Tisdall and Howland also demonstrated that the increased irritability of the neuromuscular mechanism in infantile tetany was due to a decrease in the concentration of serum calcium.

Howland and Kramer[68,69] in 1919 began a systematic study of rickets, using the innovative micromethods developed by Kramer, without which their studies of rickets would not have been possible. From their studies of rickets and tetany they discovered that the concentration of serum inorganic phosphorus in uncomplicated rickets was much lower than normal.[68] In the seventy-two cases observed, the average concentration of inorganic phosphorus was 2.0 mg/100 ml, a reduction of more than 50 percent. In the same cases, the average for calcium was 9.6 mg/100 ml, a reduction of only about 5 percent. They also noted that the determining factor in the calcification of bones in rickets was the presence of calcium and phosphorus in "such amounts that the product of their concentration in milligrams per 100 cc of serum equals a certain minimal figure which lies between 30 and 40."[69] They also discovered that calcium therapy alone would not "cure the concomitant rickets." These authors also found that the fall in the serum phosphorus could be prevented by giving the patient cod-liver oil or by employing ultraviolet rays.

Howland and Kramer[69] observed that during the process of healing, when occurring either spontaneously or as a result of administering cod-liver oil, the phosphorus content of the serum would gradually rise to a normal level; relapses were accompanied by a fall in the phosphorus concentration in the serum.

This work had immense importance in the understanding of rickets. Previously, all attention had been concentrated on the disturbances of calcium metabolism; no one had thought that the phosphorus metabolism might be affected or that the morphological changes in bone might be dependent on low phosphorus concentration in the tissue fluids.

Edwards A. Park

Following the untimely death of Howland at the age of fifty-three, Park, whose association with the Harriet Lane Home had begun with the advent of Howland, was selected to be his successor. Park had received his M.D. from the Columbia College of Physicians and Surgeons in 1903. While spending a six-month residency at the New York Foundling Hospital in 1905, he met Howland, who was an attending physician. Park then returned to the College

Figure 7–7. Edwards A. Park (1877–1969).

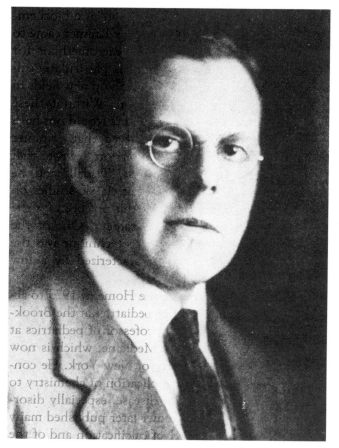

of Physicians and Surgeons as an instructor in medicine and pediatrics. He shared an office with Theodore C. Janeway (1872–1917) and worked with him for three years on a number of experimental studies, including the indirect measurement of blood pressure in man. This was Park's first venture in research. In 1912 he was invited to join Howland in Baltimore, but before moving to Baltimore he spent a year in Germany in the laboratory of the pathologist Martin B. Schmidt (1863–1949) at Marburg.[53] Here Park learned the intricacies of bone growth and how this growth was disrupted by disease. For the rest of his life he remained intensely devoted to this field of study. He was one of the very few investigators who could correlate the histological changes in bone with the clinical, biochemical, and radiological changes. Howland, Park, Kramer, Paul G. Shipley, (1888–1934), and Elmer V. McCollum (1879–1967) (Fig. 7–8) made many important contributions to the study of rickets, culminating in 1923 in the discovery of vitamin D.

Elmer V. McCollum

McCollum's[85] description of a study by the Johns Hopkins group of the cause, prevention, and cure of experimental rickets in young rats is among the most significant contributions ever made to American pediatrics. As a result of this study, physicians promptly adopted cod-liver oil as an effective means of preventing rickets in infants and children.

McCollum's[85] description of the unraveling of the pathogenesis of experimental rickets is as follows:

In September 1918, Dr. John R. Howland, Pediatrician-in-Chief of the Johns Hopkins Hospital, asked me whether I thought anyone had ever produced rickets experimentally in an animal. I expressed surprise that he, who knew all that was known about the disease, should ask the opinion of a chemist who made no pretensions to knowledge of any segment of pathology. I said, however, that we believed we had observed the rachitic state in young rats fed certain diets, and that we had such animals at that time. I invited him to the rat colony, where we exhibited two young rats which showed the deformities of the thorax and beading of the ribs on which we had concluded that the condition was indeed rickets. Dr. Howland exhibited great interest in the animals. He said

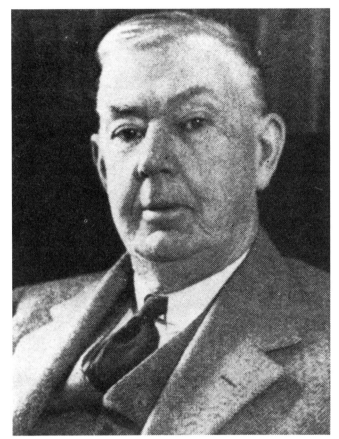

Figure 7–8. Elmer V. McCollum (1879–1967).

that what we showed him was essentially like severe grades of rickets in infants and asked how we produced it. We described the diet of cereals to which the animals had been restricted. Furthermore, I was able to show him other rats on the same seed diet modified by certain supplements, which not only showed no signs of rickets or other skeletal abnormalities, but were well developed adult animals capable of reproduction and rearing of young. Obviously we were in a position to make a searching inquiry as to the factor or factors supplied by the effective supplements which prevented the bone defects. . . .

By 1922 we had fed young rats more than three hundred experimental diets. Five or six rats from each group were delivered for histologic study. Only then did we begin to study our extensive data.

I selected perhaps a dozen group numbers, the diets of which varied in a systematic way, and Drs. Park and Shipley, Miss Simmonds, and I met for conference in the room where the sections were stored. I would call for a certain number, and the box containing the sections would be produced. A mounted section would be placed under the microscope and Drs. Park and Shipley would examine it and call attention to the amounts of resting and vesicular cartilage; the extent, if any, of provisional calcification of vesicular cartilage; the number of bone trabeculae, if any, present in the region of growth; the presence or absence of osteoid tissue surrounding bone trabeculae; the arrangement of blood vessels in the section; evidence as to whether capillaries were invading the cartilage of the diaphyseal border; and so on. We thus listened for the first time to descriptions which revealed an astonishing response of different histologic elements to abnormalities in the diet. . . .

Important conclusions were warranted, the most important of which were:

(a) That the ratio between calcium and phosphorus in the diet is of great physiologic importance. A low-phosphorus, high-calcium, or a low-calcium, high-phosphorus, ratio perverts the process of bone growth and favors the appearance of characteristics of rickets. The latter also causes lowering of serum calcium and induces tetany.

(b) That cod-liver oil contains an organic substance which exercises a profound influence in directing the processes of bone growth along normal lines even when the calcium:phosphorus ratio is unfavorable. This substance is present in butterfat but in very small amounts as compared with cod-liver oil. Lard, olive oil, and many other fats and oils exert no influence on bone growth because of the absence of the organic factor found abundantly in cod-liver oil. Both cod-liver oil and butterfat, when included in a diet, protect animals against the xerophthalmia due to vitamin A deficiency. When each of these fats was treated with a stream of hot air bubbled through the sample, vitamin A was destroyed, and neither fat so-treated prevented xerophthalmia. However, the rickets-preventing property was left unimpaired by oxidation.

Hence we concluded that the rickets-preventive factor was distinct from vitamin A. Since it was the fourth vitamin to be discovered, we called it by the corresponding letter of the alphabet, vitamin D.

Alfred F. Hess

The history of rickets during the first quarter of the century would be incomplete without mentioning the important contributions Alfred F. Hess (Fig. 7–9) made to our understanding of this disease. Besides his many clinical observations on both rickets and scurvy, he discovered that antirachitic proper-

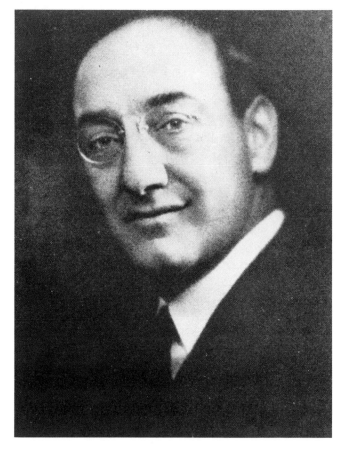

Figure 7–9. Alfred F. Hess (1875–1933).

ties could be imparted to certain oils and to food by exposing them to ultraviolet rays. He was also the first physician in this country to discover the antirachitic property of sunlight alone in the treatment of rachitic children, even in winter. Hess's book[57] *Rickets, Including Osteomalacia and Tetany* (1929) is an encyclopedic review of the subject and contains a splendid history and bibliography of this disease.

Scurvy

At the beginning of the century infantile scurvy was still largely attributed to sterilized milk and proprietary foods. However, by 1910 Henry Koplik[73] was probably the first to give up the concept of a positive etiological factor and to replace it with the concept of a deficient or negative factor. He wrote: "The very fact that breast-milk has been the exclusive article of the diet in some cases should direct attention to the fact that the affection may be caused by lack of some necessary element in the food." But just what the factor was, he was unable to say because vitamin C was not isolated until 1928, and it was not until 1933 that the first case of infantile scurvy cured by the administration of ascorbic acid was reported.

To prevent infantile scurvy, Hess[56] recommended giving orange or tomato juice to babies at one month of age rather than following the common practice of waiting until the baby was about five or six months of age before giving antiscorbutic juices. To cure infantile scurvy, orange juice was then the sovereign remedy. It was even given intravenously in severe cases or where food could not be tolerated by mouth. For intravenous use, the juice was obtained in as sterile a manner as possible, boiled for five minutes, and rendered neutral or slightly alkaline by the addition of normal sodium hydroxide just previous to its injection.

Supportive Therapy

Supportive therapy includes those procedures which might be termed physiological treatment since they are directed toward correcting physiological disturbance rather than toward eliminating the cause of disease. They involve the use of parenteral fluids such as blood, fluid, and electrolyte solutions. The infant can tolerate great physical trauma but is unable to endure fluid and salt deficits without exhibiting the train of serious symptoms associated with dehydration, electrolyte imbalance, and shock.

The pediatrician practicing in the last quarter of this century, with his modern syringes, needles, and skill, has no idea of the handicaps the physician faced less than half a century ago in performing a task so mundane as a venipuncture. Requisite technical procedures are inevitably evolved when there are definite therapeutic needs and these develop only with an understanding of the disturbances in physiological processes brought about by disease. This understanding was what was lacking fifty years ago.

The drawing of blood was facilitated by an ingenious suction apparatus devised by Blackfan[13] in 1912 (Fig. 7–10). He noted that "the methods usually employed for obtaining blood from infants are in the majority of instances extremely unsatisfactory. The veins are too small to enter and it is a tedious, difficult, and painful procedure to collect the necessary amount of blood by puncturing the fingers or toes." Blackfan had found the suction devices used in the European clinics he had visited unsatisfactory for use in most infants, and especially in the marasmic infant. He considered his modification "a simple, inexpensive device by which the necessary amount of blood could be obtained easily, with a minimum amount of discomfort to the patient and

Figure 7–10. Suction apparatus for collecting blood for the Wassermann reaction. (From K. D. Blackfan, Am. J. Dis. Child. 4:33, 1912. Copyright 1912, American Medical Association.)

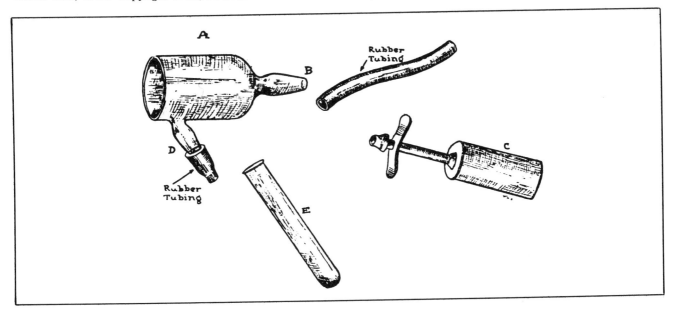

in a comparatively short space of time." The apparatus was in daily use at the St. Louis Children's Hospital in 1912 and the time spent in collecting the blood was said to have averaged about two minutes. To obtain a sample of blood, a nurse held the child in either an upright or a recumbent position and the doctor, having cleansed the area with alcohol, made an incision with a sharp-pointed scalpel in the back just below the angle of the scapula, and over the bleeding site a suction cup with attached test tube was applied. Blackfan's method of scarification, because it gave tissue juice in addition to blood, was not satisfactory for bacteriologic studies because of the possibility of bacterial contamination.

In the early decades of this century, fluids, if prescribed at all, were usually given either subcutaneously or rectally. Intraperitoneal injections of saline solution were first mentioned in the American pediatric literature by Blackfan[14] in 1918. He had used this route at the suggestion of Howland, "who saw it used as a routine measure on the service of Professor [Archibald] Garrod [1857–1936] at St. Bartholomew's Hospital, London."

Intraperitoneal fluids were prescribed extensively in the Harriet Lane Home between 1916 and 1918 with such satisfactory results that Blackfan considered the procedure a distinct improvement on any other methods that had been used. For small infants 100 to 250 ml was injected and repeated in twelve to twenty-four hours if needed; larger infants were given 300 to 400 ml, also repeated in twelve to twenty-four hours if needed.

Blackfan's use of intraperitoneal injections of salt solution was based on an earlier experimental study (1914) of Walter E. Dandy (1886–1946) and Leonard G. Rowntree (1883–1959),[25] in which they had injected solutions of phenolphthalein into the peritoneal cavities of dogs and found that 40 to 60 percent of the injected solution was absorbed in one hour; the absorption took place directly into the bloodstream and was not influenced by posture. Clinical evidence of the rapid absorption of saline solution in patients was apparent because the abdominal distension which usually followed the introduction of water intraperitoneally subsided after a short time.

Blackfan claimed, as did almost everyone else, that

because intravenous injection was so difficult, it was rarely possible by this route to inject an amount of saline solution sufficient to treat infants with severe gastrointestinal disturbances without throwing too great a burden on the circulation. He also found the subcutaneous method of fluid replacement, on which chief reliance had been previously placed, disappointing because absorption from the subcutaneous tissues was often very slow. For this reason the peritoneal route was recommended in the treatment of all cases of severe gastrointestinal disturbances in which it was impossible to introduce sufficient water by mouth or physiological saline solution by hypodermoclysis.

By 1920 intraperitoneal injections, usually of physiological saline, rarely of 5 to 10 percent glucose solution, were commonly used throughout the country in the treatment of infants and children suffering from persistent diarrhea or infantile atrophy.[45] However, the results were not particularly encouraging because the mortality in these patients remained about 50 percent. Fluids were also administered through the superior sagittal sinus.

In 1915 Henry F. Helmholtz (1882–1958)[55] wrote: "The method of obtaining blood from the veins of the scalp, from the jugular or other veins, is very difficult and open to frequent failures," but "there was one place that is far superior to any other for the purpose of obtaining blood, namely the longitudinal sinus in the area of the anterior fontanel." This route was also sanctioned for the administration of intravenous fluids. The first to use this vessel was Marfan, in 1898, for the introduction of salt solution in a case of cholera infantum.[55] In 1918 Alton Goldbloom (1890–1968), of Montreal, devised an apparatus for puncturing the superior longitudinal sinus in infants, and three years later Bret Ratner (1893–1957),[99] of New York, devised a similar apparatus which he claimed was "simple [and] inexpensive." It consisted of a small metal block ¼ inch square by 1 ¼ inches long, with an acutely beveled base. An opening of 18-gauge bore ran through the middle of the block, permitting the insertion of the needle. A thumbscrew held the needle in place after it had been adjusted to the proper length (Fig. 7–11). Others found ordinary hypodermic needles equally satisfactory. Besides using the superior sagit-

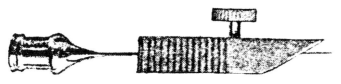

Figure 7–11. A new apparatus for puncturing the superior longitudinal sinus in infants. (From A. B. Ratner, Am. J. Dis. Child. 21:199, 1921. Copyright 1921, American Medical Association.)

tal sinus for injections of fluids and for blood transfusions, it was also used to obtain specimens of blood for the Wassermann test, blood cultures, and other diagnostic studies. In some hospitals it was a practice to give salvarsan by this route to infants with congenital syphilis, but this practice was vigorously condemned by many pediatricians because the drug was so toxic that they feared that if the sinus was transfixed, leakage of salvarsan would probably cause necrosis of the brain.

Blood transfusions were rare occurrences in pediatric practice in the early part of the century because Karl Landsteiner (1863–1943) had only recently discovered (1900) isoagglutinins in human blood capable of agglutinating other human red blood cells. These early transfusions were direct and were carried out with surgical care.

By the early 1920's intraperitoneal transfusions of citrated blood had become common because several studies had shown that blood introduced into the peritoneal cavity reappeared in the thoracic lymph stream within ten minutes.

David M. Siperstein (b. 1897)[112] postulated that erythrocytes could pass through the peritoneal mesothelium without any morphologic changes. The lymphatics draining the diaphragm were considered to be the chief portal of entrance of the transfused erythrocytes. He also documented the effective reabsorption of the transfused cells not only with red cell counts and hemoglobin determinations but also with photomicrographs showing the dual populations of hypochromic recipient and normochromic donor cells.

In 1923 James B. Sidbury (1886–1967)[111] first described transfusion through the umbilical vein in the treatment of a case of hemorrhage of the newborn. Louis K. Diamond (b. 1902)[26] in 1951, twenty-eight

years after Sidbury's report, established the umbilical route as the safest and simplest for exchange transfusion in hemolytic disease of the newborn.

Infectious Diseases

During the first quarter of the twentieth century a few diseases were brought under partial control by public health means, by immunization, or by treatment with serums, yet many others were not controlled by any of these measures. By 1925 infectious diseases were second only to malformations and diseases of early infancy as the major cause of death of American children. Of the infectious diseases, pneumonia was the greatest killer, followed by diarrheal diseases, measles, diphtheria, whooping cough, tuberculous meningitis, and scarlet fever, in that order (Table 7–1).

Diphtheria

There was an annual death toll of about 23,500 from diphtheria in the United States in 1921 in spite of the use and availability of diphtheria antitoxin.[29] The deaths from diphtheria during the 1920's were almost equivalent to the combined deaths from scarlet fever and measles. This death rate was particularly disturbing because physicians at that time fully realized that in no infectious disease, with the exception of smallpox, could so much be accomplished in the way of prevention as in diphtheria.

Knowledge of the ubiquity of the diphtheria bacillus led to vigorous campaigns to isolate patients, quarantine contacts, and disinfect anything that had been near a patient with the disease. Public funerals of children dying from diphtheria were invariably prohibited. It was also recommended that every city should establish a steam disinfecting plant where carpets, blankets, bedding, and clothes could be sent from the sickroom for disinfection.

Unfortunately, antitoxin, used so frequently as a prophylactic agent in those who had been exposed to active cases, did not protect the child for any great length of time. The breakthrough in the quest for a preparation which would offer active immunization against diphtheria began in 1907 when Theobald Smith (1859–1934),[89] an American pathologist, first suggested that immunity could be produced in human beings by mixing toxin with just enough antitoxin to make it harmless. He was aware of von Behring's* work in combining toxin and antitoxin for producing immunity in animals. Unfortunately, neither Smith nor his colleagues pursued his suggestion. In 1913 von Behring, having followed Smith's suggestion in combining toxin and antitoxin, reported that he had given such a mixture to humans and that the antitoxin had blocked the adverse reactions while the toxin produced a satisfactory antibody response.[89] Smith's achievements in other fields included his pioneer studies in anaphylaxis (1904–1905), immunization by dead vaccines (1884), differentiation of types of tubercle bacilli (1898), and the demonstration of the parasite of Texas cattle fever (1893).[89]

In 1913 Béla Schick (1877–1967), at the time a pediatrician on von Pirquet's service at the University of Vienna, published an account of the intradermal test which he had first used in 1908.[89] Schick showed that when a very small measured dose of diphtheria toxin was injected into the skin, a positive reaction, shown by a reddening at the site of the injection at the end of seventy-two hours, indicated that the subject was susceptible to the disease and a negative reaction denoted immunity to diphtheria. The Schick test, based on the antitoxin content of the blood, indicated whether or not prophylactic injections of antitoxin were necessary in children already exposed to diphtheria. It thus spared many immune children the necessity of receiving antitoxin injections.

In 1914, less than a year after the publication of von Behring's paper on the value of toxin-antitoxin, William H. Park, director of hygiene services of New York City and his associate, Abraham Zingher (1885–1927), were among the first to use toxin-antitoxin mixtures in this country.[6] Much thought was given to the best ratio of toxin to antitoxin for human use; if too much antitoxin was added, the mixture would be immunologically ineffective, and if too little, the mixture would be too toxic. In this way the beginnings of laboratory control of biological preparations were instituted.[89]

In 1919 Park started a program of performing a Schick test on every child in the New York City public schools whose parents would give permission and immunizing those with positive skin tests with

* Behring was the first recipient of the Nobel Prize for Medicine in 1901 and in the same year became known as von Behring.

his toxin-antitoxin preparation. This was the earliest large-scale practical application of bacteriologic principles in this country.

Toxin-antitoxin mixtures were not devoid of potential harm. Catastrophes in many countries from the injection of improperly prepared mixtures encouraged a search for a safer immunizing agent.[7] Park's preparations, slightly different from von Behring's remained in use in New York and most of the United States until 1924, at which time toxoid began to be substituted for it, at least in New York City.

Two reported catastrophes occurred in the United States from the use of toxin-antitoxin mixtures.[89] The first was in Dallas, Texas, in 1919 where five deaths and forty cases of severe reaction occurred after injections of toxin-antitoxin mixtures. The toxicity was caused by an error in manufacture. Instead of being added at one time, the required amount of toxin was added in fractions at two stages, allowing considerable time to elapse between additions. In accordance with a well-recognized immunological principle, a toxic mixture resulted (Danysz's phenomenon).[89]

The second catastrophe occurred in Concord and Bridgewater, Massachusetts, in 1924.[89] Although there were no deaths, a total of forty children developed severe local and marked general reactions. The children were immunized with a toxin-antitoxin mixture that contained phenol as a preservative. On investigation, it was discovered that a part of the batch had been stored below the freezing point. The alternate freezing and thawing gave rise to a local concentration of phenol, causing selective destruction of the antitoxin and leaving a toxic mixture. Other material from the same batch had not been frozen and was trouble-free on injection.

In 1923 Alexander T. Glenny (1882–1965) in England and Gaston L. Ramon (1886–1963) in France found that toxin could be made nontoxic by treatment with formalin so that it no longer caused adverse reactions while it retained its immunizing properties. This altered preparation of toxin was called toxoid. But physicians and health departments in this country were slow in replacing toxin-antitoxin preparations with toxoid. It was not until the 1930's that New York became the first state whose health department changed over entirely to the use of toxoid.[6]

Although diphtheria did not disappear during the period between 1917 and 1925, the total number of cases encountered in New York City dropped from 12,638 in 1917 to 7,500 in 1925. The deaths from diphtheria in New York City in 1917 were 1,158; and in 1925 had fallen to 425.[7]

Streptococcal Diseases

Among the most recalcitrant diseases were those caused by streptococci. The process of defining these infections and explaining how streptococci brought them about took a longer time than it had taken to comprehend typhoid fever, diphtheria, and pneumonia, mainly because streptococcal disease had so many faces.

SCARLET FEVER. One of the striking facts about the case fatality of scarlet fever for the fifty years between 1870 and 1920 had been its consistent reduction. While there was little evidence of any considerable decrease in the prevalence of scarlet fever, the death rate showed a steady decline during the first quarter of the century. The case fatality in American cities, which ran from 15 to 37 percent in the 1870's, had decreased to between 1.5 and 10 percent in the first two decades of the twentieth century.[28] There was much speculation on how to explain this observation and it was generally conceded that the virulence of scarlet fever had grown less; this factor best explained the lessened death rate. Other factors considered of importance were the more frequent hospitalization of cases, especially with the establishment of hospitals for contagious diseases, and the use of diphtheria antitoxin in cases complicated by diphtheria.[28] However, the greatest decline had occurred before diphtheria antitoxin had been introduced.[28,42]

Beginning in 1923, George Frederick Dick (1881–1967), of the University of Chicago and his wife, Gladys Rowena Dick (1881–1963), introduced a new era of scarlet fever research. When they had first become interested in scarlet fever, about 1912, there was no proof that the streptococcus was the cause of the disease. However, in 1903 streptococci had been differentiated according to their action on red blood cells in vitro. Hugo Schottmüller (1867–1936) described three distinct strains in 1903—hemolytic, green, and indifferent—and recognized that

the hemolytic strains were potentially more virulent than the other varieties. The chief advance came from the discovery that hemolytic streptococci were true toxin-producing organisms in the same way that the diphtheria and tetanus bacilli were producers of toxin. The Dicks found that the hemolytic streptococci were almost always present in scarlet fever and the clinical disease was produced when a culture of hemolytic streptococci obtained from the throat of a patient with scarlet fever was swabbed on the throat of two volunteers, one of whom developed typical scarlet fever. They were able to demonstrate a soluble toxin from hemolytic streptococci isolated from the throats of patients suffering from scarlet fever. This toxin, which was absorbed into the blood, had rash-producing or erythrogenic properties.[27] When separated from the bacteria it was capable by itself of producing the characteristic symptoms of scarlet fever, including the rash.[29] When this toxin was suitably diluted and injected intradermally, in what came to be known as the Dick test, it produced a localized rash in individuals susceptible to scarlet fever but no rash in those who were immune.[27]

Shortly after the Dicks' announcement of the rash-producing effect of toxin, Alphonse R. Dochez (1882–1964) assisted by Lillian Sherman reported an ingenious method for serum production. They introduced under a horse's skin a mass of agar and injected into the mass streptococci obtained from a patient with scarlet fever. Their thesis was that if scarlet fever was caused by a toxin, the streptococci growing in the agar would diffuse the toxin into the blood, thus enabling the animal to produce an antitoxin. The serum obtained from the horse blanched a scarlet fever rash and, when injected subcutaneously, caused marked improvement of the early symptoms of scarlet fever. In 1926 Dochez definitely established that scarlet fever streptococci could cause throat infections without a rash.[29]

The Dicks[27] claimed that the important features of the disease and most of the complications were caused by the erythrogenic toxin, but in 1926 Francis Blake (1887–1952) and James D. Trask (1890–1942), of Yale University, disproved this concept. They showed that the level of erythrogenic toxin in the blood of patients paralleled only the extent of the rash and not the duration of illness or the presence of complications. Thus the streptococcal infection itself was the prime factor in scarlet fever and caused the complications and death, whereas the rash was an incidental, although dramatic, feature.[29]

The use of scarlet fever antitoxin, which was usually prepared in horses by the inoculation of toxic filtrates in much the same way as diphtheria antitoxin, may have been of value in the treatment of the initial toxemia of scarlet fever but had no direct action on the septic complications.

The Dicks introduced a method of active immunization. Their scarlet fever prophylactic consisted of toxin and not, as in the case of diphtheria immunization, of toxoid or a preparation of toxoid. (It was unfortunate that scarlet fever toxoid could not be prepared because the addition of formalin to the toxin destroyed both its toxicity and antigenicity.[27]) An immunizing course consisted of five or more doses of scarlet fever toxin which were injected subcutaneously. The doses were graduated from 250 skin-test doses to 25,000 or even 100,000 skin-test doses. Dick-positive persons usually became negative after receiving toxin. There was much debate about the value of this procedure. The reactions were unpredictable and often severe, and for this reason the Dicks' active immunization against scarlet fever had only a limited usefulness. The Dicks also believed that scarlet fever was caused by a specific strain of streptococci. This belief was refuted when hemolytic streptococci were divided into groups and these into types beginning in 1933 by studies of Rebecca Lancefield (b. 1895).

Complications of Streptoccocal Disease

Two other illnesses, rheumatic fever and acute glomerulonephritis, both late complications or sequelae of hemolytic streptococcal infection, differ from scarlet fever because the organs principally affected are not invaded directly by the streptococci. Early twentieth-century physicians were aware that these two diseases usually developed after a latent period of approximately one to three weeks and that their incidence was not related to the severity of the initial infection.

RHEUMATIC FEVER. Rheumatic fever in the pre-antibiotic era tended to manifest itself either by arthritis or choreiform movements with carditis of varying degrees of severity more frequently than at the present time. Chorea during this period was a common manifestation of rheumatic fever. However, there was not universal acceptance of the prime role rheumatic fever played in its etiology. Chorea was seen most frequently between the ages of seven and fourteen years and it occurred twice as frequently in girls as in boys. While chorea was seen at all seasons, it was much more frequent in the spring months, at least in the early years of this century. Holt[61] found that in the cases he had followed, the largest number began in May. Overpressure in school was thought to be an important factor in the production of chorea. During this period chorea was said to develop as a sequel of any of the infectious diseases, more particularly scarlet and typhoid fevers. The immediate prognosis for chorea was favorable; however, many patients were left with severe heart disease.

It took centuries for the disparate symptoms of rheumatic fever to be recognized as a single disease. It was not until 1930 that Alvin Coburn (1899–1975) first clearly implicated the hemolytic streptococci as the sole incitants of the tissue reactions in rheumatic fever.[29]

Most studies on the etiology of cardiac disease in pediatric patients during the first quarter of this century indicated the overwhelming preponderance of rheumatic fever as a cause of cardiac disease. For example, a study reported from Boston in 1913 showed that of three hundred and four patients admitted to the Boston Children's Hospital with heart disease, 87 percent had had rheumatic fever, and only 7 percent had congenital heart disease.[33]

Until about 1920 rheumatic nodules were thought to be less commonly seen or felt in this country than in England. For example, Koplik[73] in 1910 wrote: "The so-called subcutaneous rheumatic nodules are seen in children less frequently in this country than in England," and Rachford[97] in 1912 wrote: "In England these nodules are common. . . . In America, however, they are comparatively rare." But by 1919 Joseph G. Brennemann (1872–1944),[17] who took a particular interest in looking for these nodules, had found them in about half the American patients with rheumatic heart disease, a frequency equal to that mentioned by Sir George F. Still in England. Brennemann[17] also believed that rheumatic nodules were largely confined to cases of rheumatic fever with active carditis. He summarized his conclusion about the prognostic significance of these nodules as follows: "A peculiar interest has, to my mind, always attached to the nodules found on the knuckles. The hand is the only exposed part in this condition. By a glance at the knuckles in such a case we have been able to say: 'This child has rheumatism; it is probably active; it is severe; he has an endocarditis.' "

GLOMERULONEPHRITIS. Nephritis, a frequent complication of scarlet fever during the early decades of this century, occurred in about 13 to 15 percent of cases. Efforts had been made by many writers of that period to relate the damage to the kidney to certain specific factors such as the putative cause of scarlet fever. But as there was no definite information at that time regarding the etiologic agent in scarlet fever, such discussions were largely hypothetical. Some physicians thought the child's diet played a role in the development of nephritis as a complication of scarlet fever. A commonly accepted belief was that a milk diet reduced the chances of the child's coming down with nephritis, while a liberal diet rich in meats was a likely cause.

"Taking cold" was often assigned a leading role in the etiology of nephritis. Physicians and parents alike tended to accept published reports that cold drafts directed toward the back of a patient convalescing from scarlet fever could bring on an attack of nephritis. In 1925 an American authority on infectious diseases of children wrote: "Two of our cases of severe nephritis occurred in children who during convalescence were chilled by getting out of bed and standing at open windows. The nephritis in both appeared immediately after the exposure"[122]

Pertussis

The causal agent of pertussis, *Bordetella pertussis*, was first observed by Jules Jean Bordet (1870–1961) and Octave Gengou (1875–1957) in 1900 but was not cultured by them until 1906.

Pertussis still killed more than ten thousand children per year in the United States as late as 1916. In the five-year period, 1911 to 1915 inclusive, whooping cough caused 835 more deaths than scarlet fever in New York State. The mortality was found to be consistently higher among girls than boys. For example, in the Registration Area of the United States for the years from 1900 to 1911 (inclusive), the death rate in female children from pertussis averaged 12.5 per 100,000 per year as against 10.5 for males.[41] The same female excess was also noted in the British and Bavarian statistics.[15,42] The greatest mortality and the greatest incidence occurred before the fifth year of life. Between 1900 and 1920 whooping cough caused more deaths during the first year of life than any other infectious disease.[41] Thus the death rate in Massachusetts in the first year of life was more than two and a half times the death rate in the second. Three-fourths of the deaths due to whooping cough were in children under two years of age, and two-thirds in children less than a year of age. Mortality from pertussis had not changed from 1883 to 1912 in Massachusetts. Most of the deaths were due to bronchopneumonia during the winter months and from convulsions, diarrhea, and vomiting during the summer months.[61]

TREATMENT. No disease had a larger list of remedies proposed and enthusiastically lauded as "specifics" than had pertussis.[41] Unfortunately, the therapeutic value of x-ray treatment in the management of pertussis had been highly praised beginning about 1915. Its use was based on the selective affinity of the x-ray for lymphatic tissues. The good results obtained from the use of x-rays in pertussis were attributed to the shrinking of the enlarged tracheobronchial lymph nodes so frequently present in this disease. The fact that under x-ray treatment the lymphocytes disappeared was used to support this form of treatment. It was further believed during this period that the lymphocyte was merely a manifestation of the adenopathy and "not part and parcel of the pertussis."[41]

For several years after the discovery of the pertussis organism, vaccines were prepared by various methods and used fairly widely in several countries. A few reports were published of tests on small numbers of children without control groups. The assessment of such inadequate trials was very difficult. However, it was generally assumed, rather than proved, that vaccines could be valuable.

The first use of pertussis vaccine in this country

was by Louis W. Sauer (b. 1885);[101] he began to use a vaccine prepared from freshly isolated, strongly hemolytic strains as early as 1926, and he claimed good immunity in three hundred young children vaccinated between 1928 and 1933.

Bacterial Meningitis

During the first quarter of this century several different kinds of acute bacterial meningitis in children had been defined. Meningococcal meningitis was the only form that occurred epidemically, although it often occurred sporadically. Epidemic meningitis was usually called cerebrospinal meningitis or cerebrospinal fever. The other forms of acute bacterial meningitis that were known resembled meningococcal meningitis more or less clinically and were at times confused with it. During the first part of this century tuberculous meningitis was said to be the most frequent form of meningitis in young children, except during epidemics of meningococcal meningitis.

The relative frequency of the different forms of acute bacterial meningitis—as seen apart from epidemics—in children under three years of age at the Babies Hospital in New York City in the first one and a half decades of this century was as follows:[61]

Diseases	Cases
Tuberculous meningitis	157
Pneumococcal meningitis	23
Meningococcal meningitis	24
Staphylococcal or streptococcal meningitis	11
H. influenzae	5
E. coli	1

At the meeting of the American Pediatric Society in 1907 Adams[2] discussed "grip meningitis" and reported a nicely documented case of meningitis due to the influenza bacillus in which the organism was recovered from the cerebrospinal fluid. This was the first well-documented American case of *Hemophilus influenzae* meningitis, although Adams had noted more than twenty other cases reported in the foreign literature.

The degree of communicability of meningococcal meningitis when compared with the common contagious diseases was found to be slight. Holt claimed that in 75 percent of the cases studied during the New York epidemic in 1904–1905 only one person in the home was affected, although no effort at isolation was made. Cerebrospinal, or meningococcal, meningitis was not included among the communicable diseases listed by New York City until about 1915. Holt also wrote that he had never known the disease to originate in a hospital patient, although in New York hospitals cases of cerebrospinal meningitis had been received into the general wards with other patients until 1915.[61]

The mortality was much higher in epidemics than when the disease occurred sporadically. The average mortality rate prior to treatment with serum was about 70 percent. During the last year of the New York epidemic of 1904–1905 the mortality was 76 percent. There was no recorded epidemic in which the mortality was less than 50 percent. However, not all of those who survived could be classed as recoveries, for in at least 25 to 50 percent serious sequelae remained.

TREATMENT. In 1907 Simon Flexner, of the Rockefeller Institute, reported that he had produced meningitis in monkeys with strains of meningococci obtained during the 1904–1905 epidemic in New York City.[29] He passed the infection from monkey to monkey and then protected monkeys from experimental meningococcal meningitis by injecting a serum produced by immunizing horses with meningococci.

At the annual meeting of the American Pediatric Society the following year, Flexner and James W. Jobling,[36] then also of the Rockefeller Institute, presented a study in which they analyzed about four hundred cases of epidemic meningitis treated with their antimeningococcal serum given intrathecally. The results were considered highly encouraging because after they had substracted seven moribund and fulminating cases, 75 percent of those given serum recovered, and of these the great majority were said not to have had serious sequelae. The only persistent defect noted was deafness; the number so affected was not mentioned.

In the discussion of this paper, Holt stated that in the pre-serum New York epidemic of 1904, 75 percent of the 2,350 patients died and that of 83 infants under one year of age all died. With the use of Flexner and Jobling's antimeningococcal serum, the 75 percent mortality and 25 percent recovery noted in pre-serum days were approximately reversed.

The serum was administered intrathecally after withdrawing by lumbar puncture all the cerebrospinal fluid that would flow freely. The serum, warmed to body temperature, was injected slowly by gravity, using a rubber tube and small funnel. The initial dose was between 10 to 25 ml, repeated in twenty-four hours, and then daily until four or five doses had been given. An immediate effect of the injection was seen in the cerebrospinal fluid with marked reduction of the polymorphonuclear cells and in the number of meningococci. During this period lumbar puncture per se was thought to have some therapeutic value by virtue of relieving intracranial pressure and reducing the number of microorganisms in the cerebrospinal fluid.

TREATMENT. Bromides, chloral, sulfonal, and trional were variously prescribed for delirium and sleeplessness. Stimulants such as caffeine, digitalis, or strophanthus were recommended if the pulse was weak, rapid, or irregular.

Serum therapy soon became established in the United States and in many other countries. Although the Germans were pioneers in this form of therapy, the main credit for developing this project and for the early assessment of its value belongs to Flexner and his colleagues.

Tuberculosis

In 1921 Charles Hendee Smith (1876–1968)[113] wrote:

There is widespread belief among the physicians in this country that practically all children are infected with tuberculosis before adolescence and that, since the infection is so nearly universal, a positive skin reaction has no diagnostic significance after early infancy. This has been taught medical students largely as the result of the work of [Franz] Hamburger and others in Vienna, which is notoriously the most tuberculous city in Europe. This view has been questioned by only a very few writers in America, and their findings are distinctly at variance with it.

Although in the American experience childhood tuberculosis was less frequent than in Europe, the incidence of tuberculosis, as determined by the percentage of positive skin reactions on a series of children from St. Louis in 1915, showed that by three years of age 25 percent of the children were tuberculin positive and by age seven this figure had risen to 40 percent.[113] The incidence of tuberculosis, as determined by positive skin tests in a series of children in three American and five European cities during the period 1910–1920, is shown in Figure 7–12.

The importance of the early diagnosis of tuberculosis in children was constantly stressed because it was claimed that "tuberculous children do wonderfully well if they are treated carefully. They do very badly if neglected." If the tuberculin skin test was positive, immediate efforts were made to determine whether or not the disease was active. The signs of activity of tuberculosis were fever, languor, malnu-

Figure 7–12. Incidence of tuberculosis as determined by positive skin tests in a series of children in three American and five European cities, 1910–1920. (From C. H. Smith, Trans. Am. Pediatr. Soc. 33:246, 1921. Reprinted by permission.)

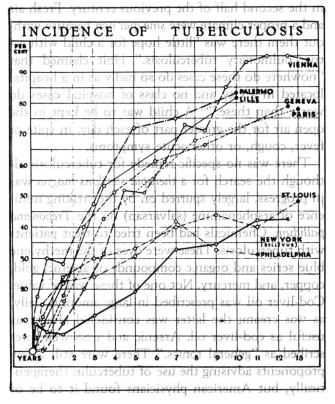

trition, anemia, and hypertrichosis. The last-named sign was said to be particularly helpful because "long lashes proverbially suggest tuberculosis" and "hypertrichosis before puberty gives rise to a suspicion of tuberculosis."[113]

Several authors of this period noted that mistakes were often made in diagnosing other chronic lung conditions as tuberculosis, with or without bronchiectasis. Smith claimed that pulmonary fibrosis in children, with or without bronchiectasis, was seen more often than was pulmonary tuberculosis and that many of the children with bronchiectasis were sent to tuberculosis sanitariums even with negative tuberculins. One wonders how many of these children may have had cystic fibrosis rather than tuberculosis.

During this period the prevention, diagnosis, and cure of tuberculosis were still among the most demanding problems of medicine. The National Tuberculosis Association in 1916 placed the annual death rate from all forms of tuberculosis in the United States at a hundred and fifty thousand, the diagnosed active cases at one million, and the unsuspected cases at 2 million.[6]

TREATMENT. This remained the same as it had been in the second half of the previous century. Fresh air and a proper climate were *sine qua non* because without them there was "little hope for a child with active pulmonary tuberculosis." Holt claimed that "nowhere do these cases do so badly as in a hospital located in a city and no class of hospital cases do worse than these."[61] A child was to be kept in the open air for the greater part of each day, in spite of fever, cough, or other acute symptoms.

There was no specific remedy for tuberculosis although the search for a *therapia sterilans magna* was in progress, largely spurred on by the striking influence of arsphenamine (salvarsan) on the *Treponema pallidum*. Chemicals had been tried to treat patients with tuberculosis. These were dyes of the methylene blue series and organic compounds of arsenic, gold, copper, and mercury. Not one of these was of value. Cod-liver oil was prescribed in large amounts daily, as was cream; the latter was considered almost as useful as cod-liver oil. Arsenic and iron were prescribed as "general tonics." There were still a few proponents advising the use of tuberculin therapeutically, but American physicians found it to be of little or no value. However, tuberculin treatment was employed extensively in the treatment of cervical adenitis due to tuberculosis. It was the consensus that this method of treatment was of benefit and that it diminished the tendency to softening of the cervical nodes and promoted resolution; but it usually did not take the place of operative measures.

Pneumonia

During the first quarter of the century, pneumonia was very common as a primary disease in children and ranked first as a complication of the various forms of acute infectious diseases of children. It was one of the largest factors in the mortality of infancy and childhood.

Pneumonias were divided into two major categories: bronchopneumonia, also known as catarrhal or lobular pneumonia; and lobar pneumonia, also known during this period as either croupous or fibrinous pneumonia.

Studies of three hundred and seventy cases of acute pneumonia at the New York Infant Asylum showed that during the first two years of life, 25 percent were lobar and 75 percent were bronchopneumonia.[61] The latter was essentially the pneumonia of infancy. Under two years, the great majority of the cases of primary pneumonia were of this variety, and throughout childhood nearly all the cases of so-called secondary pneumonia. Bronchopneumonia had a more serious prognosis than did lobar pneumonia. Before the advent of the sulfonamides, the mortality from bronchopneumonia during the first year of life was 66 percent; this fell to 33 percent by the third year, and to 16 percent by the fourth year.

TREATMENT. For bronchopneumonia the treatment included counterirritation by means of mustard paste, used three to six times daily. It was considered to be of greatest value in the early stage of acute pulmonary congestion, and during attacks of cardiac or respiratory failure. Alcohol was felt to be of benefit, although there was considerable doubt as to its mode of action. Of the circulatory stimulants; caffeine, camphor, and digitalis were recommended in the order named.

After the third year of life lobar pneumonia was more frequent than bronchopneumonia and most of the cases occurred in March and April. Physicians of the period noted that there was probably no disease in children over three years of age in which the patient appeared so ill and yet so often recovered completely. Of 1,295 cases of lobar pneumonia reported by Holt, chiefly from hospital practice, there were only 39 deaths, a mortality of 3 percent, and in only one of the fatal cases was the child over two years old.[61]

In the majority of cases the treatment of lobar pneumonia was essentially hygienic because it was considered a self-limiting disease with a strong tendency to recovery in the great majority of cases regardless of the treatment adopted. Cold air and wide-open windows, even though the room temperature was kept constantly as low as 50° F, were advocated. Cold sponge baths, cold packs, or ice bags applied to the chest were considered the best antipyretics.

Typhoid Fever

Typhoid fever in the infant was a relatively rare disease during this period, but it was by no means rare in children. After the fifth year it occurred frequently. Because of the relative mildness of the disease in children under two years of age, the newer methods of diagnosis, such as the serum agglutination reaction of Georges F. Widal (1862–1929), were needed to bring it to light. Typhoid fever could be transmitted to the infant through the mother's breast milk.[54] It was also known that when a pregnant woman developed typhoid fever, infection of the child in utero was a frequent but not invariable occurrence. The most common result was death of the fetus and consequent abortion.

Griffith[50] claimed that in 1899 "the wards of the Children's Hospital in Philadelphia were so full of these cases [typhoid fever] that it was difficult to get enough cases of other diseases to present to the class." Holt,[61] on the other hand, claimed that typhoid fever was a relatively rare disease in children because in over 14,000 admissions to Babies Hospital, New York, covering a period of thirteen years, only 11 children under two years of age were admitted with this disease and but 5 cases of one year or under; the youngest case was in a child of eight months. However, during the fall of 1913 an epidemic of typhoid fever occurred in New York City with 521 reported cases, of which 221 were in children under fourteen years of age. Osler, in a review

of 1,500 cases of typhoid fever admitted to the Johns Hopkins Hospital, found that 231, or 15 percent, were under fifteen years of age. The New York City Health Department in 1912 reported that approximately one-fourth of the cases of typhoid fever occurred in children under twelve years of age.[21]

PROGNOSIS. In 2,623 cases in children collected in 1917 by Holt[61] from the reports of twelve different writers, the mortality was 5.4 percent. Death seldom resulted from the disease itself but usually from some accident or complication, the most frequent being pneumonia and intestinal hemorrhage or perforation. In Griffith's[50] collection of cases in Philadelphia, the death rate for the first year of life reached nearly 50 percent.

TREATMENT. It was the policy to put to bed every child with typhoid fever during the febrile period (which usually lasted three weeks), and a few days beyond it, no matter how mild the attack. The diet consisted of sterilized milk, broth, cereal gruels, milk toast, soft eggs, custard, and plain ice cream. These were to be given liberally every four or five hours.[21]

Diarrhea was not treated unless there were more than four or five bowel movements a day. Opium and bismuth were considered the best means to control excessive diarrhea.

Temperature over 104° F called for antipyretic measures or cold or tepid sponging. The preferred method, advised by Holt,[61] was the so-called graduated bath; the child was placed in the tub with water at a temperature of 95° to 100° F; this was gradually lowered to 95°, 90°, or even 85° F, but seldom lower. The child's body was to be actively rubbed while he was in the bath "to prevent shock and cardiac depression." The bath was repeated every three to six hours.

Epidemic Vulvovaginitis in Young Girls

In the pre-antibiotic era, epidemic gonorrheal vulvovaginitis in young girls was a serious and frustrating disease. During the first third of the century it was one of the most prevalent infections in most of our large cities. This was especially true in hospitals and other institutions that cared for female children. The prevalence of this disease and its intractability to treatment coupled with its defiance of ordinary quarantine regulations made it an extraordinarily difficult contagious disease to control.[34]

Jacobi,[70] for example, wrote: "There is nothing more dangerous than [gonorrheal vulvovaginitis].... It can be treated easily, but cured with difficulty, and sometimes treated with no result at all." He also claimed that he had "seen cases lasting for years, relapsing from time to time, seemingly absolutely incurable.... That is why I fear vaginitis more than anything else."

Epidemics of gonococcal vulvovaginitis in institutions for children, including children's hospitals, spread widely through nonvenereal contact. Possible sources of contagion were toilet seats, towels, bed linen, and common thermometers. Epidemics of this disease were often spread through the use of inadequately sterilized diapers.[34] The prevalence of the disease was in part attributed to the peculiar susceptibility of the prepubertal vaginal mucosa to gonorrheal infection.[98]

Vulvovaginitis was said to have occurred in approximately 20 percent of hospital cases and 5 to 10 percent of patients in private practice in the early part of this century.[34] Among six hundred admissions to Babies Hospital in New York City in one year, there were seventy cases of vulvovaginitis and ten cases of arthritis due to the gonococcus.[34] The disease showed itself as a vulvovaginal irritation or as a purulent vaginal discharge cause by the gonococcus. Complications were rare, although ophthalmia, salpingitis, and lymphadenitis were reported. During this period almost every case of vaginal discharge in young girls was attributed to gonococcal infection, with the possible exception of the vaginitis that sometimes accompanied measles.[98]

Koplik[73] emphasized the distressing nature of the disease and its seriousness, having seen several deaths from peritonitis. Many reports attested to the disease's chronicity; the average time until cure—if attained—was given in weeks or months.

Prophylaxis was very strictly observed, especially in institutions and children's hospitals. At many children's hospitals at least three negative smears on consecutive days had to be obtained before girls were admitted to general hospital wards.[98]

Local treatment consisted of daily tub baths and intravaginal instillations of preparations such as 1 percent Dakin's solution in olive oil, 1–2 percent mercurochrome solution, or 1 percent silver nitrate incorporated in an ointment of equal parts of lanolin and petroleum jelly. Solutions of boric acid or potassium permanganate were also widely used. Treatment was usually continued for at least twelve weeks. But on the whole the results of treatment in cases which had become chronic were unsatisfactory. Relapses were exceedingly common, even when there had been no discharge for weeks and even months. Vaccine therapy, either autogenous or stock, were valueless in the treatment of this disease.[61,98]

Congenital Syphilis

During the first ten years of the twentieth century more was added to our knowledge of syphilis than during the three previous centuries. In 1903 Elie Metchnikoff (1845–1916) and Pierre Roux were able to transmit the disease from man to the higher apes, thus opening the opportunity for experimental studies. Three years later, August von Wassermann (1866–1925) described the so-called Wassermann reaction, and on March 3, 1905, Fritz R. Schaudinn (1871–1906) discovered the causal organism of syphilis. Finally, in 1909 Paul Ehrlich (1854–1915) and Sahachiro Hata (1873–1938), after many experiments on the action of synthetic drugs upon spirochetal disease, discovered salvarsan ("606"), which proved to be a specific agent in the treatment of syphilis and yaws.

INCIDENCE. The available data for the first quarter of the century are too inexact to provide an accurate estimate of the incidence of this disease because most of the studies dealt with selected groups. In the United States Registration Area, for the years 1910 to 1913, 1 percent of the infant deaths was due to syphilis, and it was responsible for 0.8 percent of the total deaths under ten years of age. These were considered minimum figures because many infants delivered at home were not included in these reports. Such figures as had been gathered showed that in the United States about 10 percent of the adult male population had syphilis. Philip C. Jeans (1883–1952),[71] by collecting studies made in several different American cities, found that of over five thousand pregnant married women in hospitals slightly under 10 percent were syphilitic.

Borden S. Veeder (1883–1970) and Jeans[121] noted that approximately one-half of the pregnancies in syphilitic families ended in death before term or during infancy. Of the one-half with surviving children only a third led to healthy offspring, and the rest resulted in children with congenital syphilitic infection.

TRANSMISSION. By 1920 it was generally accepted that the mother was infected in every instance of transmission to the second generation. No study published during this period purported to prove that the infection could be transmitted directly from the father to the offspring. Thus, for the first time, physicians now conceded that syphilis in the father could not be transmitted to the child in utero without the mother's becoming infected at the same time. The Wassermann reaction proved that almost all the "apparently healthy" mothers had syphilis.

J. Whitridge Williams (1866–1931)[124] in 1922 found that 48.5 percent of the children born to untreated syphilitic mothers were syphilitic, while with treatment of the mother, the proportion of infected children fell to 6.7 percent. Prematurity was also reduced to one-half, stillbirths to one-third, and infant mortality to one-ninth of that found in untreated syphilitic mothers.

Jean V. Cooke (1883–1956) and Jeans,[23] also in 1922, found that prophylactic treatment during the mother's pregnancy would as a rule protect the infant against infection. They noted that in the average case surprisingly little treatment was sufficient to protect the infant.

TREATMENT. Two years after the introduction of salvarsan by Ehrlich and Hata, LaFétra[78] published the first American account of the use of this drug in the treatment of infants and young children with congenital syphilis. He gave the drug, also known as arsphenamine (a compound of arsenic with aminobenzene in which the arsenic is trivalent), intravenously to ten children, ranging in age from six weeks to five and a half years, with great benefit. LaFétra administered the drug intravenously and "nearly always after having cut down and exposed a vein at the bend of the elbow," because "to plunge the needle through the skin and subcutaneous fat and into the vein is not easy in infants, since the vein slips away or else is pierced clear through." Holt[78] described twenty-four patients at Babies Hospital who had received one or more intravenous injections of

salvarsan. Like LaFétra, he also found that "the introduction of the needle into the vein of an infant had been found extremely difficult and unsatisfactory." He resorted to "a dissection of the vein . . . and for this general anesthesia was desirable." He tried local anesthesia but found it unsatisfactory.

In 1922 sulpharsphenamine was introduced as an antiluetic agent; it had an advantage over salvarsan because it could be given intramuscularly, whereas administration of salvarsan by this route not only was extremely painful but also caused tissue sloughing.

Poliomyelitis

The first epidemic of poliomyelitis of any size in the United States appeared in 1894, involving 132 cases in Rutland County, Vermont. This epidemic was reported in detail by Charles S. Caverly (1856–1918), public health officer of that state.[92] He called it a new disease because nothing like it had ever been seen previously by him or other physicians in Vermont. Actually, this epidemic turned out to be the largest one that had ever been reported in one year anywhere in the world.[92] Karl Oscar Medin (1847–1927) had described 44 cases in Stockholm in 1887, which was the largest reported epidemic anywhere prior to the 1894 epidemic in Vermont.[92] Increasingly larger epidemics followed, culminating in 1916 in an epidemic in the Northeastern part of the United States of at least 29,000 cases with slightly more than 6,000 deaths. The mortality rate was about 22 percent and over two-thirds of the cases occurred in New York City alone.

Up to 1907 there were records of thirty-three worldwide epidemics with a total of 1,942 reported cases, of which, 1,053, or more than half the entire number, had occurred in the Scandinavian epidemic of 1905 and 1906.[92] But by the 1907 epidemic in New York City and vicinity alone the number of cases was estimated at from 2,000 to 2,500. The mortality rate in various epidemics varied from 6 to 20 percent, with the modal rate being about 6 percent.[92]

The epidemic of 1916, the largest up to that year of all epidemics of this disease,[92] so far outstripped the earlier ones that the U.S. Public Health Service had to come to the aid of the overtaxed municipal services. An extraordinary degree of anxiety gripped the public, the medical profession, and the staffs of hospitals and public health agencies alike, all of whom were unprepared to cope with the harrowing problems of a sudden epidemic of this magnitude. Up until the time of this epidemic the maximum annual rate of reported cases in the United States had never exceeded 7.9 per 100,000 population but, in 1916, within the epidemic area, it reached an all-time high of 28.5. In New York City alone there were over 9,000 cases with an urban rate of over six times that in the total epidemic area.[92]

Haven Emerson (1874–1957), the health commissioner of New York City, set in motion a rigorous plan to control the epidemic. Orders were given that all premises housing a case of poliomyelitis should be placarded and the family quarantined; the windows were to be screened and the bed linen disinfected; and household pets were not allowed in any patient's room as they too were considered suspect.[92] Travel was severely restricted. Children under sixteen years of age were not permitted to leave New York City from July 18 until October 3, 1916, unless a certificate was produced indicating that the premises they occupied were free from poliomyelitis. This measure failed to check the epidemic because, as was later shown, most of the spread is from person to person with mild or completely symptomless infections. By the end of October the epidemic was over.[92]

Landsteiner and Erwin Popper in Vienna made an important advance in the study of poliomyelitis in 1909 when they transmitted it to monkeys by intraperitoneal injections of a saline emulsion of the spinal cord of a child who had died during the fourth day of an attack.[92] The transmission was viewed as surprising, since poliomyelitis was not known to occur in any animal other than man. Landsteiner eventually settled in the United States and became a member of the staff of the Rockefeller Institute. In 1930 he was awarded the Nobel Prize for his discovery of the human blood groups.

Simon Flexner and Paul A. Lewis (1879–1929), of the Rockefeller Institute, also in 1909, extended Landsteiner and Popper's observations by infecting monkeys not only by the intraperitoneal route but also subcutaneously, intravenously, intracerebrally, and by the path of the larger nerves. They were also able to produce the disease by using Berkefeld filtrates from the nasopharyngeal washings from a patient.[37] This led them to suspect the olfactory nerves as a probable portal of entry of the virus—a view which was later disproved.

The following year, Flexner and Lewis demonstrated neutralized substances in the serum of monkeys that had recovered from poliomyelitis; paralysis in monkeys could be prevented by intrathecal injection of this convalescent serum within twenty-four hours of infection.[92] Recovery from an attack of experimental poliomyelitis also provided protection against a second inoculation. Antibodies were also detected in the serum of human beings who had recovered from an attack of poliomyelitis.[92]

TREATMENT. Spurred on by a French report in 1915 of favorable responses from the use of convalescent poliomyelitis serum in thirty-four cases of the disease, the first of several therapeutic trials in humans to be reported in the United States was carried out in 1916. This series of twenty-one cases treated with convalescent serum suggested a dubious therapeutic value.[107] Far more extensive trials were under way in 1916, including one by the New York City Department of Health under the direction of W. H. Park. Serum was collected from patients convalescing from poliomyelitis at New York City's Willard Parker Hospital and in some instances from patients at other hospitals.[92]

In 1916 the administration of convalescent serum was cumbersome and time-consuming. The recommended method was to administer it intrathecally in a manner similar to that employed in the treatment of meningococcal meningitis.[36]

The dose was to be repeated every twenty to twenty-four hours until two or three had been given. Since this procedure was meant solely as treatment of an affected patient, a major problem was to decide which patients were to be treated. Hence the crucial point was the detection of a "positive" spinal fluid. This was considered mandatory for the initiation of serum treatment. But this made it difficult, according to John R. Paul (1893–1971),[92] "to assemble a group of untreated controls, for any physician who performed a lumbar puncture and found the characteristic spinal fluid changes was more than likely to use the serum and equally likely to incur the wrath of the patient's parents if he withheld it." These tests failed because of the failure to arrange for carefully matched treated and control groups.

In Boston, Francis W. Peabody (1881–1927)[93] treated a series of fifty-one cases during the 1916 epidemic by giving only one intrathecal injection. Peabody's trial was of necessity an emergency measure; he recognized its inadequacies and was cautious about the significance of his results:

For the proper interpretation of the results of treatment it is essential that we should have a much more complete knowledge of the natural history of the disease. At the present time we have only an imperfect idea as to what proportion of persons affected with the disease became paralyzed even if no treatment is instituted. Nevertheless, there is apparently general agreement among those who have used immune serum as to its harmlessness, and as to the fact that in certain, possibly in numerous instances, its administration is beneficial.

As time progressed and with more carefully controlled studies, the value of convalescent serum in the treatment of poliomyelitis was discounted. Once the diagnosis was made, it was too late to give serum.

No specific drug therapy for poliomyelitis has ever been discovered. Since the turn of the century wise medical opinion has held that powerful drugs or drastic therapeutic methods in the acute stages of poliomyelitis were harmful. Osler in 1892, in the first edition of his famous textbook, *The Principles and Practice of Medicine*, advocated the sensible policy that it was far better to use the least innocuous of remedies or even to do nothing than to run the risk of aggravating the disease by drastic treatments. He wrote: "No drugs have the slightest influence upon acute [polio]myelitis. . . . The child should be put to bed and the affected limb or limbs wrapped in cotton."

CONSTITUTIONAL FACTORS. Within a year after the epidemic of 1916 George Draper (1880–1959)[30] published his small book entitled *Acute Poliomyelitis*, in which he added some novel ideas to the literature of poliomyelitis; these centered on constitutional factors in relation to disease in general and to poliomyelitis in particular. He maintained that susceptibility to a number of diseases could be detected by the presence of certain physical traits. For example: "The type of child which seems most susceptible to the disease [poliomyelitis] is the large, well-grown, plump individual who has certain definite characteristics of face and jaws, is broad browed, and broad of face. The teeth are particularly interesting. . . . The wide spaced dentition has been a striking feature and frequently involves all the single teeth of both jaws, so that each tooth stands entirely free." Most physicians who came before and after Draper were unable to perceive these subtle physical features that were supposed to indicate susceptibility to poliomyelitis. Although Draper's theories have not stood the test of time, they went along with a growing body of evidence that of all the factors involved in familial clusters of certain diseases, the genetic influence is one which is most pervasive.

The concept of constitution and disease was not unique to Draper, and even Osler believed there was a certain type of patient particularly susceptible to tuberculosis (p. 126). There was a widely accepted belief in the early decades of this century that children who were fat, flabby, overnourished, and pasty were more likely to bear scarlet fever badly. And in England, Still was convinced that there was an "association of red hair with rheumatism and rheumatic heredity."

Roseola

John Zahorsky (1871–1963)[126] in 1910 described a previously unreported exanthematous disease of early childhood which he termed roseola infantilis, and in a second paper published three years later, he changed the name of the disease to roseola infantum.[127] In the first paper Zahorsky described the syndrome; in the second he presented brief histories of twenty-nine cases observed during a period of three years. Of these all but two occurred in children under two and a half years of age. All of the patients had a high fever that lasted several days, followed by a morbilliform rash that developed as the patient's temperature fell.

In 1921 Veeder and Theodore C. Hempelmann (1885–1943)[120] presented their findings in more than twenty patients with the symptom complex first described by Zahorsky. They noted, as he had, the apparent absence of contagiousness of this disease and its striking predilection for affecting infants rather than older children. Veeder and Hempelmann were the first to report blood counts on patients with this disease; leukopenia was present in all of their patients, falling as low as 3,200 cells per cubic millimeter in two cases. In all but one of the eight patients in whom blood counts were done there was also a relative lymphocytosis, amounting to from 80 to 90 percent of the total number of white cells.

Veeder and Hempelmann[120] did not consider rose-ola infantum an appropriate name for this disease after they discovered that the same name "was formerly used to describe a large indefinite group of diseases by older authors and dermatologists." In its place they suggested the name exanthem subitum "as being descriptive of the most striking clinical symptom, namely the sudden, unexpected appearance of the eruption on the fourth day."

It is of interest that Holt[61] in the seventh edition of his textbook, published in 1917, failed to mention this exanthem.

Herpangina

Zahorsky[128] in 1920 first described another "new" disease which he termed herpetic sore throat; in 1924 he suggested changing the name to herpangina, because the name herpetic sore throat might "readily be confused with other diseases of the mouth and fauces."[129]

His description of herpangina as a specific febrile disease, characterized by the appearance of minute papules, vesicles, and ulcers in the throat, is a model of clarity. The only omission was the etiology of the disease, which was added by Robert J. Heubner (b. 1914) and his associates in 1951, when they proved that herpangina was etiologically associated with Coxsackie A viruses.

Zahorsky[128] described the clinical findings observed in herpangina in this way:

The disease begins suddenly as an acute febrile movement. The temperature often rises to 104°. A convulsion may occur. Vomiting is often present. Anorexia and prostration are sometimes marked. The throat and posterior part of the mouth show minute vesicles or, if these have ruptured, small punched-out ulcers. They occur on the anterior pillar of the fauces, the tonsils, the pharynx and edge of the soft palate. The number of lesions varies from ten to twenty. Dysphagia is often marked. The general and local symptoms disappear in a few days. The disease may be confused with ulcerative stomatitis which some-times begins in the throat. The prognosis is favorable and the treatment is symptomatic.

The Newborn Infant

Full-Term Infants

During the first decade and a half of this century, save for infant feeding studies, little scientific attention had been directed toward the newborn infant, despite the remarkable progress of pediatrics in general during that period. The first edition of Max Runge's (1849–1909) book about the diseases of the newborn period, *Die Krankheiten der ersten Lebenstage*, was published in 1885, and Budin in France published many of his lectures at the turn of the century, but these publications concerned purely clinical phases and were written largely from the standpoint of obstetrics.

The first comprehensive book on the diseases of the newborn was published in Vienna in 1914 by August von Reuss (1879–1954); an English translation appeared in 1922. His book was primarily concerned with diseases but did outline normal growth and development and the meager knowledge then available about the physiology of the newborn infant.

From 1900 to 1925 the number of prenatal clinics increased markedly and a growing number of American mothers decided to have their babies in hospitals; this trend led to the establishment of newborn nurseries in American hospitals. While less than 5 percent of American women had delivered their infants in hospitals in 1900, the percentage greatly increased in the 1920's. By 1921 more than half the births in many large American cities took place in hospitals, varying from a high of 85 percent in San Francisco to a low of 9.2 percent in New Bedford, Massachusetts. The development of newborn nurseries in hospitals and the need for someone to direct them stimulated more than anything else an interest in the medical care of the newborn.

This interest in the neonate was further heightened by the nationwide mortality figures published by the newly created Children's Bureau (pp. 156–157). These studies, while indicating a favorable trend in lowering the death rate among infants in general, clearly pointed out that the infant mortality

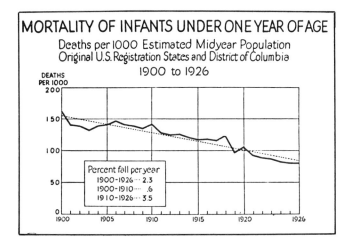

Figure 7–13. Mortality of infants under one year of age—original U.S. Registration States and District of Columbia, 1900–1926. (From L. K. Frankel. The Present Status of Maternal and Infant Hygiene in the United States. *New York: Metropolitan Life Insurance Co., 1927. Reprinted by permission.*)

in the first month of life had remained practically stationary during the twenty-year period from 1900 to 1920.

In 1914 one infant in every twenty-five died in the first four weeks of life and almost a third of the total number of deaths occurred in this four-week period.[74] The largest single cause of death was called congenital debility, which included prematurity; this category amounted to half of the total mortality for this age. Next in importance were deaths from birth injuries, sepsis, and cerebral hemorrhage, followed by congenital malformations and syphilis.

As the first quarter of the century ended, the reduction of infant mortality between 1900 and 1926 was considerable. For the ten original Death Registration States and the District of Columbia, the infant mortality rate in 1900 was 162 per 1,000 live births. by 1926 the rate was approximately 80 per 1,000 (Fig. 7–13), or about half that of 1900. However, most of the improvement had taken place since about 1910. Comparing the points on the trend line shown in Figure 7–13 for the years 1900 and 1910, the infant mortality during these years declined by only 6 percent, or an average fall of 0.6 percent per year. Between 1910 and 1926, it declined at an average of about 3.5 percent per year. Averaging the gains and losses over the whole period, the infant mortality rate declined on the average about 2.3 percent per year.[38]

Between 1918 and 1925, in infants beyond one month of age, there was a fall of 41 percent in the mortality rate, or an average of 7.4 percent per year. It was in this period of life that most of the saving of infants' lives had taken place. Under one month of age, the death rate declined less than 15 percent between 1918 and 1925, or on the average about 1.8 percent per year (Fig. 7–14). Furthermore, most of the reduction of mortality in the first month of life occurred in the second, third, and fourth weeks, where the decline was about 4 percent per year. Within the first week of life, excluding the first day, the reduction was only 1.3 percent per year. And worst of all, the mortality during the first day of life had not decreased at all between 1918 and 1925[38]

In 1925 the four most important causes of infant mortality were prematurity (congenital weakness), congenital malformations, birth injury, and congenital syphilis (Fig. 7–15). Between 1918 and 1925 the death rate from prematurity was about 19 per 1,000 infants, remaining about the same each year. In 1925, prematurity accounted for 24.1 percent of the infant deaths under one year; for 36 percent of the deaths in the first week, excluding the first day; and for 62.6 percent of the deaths on the first day of life.[38]

The death rate from congenital malformations de-

Figure 7–14. Infant mortality by age intervals—U.S. Birth Registration Area of 1917. (From L. K. Frankel. The Present Status of Maternal and Infant Hygiene in the United States. *New York: Metropolitan Life Insurance Co., 1927. Reprinted by permission.*)

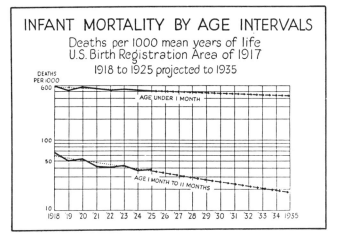

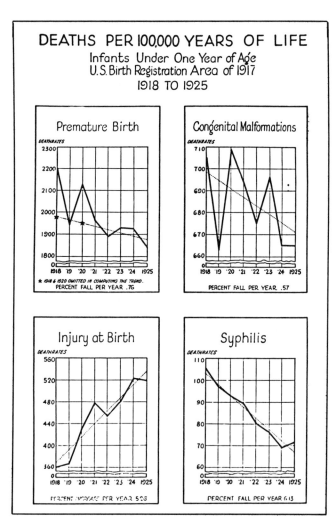

DEATHS PER 100,000 YEARS OF LIFE
Infants Under One Year of Age
U.S. Birth Registration Area of 1917
1918 TO 1925

Premature Birth

DEATHRATES

2300
2200
2100
2000
1900
1800
0

1918 '19 '20 '21 '22 '23 '24 1925
* 1918 & 1920 OMITTED IN COMPUTING THE TREND.
PERCENT FALL PER YEAR .76

Congenital Malformations

DEATHRATES

710
700
690
680
670
660
0

1918 '19 '20 '21 '22 '23 '24 1925
PERCENT FALL PER YEAR .57

Injury at Birth

DEATHRATES

560
520
480
440
400
360
0

1918 '19 '20 '21 '22 '23 '24 1925
PERCENT INCREASE PER YEAR 5.06

Syphilis

DEATHRATES

110
100
90
80
70
60
0

1918 '19 '20 '21 '22 '23 '24 1925
PERCENT FALL PER YEAR 6.13

Figure 7–15. Deaths per 100,000 years of life: Infants under one year of age. U.S. Birth Registration Area of 1917, 1918 to 1925. (From L. K. Frankel, The Present Status of Maternal and Infant Hygiene in the United States. Metropolitan Life Insurance Co., New York City, 1927, with permission.)

clined about 0.6 percent per year between 1918 and 1925. This comprised 16.2 percent of the deaths in the first week, excluding the first day, and 9 percent of the deaths on the first day.

A startling fact observed during the period between 1918 and 1925 was the sharp increase in the death rate of infants from birth injuries. Between 1918 and 1925, this death rate increased more than 5 percent per year. Injuries at birth made up 14.5 percent of the deaths on the first day of life in 1925 and 16.7 percent of the deaths in the first week, excluding the first day.[38] This increase was never satisfac-

torily explained and it seems difficult to believe that it was entirely due to better birth registration data.

The infant mortality from syphilis fell from 105 per 100,000 births in 1918 to 72 per 100,000 in 1925.[38] Concentrated efforts to discover syphilis early in pregnancy and then to treat the affected mother materially reduced the infant mortality from this cause. One study found that only 7 percent of the infants of syphilitic mothers died within the first two weeks or were stillborn when satisfactory antiluetic treatment was given, as compared with a mortality of 52 percent within the first two weeks when such treatment was not given.[124]

AVERAGE BIRTH WEIGHT OF INFANTS. During this period a number of studies on the average birth weight of American infants were published. These ranged from a low of 3,228 grams to a high of 3,965 grams. However, the latter figure was only for infants in well-to-do families. The upper limit of weight was about 4,500 grams.[51] The references to much larger infants prior to the twentieth century were thought to have been the result of inaccurate weighing. However, an infant weighing 11,360 grams (25 pounds) and accurately weighed at birth was reported in 1916.[11]

FEEDING THE NEWBORN INFANT. Breast-feeding was strongly recommended because it was still felt that the life of the infant depended to such a great extent upon whether or not the mother could nurse it. In a thorough review of the literature, Griffith in 1912 noted that "breast-fed babies have a least five times the chance of living than the bottle-fed babies possess." Fourteen years later Grulee[51] wrote that "only an extremely small percentage, certainly less than 1 percent of newly born infants, should be fed artificially from birth on. Certainly the number of mothers who cannot secrete any breast milk for their newly born infants is extremely small." Grulee, like many others during the 1920's, had been greatly impressed with Julius P. Sedgwick's (1876–1923)[109] campaigns to promote breast-feeding in Minneapolis in 1917 and again in 1920; this was probably the most successful breast-feeding crusade in America and undoubtedly the last on so large a scale. For a period of nine months Sedgwick followed the mothers of practically every infant born in Minneapolis in 1919 and 1920. If the mothers were not successful in nursing their babies directly, they were taught manual expression of milk. According to the ages of the infants, 98 percent were breast-fed at one month, 95 percent at two months, 92 percent at three months, and 79 percent at eight months. Sedgwick also noted that as a result of the breast-feeding campaign the infant mortality dropped significantly.

If the newborn infant, for one reason or another, had to be bottle-fed, Grulee[51] favored undiluted albumin milk. If that was not available, he recommended a simple milk dilution consisting of half cow's milk and half water. The amount to be given was approximately three ounces per pound of body weight in twenty-four hours, to which was added one-half ounce of dextrin-maltose mixture for the twenty-four-hour feeding. He warned, however, that "when the child is fed altogether on artificial food from birth on, we cannot expect the same nutritive results, of course, as where it is given its natural nourishment." But he did qualify this by noting that "under favorable conditions, the immediate results, however, are not so bad as a rule."

Premature Infants

In 1922 Julius H. Hess (1876–1955),[58] of Chicago, published the first book ever written dealing solely with premature and "congenitally diseased" infants. The foundation of his work was mainly the researches of European physicians such as Étienne Tarnier (1828–1897) and Budin, of France, and of Finkelstein and Leo Langstein (1876–1933),[32] of Germany. The influence of the French and German centers for premature infant care played a significant role in the development of such centers in other countries. For example, Hess, who founded the first premature infant center in the United States at the Michael Reese Hospital in Chicago, spent several years in Germany and Austria studying the care and feeding of premature infants.

In the preface of his book Hess[58] wrote: "In the United States the care of premature infants has not received the general attention of the medical profession which it merits. Facilities for the care of such infants are lacking; first, because special obstetrical hospitals in most instances decline outside cases, and, second, because comparatively few general hospitals are properly organized to undertake the special

care required. Proper handling of these infants demands a thorough knowledge of their immediate needs."

In the early part of this century a premature infant was defined as one born prior to the usual two hundred and eighty days or before the end of the fortieth week of pregnancy, but in common usage it usually referred to those infants who had undergone a gestation period of two hunded and sixty days or less.

Another class of infants who were considered in the same category as the premature infant were the so-called weaklings, infants born possibly at term, or nearly so, yet who were thought to have suffered more or less severely in utero through factors that interfered with their nutrition and consequently their development. They were classed as congenitally diseased or debilitated. For practical reasons, premature and congenitally debilitated infants were grouped together for statistical and therapeutic purposes.

The diagnosis of prematurity on the basis of birth weight was first described by Alexandre Gueniot (1832–1935) in 1872 as "not over 2,300 gm and may be below 1,500 gm."[32] The criterion of 2,500 grams to distinguish a premature from a mature infant was used for the first time by Nikolay F. Miller (1847–1897), of Moscow. This standard was also used by Budin in 1888.[32] However, it was not until 1935 that the American Academy of Pediatrics adopted such a definition and not until 1950 that the World Health Organization recommended this figure for use by member nations.[32]

ETIOLOGY. The most frequent cause of premature birth during this period was chronic disease in the mother, of which syphilis played the leading role; it was estimated as being a factor in from 50 to 80 percent of all cases of prematurity.[51, 58] Chronic nephritis was also a common cause. The puny offspring of these mothers were attributed either to the systemic effect of a chronic disease on the mother or to impaired nutrition of the fetus from placental hemorrhages and infarcts. Primary tuberculosis was a less frequent cause of premature labor, but the infants of tuberculous mothers, even at term, were often found to be small and weak. Maternal infections due to smallpox, diphtheria, measles, typhoid fever, scar-

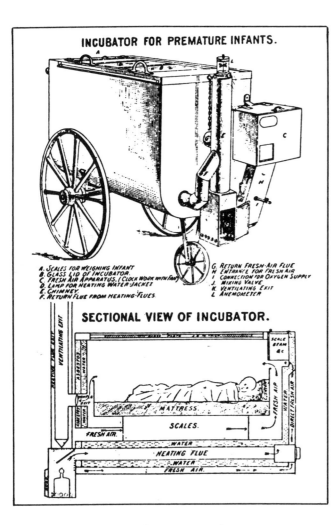

INCUBATOR FOR PREMATURE INFANTS.

A. SCALES FOR WEIGHING INFANT
B. GLASS LID OF INCUBATOR.
C. FRESH AIR APPARATUS. (CLOCK WORK WITH FAN)
D. LAMP FOR HEATING WATER-JACKET
E. CHIMNEY.
F. RETURN FLUE FROM HEATING-FLUES.

G. RETURN FRESH-AIR FLUE
H. ENTRANCE FOR FRESH AIR
I. CONNECTION FOR OXYGEN SUPPLY
J. MIXING VALVE
K. VENTILATING EXIT
L. ANEMOMETER

SECTIONAL VIEW OF INCUBATOR.

Figure 7–16. Rotch incubator (From Thomas Morgan Rotch. Pediatrics (4th ed.). Philadelphia: Lippincott, 1903.)

let fever, and influenza were also cited as frequent causes of prematurity.

PRINCIPLES OF CARE. Budin[32] was the first to outline the special care needs for premature infants that still prevail. He wrote that "with weaklings we shall have to consider three points: (a) their temperature and their chilling, (b) their feeding, and (c) the diseases to which they are susceptible."

The first and most immediate need was to keep the infant warm. The inability of the premature infant to maintain its body temperature was a well-known fact, and the need for an artificial means to overcome this handicap led to the development of incubators. The first practical incubator was designed by Tarnier[117] in 1889 for use at the Paris

Maternity Hospital. Rotch's incubator was the first manufactured in the United States (Fig. 7–16) but it was too expensive and cumbersome to be of general use. To meet the need for a practical model, Hess designed a water-jacketed incubator in 1914 (Fig. 7–17); the Hess incubator was widely used in the United States for the next twenty-five years.

Not all American pediatricians viewed the use of the incubator with favor. For example, LeFétra,[79] in a detailed review published in 1916 of the hospital care of two hundred and seventy-eight premature infants at Bellevue Hospital in New York, wrote that his experience with most incubators and their methods of management had led him to adopt a decidedly negative view of their usefulness. He claimed that there were "so many disadvantages in the use of incubators, as compared to their advantages, that the plan of setting aside a small room as an incubator room and having that kept at the proper temperature is much more satisfactory in every way."[79]

LaFétra's premature room at Bellevue Hospital had a capacity of ten cribs, with airspace of 1,000 cubic feet per crib. The air was kept moist by keep-

Figure 7–17. Hess incubator, c. 1920.

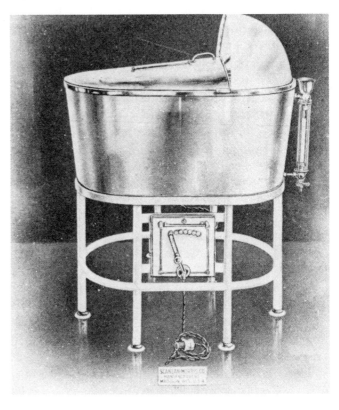

ing a large pan of water simmering on an electric stove. The room temperature was kept from 76° to 80° F with the relative humidity maintained between 60 and 70 percent. Very feeble infants were not only wrapped in cotton but hot water bottles were put at the bottom and sides of the crib until the infant developed sufficiently to maintain an even body temperature without them.

Walter L. Carr (1859–1942),[20] writing in 1921 about his experiences in caring for premature infants at the Manhattan Maternity and Dispensary Hospital, also favored an incubator room in preference to incubators. His incubator room was 6½ feet by 7 feet with a ceiling 12 feet high. The air intake was from a window by a means of a flue 9 by 2 inches and the air was warmed by being carried in back of a radiator. The room temperature was kept at 80° F. No mention was made of the relative humidity.

FEEDING THE PREMATURE INFANT. Human milk was considered by most pediatricians of the utmost importance in feeding premature infants, and a few believed that even breast milk should diluted and even predigested for feeding the infant weighing less than 1,500 grams. If breast milk was unavailable, Hess recommended buttermilk, or skimmed milk with added carbohydrates, for the first three weeks, at which time some whole boiled milk was added to prevent fat inanition. Grulee[51] favored albumin milk.

During the early years of this century the number of calories per kilogram per day required by premature infants was believed to be between 120 and 150. These figures were derived from German studies inaugurated by Heubner in Leipzig in 1894 from his work with the respiration calorimeter designed for infants.

LaFétra,[79] as early as 1916, had noted that as the premature infant gained weight and its subcutaneous fat increased, the caloric requirement diminished, "so that by the time the weight of five pounds is reached the calories may generally be safely reduced to 110 or 120 per kilogram [per day]."

Premature infants were fed by gavage or by using a Breck feeder* if they were too weak to nurse. In the premature wards in Bellevue Hospital breast milk was diluted one-half with whey for the first few

*Designed by Samuel Breck (1862–1926), the first superintendent of the medical department of the Boston Floating Hospital.

days, one ounce being given every one and a half to two hours, depending on the size of the baby. The infants were initially given 120 to 150 calories per kilogram[79] per day.

Not everyone considered breast milk the ideal food for premature infants. Rotch, at one time, believed that the best way to feed them was by means of a modified milk formula carefully prepared at milk laboratories. He believed that this method of feeding premature infants was "far superior to even breast feeding, and . . . will result in a decided reduction in their mortality." The advantages he saw in this method were its sterility, its properly balanced constituents, and the ability to vary the percentages of carbohydrate, protein, and fat in the milk formula at will, in addition to which the infant could be fed without being removed from the incubator. The formula recommended by Rotch for a twenty-eight-week-old infant contained "1 percent fat, 3 percent sugar and 0.5 percent protein."

PROGNOSIS. In 1916 LaFétra[79] reported that of the last 200 premature infants admitted to the infants' ward at Bellevue Hospital only thirty survived long enough to be discharged home (15 percent). Ninety of the two hundred infants died on the first day, many within an hour or so of the time of admission; twenty-eight died on the second and third day. The smallest surviving infant weighed 2 pounds 13½ ounces. This baby remained in the hospital for seven months and weighed 5 pounds 6½ ounces at the time of discharge.

Herman Schwarz (1876–1945) and Jerome Kohn (1893–1964),[108] in their study reported in 1921, found that among the infants of low birth weight (2,500 grams or less), 10.5 percent died within the first twenty-four days, and 14 percent in the first week. From a survey of the statistics of others, included with their own, these authors found that 30 percent of infants under 2,500 grams died in the first month of life. The mortality increased as the weight decreased. For those under 1,000 grams, 94 percent died; 1,000 to 1,500 grams, 69 percent; 1,500 to 2,000 grams, 41 percent; and 2,000 to 2,500 grams, 11 percent. They also emphasized the importance of prematurity in determining the infant mortality rate because among 1,000 premature infants, 425 died, while of 1,000 full-term infants, only 233 died.

In 1905 DeWitt Sherman (1864–1940),[110] of Buffalo, published the following table showing the number of premature infants saved according to weight in his institution:

Birth weight	Percentage saved
2 to 2½ pounds	25.0
2½ to 3 pounds	50.0
3 to 3½ pounds	42.8
3½ to 4 pounds	50.0
4 to 4½ pounds	75.0

Maynard Ladd (1873–1942),[77] in a study published in 1910 on premature infants fed modified cow's milk formulas and without the benefit of incubators, revealed that of 125 infants, 82, or 62.5 percent, died; the mortality rate for those weighing from 1,200 to 1,500 grams was 71.9 percent and from 1,500 to 2,000 grams, 44.2 percent. No infant of less than 1,200 grams survived. "Modified milk, however carefully given and supervised," Ladd claimed, "must be considered an unsatisfactory food for premature infants, and should be used only when breast milk was not available." The mortality rate in infants fed on breast milk was not stated.

Paul Cook[22] in 1921, in an effort "to get a clearer idea of the management of prematurity," analyzed the data he had collected on 77 premature infants. There were 33 deaths among the 77 cases, or a gross mortality of 43 percent. Of the total number of deaths, 19, or 57.5 percent, occurred on the first day of life. In the remaining 58 cases, the mortality was 24 percent. But after the first three days, the death rate dropped to 15 percent. The smallest survivor in this series weighed 1,250 grams and was 38 centimeters in length.

The smallest reported premature infants born in the United States to have survived the neonatal period during the period between 1900 and 1925 were two survivors of a triplet delivery cared for by Hess[58] in Chicago. They were two girls born of a Greek mother at six and a half months of gestation, weighing 740 and 690 grams at birth. They survived for seventy-two and seventy-one days, respectively, and both succumbed during attacks of cyanosis due in all probability, according to Hess,[58] to overfeeding.

During the first quarter of this century physicians caring for newborn infants were concerned primarily with how best to feed such infants, especially if breast milk was not available. However, there were three additional concerns about which much was written: inanition fever, icterus neonatorum, and hemorrhagic disease of the newborn.

Inanition Fever (Transitory Fever)

In 1895 Holt[59] described a transitory fever he termed inanition fever, which occasionally occurred from the second to the fourth day of life, at a time when the infant's weight had reached its lowest level. Although Holt did not like the term, it was adopted nonetheless, because it emphasized the "very close connection between the elevation of temperature and the condition of inanition or starvation." The condition was apparently common, since so much was written about it during this period. Many pediatricians accepted it as a definite entity, although there was a difference of opinion regarding the cause of the fever.

Most believed it was caused by a loss of body water during the first few days of life coupled with the fact that the infant got very little, frequently nothing at all from the breast during this time. But Grulee and Barnet E. Bonar (1894–1937)[51] were unable to find a relationship between 'inanition fever and the quantity of fluids ingested by the infant, nor was there any relationship between the percentage of weight loss and the fever." They were inclined to explain the condition on the basis of a "bacterial infection of the bowel due to the moistening of the meconium," which, they believed, "made that material a good medium for the growth of bacteria." The absorption from the intestines of bacteria or their products, which these authors felt could be fever-producing, would be overcome "by the ingestion of breast milk or other food that would change the character of the bacterial nutritive medium."

Harry Bakwin (1894–1972)[8] in 1922 claimed that plasma water was decreased in infants suffering from this type of fever and that coincident with the fall of the infant's temperature, there was an increase in plasma water. In a later paper (1924) Bakwin[9] wrote that when the infant with inanition fever was offered "water in the amount of 40 cc/kg/body weight by mouth, the temperature fell rapidly to normal within 30–90 minutes."

The only worrisome symptom was the fever. The temperature of affected infants varied from 100° to

105°, with the peak occurring on the first day of fever; as a rule the temperature returned to normal within twenty-four hours after fluid had been offered to the infant. When the temperature started to fall, it nearly always dropped to normal almost immediately. The only other symptom reported was that some infants were slightly more languid than normal. The most noticeable observation, however, was that there were so few findings in comparison with the height of the fever.

Treatment was simple. The mere giving of a little extra milk or water resulted in an almost immediate drop of the temperature. On the average, one and a half ounces per feeding was said to be sufficient to lower the infant's temperature. Nor did there seem to be any tendency after having offered fluid to the infant for the temperature to rise again.[9]

Icterus Neonatorum

There was much disagreement about the frequency of icterus neonatorum. It had been described in as high as 90 percent and as low as 20 percent of newborn infants.[51] Some thought it occurred in epidemics; this was vigorously denied by others.

Three distinct forms of icterus neonatorum were described: the simplex, the prolongata, and the gravis. Much discussion was focused on the nature of the gravis form; some believed that it was always the result of sepsis, although when attempts to grow bacteria from tissues at autopsy were tried, the results were usually negative. Others considered the gravis form to be the result of congenital syphilis, but this was a period when almost every puzzling clinical finding was attributed to syphilis. Some thought the gravis form was caused by a powerful but unknown poison, while others incriminated chloroform as playing a large role in its development.

Abt,[1] writing in 1917, doubted the septic nature of what he termed familial icterus (icterus gravis); nor did he believe there was any hereditary influence, a history of birth injury, or toxemia of pregnancy.* He also had noted that in familial icterus the first or second child often survived while "later

*Although a familial form of icterus neonatorum was known, in which several children of the same family had been affected, it was usually considered unrelated to what was then termed nuclear icterus, or kernicterus.

children die a few days after birth as the result of a grave and progressive icterus." He wrote that "at the onset there may be hyperemia of the skin," but if the disease continued, "hemorrhages from the various mucous surfaces and into the skin, as well as from the umbilicus, occurred." Atonic convulsions, particularly of the upper extremities, as well as opisthotonus were frequently observed.

In icterus simplex, no treatment was necessary. Cholagogues were not recommended because it was generally believed that the condition was not associated in any way with obstruction of the bile ducts. For icterus gravis, no treatment was thought to be of any value. However, Paul Klemperer (1887–1964)[72] in 1924 suggested the use of glucose transfusion, though he did not explain why.

Hemorrhagic Diseases of the Newborn

Although it was recognized that bleeding in the newborn infant could result from a number of causes such as infection and trauma, it was also known that even after hemorrhages from these causes had been accounted for, there still remained some that were idiopathic in nature. Hemorrhagic disease of the newborn was looked upon as a very serious problem in the early years of the century, when 60 percent of the patients died, half of them in the first twenty-four hours after the onset of bleeding.[46] If they survived a week, they almost invariably recovered.

The most effective treatment was the use of blood and blood serum. The use of human blood was considered the most rational measure because it supplied the materials lacking for coagulation. (Of course, this was before the role of the Rh factor in possibly sensitizing Rh-negative patients was appreciated.) Blood was given as whole blood, or blood serum, or both. It was usually given either subcutaneously or intramuscularly. The preferred method was to take the blood directly from the donor's vein and to inject it deep into the infant's buttocks. The amount of blood given this way was usually between 15 and 30 ml.[51] If the human blood or serum was given intravenously, which was done in rare cases, the superior sagittal sinus was the preferred route of administration.

Diatheses and the Thymus

Two other conditions that concerned pediatricians during the first quarter of this century were the diatheses and, especially, the role of the thymus as a cause of sudden, unexplained death.

Diatheses

A diathesis was defined as a bodily condition or constitutional anomaly which predisposed to other pathological conditions.[19] To explain this a peculiarity of constitution had been assumed. A corollary of this assumption was the theory of organic inferiority. Constitutional differences were often given as the reason why some infants failed to thrive under the best of care and also why vastly different methods of artificial feeding might give either good or bad results in the hands of the same investigator. Before the development of bacteriology this concept was generally accepted to explain a disease such as scrofula. When it became obvious that many of the symptoms of scrofula were symptoms of tuberculosis, the concept was gradually given up. But three so-called diatheses lingered on for most of the first third of the century. These were the exudative, the neuropathic, and the lymphatic diatheses. (The last-named is described below in the discussion of the thymus, with which it was thought to be associated.)

The symptoms of the exudative diathesis, popularized especially by Czerny, developed early in life and were largely confined to lesions of the skin and mucous membranes. Infants with this condition tended to show early seborrhea of the scalp, prurigo, and intertrigo and to be particularly liable to eczema. There were usually well nourished, even obese, with flabby musculature. Anemia and a great tendency toward rhinopharyngitis were also common findings. The pathogenesis of this diathesis was variously attributed to a number of nebulous causes such as faulty metabolism, autointoxication, and faulty assimilation.

The neuropathic or vagotonic diathesis was defined as a morbidly exaggerated tonus of the autonomic nervous system. The vagotonic disposition was thought to be either general, in which case it was characterized by nervousness, or local and characterized by localized spasms. The symptoms of vagotonia in children were said to have been salivation, sweating, laryngospasm, stomach and bowel unrest, nervous diarrhea, spastic constipation, polyuria, and reflex anuria.

The Thymus and Status Thymicolymphaticus

Until about the mid-1930's the thymus gland, especially if it was thought to be enlarged, evoked enormous concern and fear. It was a gland that stood accused of unphysiological activities and was alleged, as Gamble[43] wrote, "to be dangerously subversive of the steady state . . . with the malign intent of causing sudden and violent death of infants." Many physicians believed that a large thymus was capable of causing suffocation from pressure on the trachea, the so-called mors thymica, first described in 1614 by Felix Platter (1536–1614).[94] Others were convinced that it played a dominant role in so-called status thymicolymphaticus, also known as status lymphaticus or the lymphatic constitution or diathesis.

The clinical picture caused by the putative pressure of a "persistent" or "enlarged" thymus in infants included one or more of the following symptoms: a paroxysmal or a dry and hacking nocturnal cough, intermittent inspiratory stridor, continuous or remittent dyspnea, choking while nursing, spells of cyanosis, and head retraction. All these symptoms were said to be frequently relieved by lying on the side with the head back and to be intensified by flexing the head on the chest. There was considerable controversy about the relationship of the width of the thymic shadow on the x-ray film to the reputed thymic symptoms. Equally controversial were two other matters: first, at what point the shadow signified an enlarged thymus; and second, how large the shadow should be before treating the child with x-rays or radium to decrease the gland's size.

The supposed mechanical effects due to thymic hyperplasia were thought to be independent of status thymicolymphaticus, an entity first described by Arnold Paltauf (1860–1893)[88] in 1889; he persistently maintained that the marked lymphoid hyperplasia associated with an enlarged thymus was anatomic evidence of a constitutional weakness or diathesis. Just why this should be so was not explained. In such cases the patient was thought to be so constituted that he could be killed by insignificant causes as compared to those required to bring about the death of a normal person. Paltauf based his hypothesis on a rather sketchy analysis of only five cases; the weights of the thymuses in these five cases were not recorded. As Edith Boyd (1895–1978)[16] has noted: "This work seems hardly an adequate basis for a new pathologic entity." Nevertheless, Paltauf's hypothesis was widely accepted by many pediatricians during a good part of this century; it was often uncritically mentioned as the cause of sudden death in any person with a thymus that weighed more that 15 grams and containing lymphoid tissue which the pathologist might claim was "enlarged." Paltauf described his subjects as pale, overweight, rachitic infants who were found dead, or as young, well-nourished adults who dropped dead while in swimming. The common feature in almost every case of status thymicolymphaticus was sudden death.

From Paltauf's short paper, published in two installments, there sprung an enormous "literature" amounting to more than eight hundred papers by 1922. A review of these papers provides the reader with a splendid example of the luxuriant growth and tenacious vitality of a medical myth. Park[90] said there was something about the thymus that made it "a kind of fabulous island of romance which must have been inhabited by sirens when visited by some investigators, for treasures were loudly proclaimed which have turned out on analysis to be indifferent stone." Irradiation of the supposedly enlarged thymus gland was unfortunately introduced in clinical medicine by Alfred Friedlander (1871–1939) in 1917 as a result of Herman Heineke's (1873–1922) demonstration of the rapid atrophy of the thymus in small animals following roentgen exposure.

Skepticism about the relation between the supposedly enlarged thymus and lymph nodes and the symptoms they were said to have caused developed haltingly because the more one tried to pinpoint the pathogenesis of status thymicolymphaticus the more nebulous the entity became. Acceptance of the condition was strengthened perhaps because respected academicians such as Howland and Holt had accepted it, at least initially. Howland[63] in 1907 reported twenty-five cases of sudden death due, as he then thought, to an enlargement of the thymus above 15 grams, which he set as the upper limit of normal. The cases were divided into two classes: those in whom sudden death had occurred without

any previous symptoms and those in whom a high fever (up to 109° F) had developed suddenly, associated with rapid breathing, cyanosis, convulsions, and coma, with death in thirty-six to forty-eight hours. The striking points found in the latter group, according to Howland, were the presence of marked dyspnea and cyanosis without sufficient pulmonary involvement to explain them, plus convulsions and an extremely high temperature.

Holt[61] wrote that status lymphaticus was "applied to a very definite pathological condition which was associated with clinical manifestations, less constant and not characteristic." These qualifications would seem to weaken his assertion that it was "a very definite pathological condition." He further claimed that in status lymphaticus the thymus was often five to ten times larger than normal; weighing as much as 30 to 40 grams, but more usually 15 to 20 grams. However, J. A. Hammer[52] had shown that in well-nourished infants between one and two years of age the thymus could weigh as much as 36 grams and even as much as 40 grams in some well-nourished adolescents.

Edith Boyd,[16] in her meticulously documented paper published in 1927, should have destroyed the myth of the thymus as a cause of sudden death, but the myth lingered on for several more years. Her skepticism about status thymicolymphaticus was aroused by this case:

I was consulted on a coroner's case of a 5-year-old boy who had died in convulsions ten minutes after the onset. I found nothing to account for the death. The lymphoid tissue was prominent, and the thymus weighed 50 gm. The microscopic sections showed prominent lymph nodules in the lungs and in the spleen. I could find no evidence of infection, and finally committed myself by saying that this was the anatomic picture of status thymicolymphaticus. Since it was a coroner's case, I brought the contents of the stomach to the state toxicologist. Two months later I was called to testify in a murder trial for strychnine poisoning, about 25 mg. of strychnine having been recovered from this boy's stomach. From these and similar cases, in which there was early pneumonia, I became skeptical of the diagnosis of status thymicolymphaticus.

Griffith[48], of Philadelphia, published a report in 1919 of seven sudden infant deaths in one family which he labeled "the so-called thymus death." However, he was troubled with this explanation because he found it intellectually unsatisfactory and also because he was aware that in many postmortem examinations of infants who had died suddenly, no satisfactory cause of death was discovered. He wrote:

Certainly as far as my own experience and reading of literature goes, I feel convinced that whereas there are cases in which death results from pressure of the thymus gland upon the trachea, these are exceptional, and warning in such cases is given by symptoms of strangulation gradually increasing in severity. The cases of actually sudden, or at least rapid, death, I think depend upon a neurosis which may be associated with lymphatic and thymic enlargement as its anatomic manifestations, but is not necessarily so. It is only on the supposition of some such neurosis as a result of which cardiac inhibition takes place from insignificant cause, that a reasonable explanation is to be found for the sudden death sometimes occurring in eczema following plunging into cold water, and giving of hypodermic injections, the puncturing of the pleural cavity, and the like.

The banal denouement of the thymus story, which came about chiefly as a result of the careful studies by Hammer[52] on the growth and involution of the thymus, was that the anatomic picture that Paltauf had described as that of status thymicolymphaticus represented merely the normal thymus and lymphoid tissue of the well-nourished child. Perhaps because status thymicolymphaticus was polysyllabic, had Latin endings, and sounded impressive it found acceptance for many more years than it deserved. The final devastating blow came in 1950 when it was shown that thyroid carcinoma can be a late sequel of "preventive" irradiation for the supposedly enlarged thymus.

Endocrine Disorders

The only two pediatric endocrine disorders during this period for which effective treatment was available were diabetes and hypothyroidism (sporadic cretinism or myxedema).

Sporadic Cretinism

Sporadic cretinism, as distinct from the endemic variety, first described by Charles H. Fagge (1838–1883) in 1871, was well known to physicians in the early part of this century, as was hypothyroidism and its many symptoms. Treatment of both of these diseases with desiccated thyroid gland gave dramatic results, especially in sporadic cretinism. In fact, in sporadic cretinism the change was so dramatic that Osler[87] wrote: "Not the magic wand of Prospero nor the brave kiss of the daughter of Hippocrates ever effected such a change as that which we are now enabled to make in these unfortunate victims, doomed heretofore to live in hopeless imbecility, an unspeakable affliction to their parents and to their relatives."

Diabetes

David M. Cowie (1872–1940) and John P. Parsons[24] in 1923 published a long and detailed report on the use of insulin in diabetes based on five adults and six children; this was probably the first report in the pediatric literature on the use of insulin in children, since the original paper by Sir Frederick G. Banting (1891–1941) had been published only a year before.

Until the discovery of insulin it could be truthfully said that in few diseases had the prognosis been so bad as in juvenile diabetes. The course of the disease had been almost invariably steadily and progressively downhill; almost all diabetic children died of diabetic coma within months or a year or two after the diagnosis had been made.[115]

In diabetic children, insulin proved strikingly beneficial. For the first time, children with diabetic acidosis and even coma were brought back to health. Despite the introduction of insulin as a "specific" for diabetes mellitus, a fear of the disease as life-threatening still remained for a few years after the discovery of insulin.

Allergy

The word *allergy* was coined by von Pirquet, who recognized the common denominator that links immunity to hypersensitivity. In 1912 Schloss[102] made a major contribution to modern medicine with his report "A Case of Allergy to Common Foods." Under this simple title, he described an eight-year-old boy who developed urticaria on ingestion of eggs, almonds, or oatmeal. Schloss, aware of the concepts developed by von Pirquet and Schick on tuberculin allergy (1907), demonstrated that cutaneous inoculation of any one of these foods produced an immediate urticarial wheal at the site of inoculation. He showed further that the urticarial wheals were produced only by the protein constituents which he extracted from these foods. Harry Gordon (b. 1906)[47] wrote: "Although H. L. Smith reported at approximately the same time local and general reactions to cutaneous application of buckwheat in a case of buckwheat poisoning . . . it is fair to say that Dr. Schloss' elegant experiments supplied the basis for the use of skin testing with allergens as a diagnostic measure in pediatric practice."

In 1915 Schloss again reported on allergy to common foods. As Faber and McIntosh[35] noted, Schloss "made cutaneous tests, including intracutaneous, and discovered several cases of egg sensitivity. In two of these, in one of sensitivity to milk and in one [of sensitivity] to oats, he succeeded in passive transfer to sensitivity with the patient's serum to a normal individual." He also described several cases in which eczema was relieved by elimination of offending foods, and a few with similar results in asthma. This paper, according to Faber and McIntosh, was an important milestone in the study of human allergy. A year later, Schloss[106] demonstrated the permeability of the gastrointestinal tract to undigested protein in some infants with nutritional or "gastro-enteric disorders." In these infants he noted that "foreign protein may be absorbed in an undigested or partially digested state and appear in the urine."

In 1923, Arthur F. Anderson and Schloss,[3] in their review of allergy to cow's milk in nutritional disorders of infants, demonstrated that circulating precipitins were present in eighty of ninety-eight "atrophic" infants. They were also able to show that cow's milk protein was absorbed in the course of diarrhea.

Infantile eczema during this period was considered the most frequent and most important disease of the skin in early life.[61] By 1925 some thought that it was almost exclusively due to sensitivity to foods. Talbot and Schloss, however, believed that there were many causes, not always food.[35] Two commonly held beliefs prior to 1925 was that the severity of infantile eczema bore a direct relation to the fat in the food and that it was also one of the manifestations of the so-called exudative diathesis. Eczema was said to be especially prevalent in fat, healthy-looking infants.

New Publications

American Textbooks of Pediatrics, 1900 to 1925

A flood of new textbooks of pediatrics appeared between 1900 and 1925. The following is a chronological listing of these textbooks (new editions of these or of the older pediatric textbooks previously described are not included):

1900   Nathan Oppenheim   The Medical Diseases of Childhood

1901   John Madison Taylor and William H. Wells   Manual of the Diseases of Children

1902   Henry Koplik   The Diseases of Infancy and Childhood

1905   John Ruhräh   A Manual of the Diseases of Infants and Children

1906   Walter L. Carr (ed.)   Practice of Pediatrics in Original Contributions by American and English Authors

1906   Alfred Cleveland Cotton   The Medical Diseases of Infancy and Childhood

1907   Charles Gilmore Kerley   Treatment of the Diseases of Children

1907   LeGrand Kerr   Diagnostics of the Diseases of Children

1907   Louis Fischer   Diseases of Infancy and Childhood

1909   Henry Dwight Chapin and Godfrey Roger Pisek   Diseases of Infants and Children

1911   John Lovett Morse   Case Histories in Pediatrics

1912   Benjamin K. Rachford   Diseases of Children

1914   James H. McKee and William H. Wells   Practical Pediatrics (2 vols.)

1914   Charles Gilmore Kerley   The Practice of Pediatrics

1916   Edwin E. Graham   Diseases of Children

1917   Charles Hunter Dunn   Pediatrics: The Hygienic and Medical Treatment of Children (3 vols.)

1917   George M. Tuttle and Phelps G. Hurford   Diseases of Children

1919   J. P. Crozer Griffith   The Diseases of Infants and Children (2 vols.)

1922   Langley Porter and William E. Carter   Management of the Sick Infant and Child

1923–1926   Isaac A. Abt (ed.)   Pediatrics (8 vols.)

The only new pediatric journal to appear during this period was the *American Journal of Diseases of Children*, which began publication in 1911 with Frank Spooner Churchill (1864–1946) as its first editor. This journal remains one of our major pediatric publications and is read and respected throughout the world.

The first article, written as an editorial by Jacobi, explained that this new pediatric journal would serve as a companion and ally to the *Archives of Internal Medicine* and as such would publish original manuscripts on the pediatric aspects of "anatomy—both embryonal and postnatal—physiology, biochemistry, nosology, and therapeutics." Jacobi visualized the *American Journal of Diseases of Children* "as one of the number of strictly scientific magazines which, since the first appearance of the *Journal of Experimental Medicine* and its followers, have given American medical journalism its standing as an equal coworker in the modern world of Medicine."

The progress made by American pediatrics from 1900 to 1925 was so rapid that by 1925 it had taken over the predominant role held by German pediatrics for more than half a century. Proof of this is evident in the comment made in 1927 by an outstanding German pediatrician, *"Sie stehen heute in Amerika in der Pädiatrie ober an"* ("You in America are now in the forefront of pediatrics").

As the second quarter of this century began, American pediatrics was on the threshold of even greater world recognition.

References

1. Abt, I. A. Familial icterus of new-born infants. *Am. J. Dis. Child.* 13:231, 1917.
2. Adams, S. S. Grip meningitis. *Trans. Am. Pediatr. Soc.* 19:145, 1908.
3. Anderson, A. F., and Schloss, O. M. Allergy to cow's milk in infants with nutritional disorders. *Am. J. Dis. Child.* 26:451, 1923.
4. Baker, S. J. The reduction of infant mortality in New York City. *Am. J. Dis. Child.* 5:151, 1913.
5. Baker, S. J. Why do our mothers and babies die? *Ladies Home J.* 40:212, 1923.
6. Baker, S. J. *Child Hygiene.* New York: Harper, 1925.
7. Baker, S. J. *Fighting for Life.* New York: Macmillan, 1939.
8. Bakwin, H. Dehydration fever in new-borns II. *Am. J. Dis. Child.* 24:508, 1922.
9. Bakwin, H., Morris, R. M., and Southworth, S. D. The effect of fluid on the temperature and blood concentration in the new-born with fever. *Am. J. Dis. Child.* 27:578, 1924.
10. Beaven, P. W. History of the Boston Floating Hospital. *Pediatrics* 19:629, 1957.
11. Belcher, D. P. A child weighing twenty-five pounds at birth. *J.A.M.A.* 67:950, 1916.
12. Benison, S. Poliomyelitis and the Rockefeller Institute. *J. Hist. Med.* 29:74, 1974.
13. Blackfan, K. D. Apparatus for collecting infants' blood for the Wassermann reaction. *Am. J. Dis. Child.* 4:33, 1912.
14. Blackfan, K. D., and Maxcy, K. F. The intraperitoneal injection of saline solution. *Am. J. Dis. Child.* 15:19, 1918.
15. Bolt, R. A. The Mortalities of Infancy. In Isaac A. Abt (ed.), *Pediatrics*, vol. 2. Philadelphia: Saunders, 1923.
16. Boyd, E. Growth of the thymus. *Am. J. Dis. Child.* 33:867, 1927.
17. Brennemann, J. The incidence and significance of rheumatic nodules in children. *Trans. Am. Pediatr. Soc.* 31:201, 1919.
18. Caillé, A. The influence of the American Pediatric Society in promoting the welfare of American children: *Trans. Am. Pediatr. Soc.* 16:6, 1904.
19. Caillé, A. Diatheses in their clinical aspect. *Arch. Pediatr.* 34:16, 1917.
20. Carr, W. L. A clinical report of simple methods in the care of premature babies. *Trans. Am. Pediatr. Soc.* 33:70, 1921.
21. Chapin, H. D. A clinical study of typhoid fever in children. *Am. J. Dis. Child.* 8:130, 1914.
22. Cook, P. A clinical study of the premature infant. *Arch. Pediatr.* 38:201, 1921.
23. Cooke, J. V., and Jeans, P. C. The transmission of syphilis to the second generation. *Am. J. Syph.* 6:569, 1922.
24. Cowie, D. M., and Parsons, J. Clinical observations on the use of insulin in the treatment of diabetes in adults and children with particular reference to the state of hyperinsulinaemia: A consideration of insulin and renal glycosuria. *Trans. Am. Pediatr. Soc.* 35:217, 1923.
25. Dandy, W. E., and Rowntree, L. G. Peritoneal and pleural absorption, with reference to postural position. *Ann. Surg.* 59:587, 1914.
26. Diamond, L. K., Allen, F. H., Jr., and Thomas, W.

O., Jr. Erythroblastosis fetalis, VII—Treatment with exchange transfusion. *New Engl. J. Med.* 244:39, 1951.

27. Dick, F. D., and Dick, G. R. *Scarlet Fever.* Chicago: Year Book Publishers, 1938.

28. Donnally, H. H. Scarlet fever, morbidity and fatality. *Am. J. Dis. Child.* 12:205, 1916.

29. Dowling, H. E. *Fighting Infection.* Cambridge, Mass.: Harvard University Press, 1977.

30. Draper, G. *Acute Poliomyelitis.* Philadelphia: Blakiston, 1917.

31. Duke, E. *Infant Mortality—Results of a Field Study in Johnstown, Pa.* Washington, D.C.: U.S. Children's Bureau Publication #9, 1915.

32. Dunham. E. C. Evolution of premature infant care. *Ann. Paediatr. Fenniae* 3:170, 1957.

33. Dunn, C. H. Cardiac disease in childhood, with special reference to prognosis. *Trans. Am. Pediatr. Soc.* 25:237, 1913.

34. Editorial: Gonorrhea and vulvo-vaginitis in children. *Pediatrics* (New York) 22:220, 1910.

35. Faber, H. K., and McIntosh, R. *History of the American Pediatric Society.* New York: McGraw-Hill, 1966.

36. Flexner, S., and Jobling, J. W. An analysis of four hundred cases of epidemic meningitis treated with the antimeningitis serum. *Trans. Am. Pediatr. Soc.* 20:17, 1908.

37. Flexner, S., and Lewis, P. A. The transmission of acute poliomyelitis to monkeys. *J.A.M.A.* 53:1639, 1913.

38. Frankel, L. K. *The Present Status of Maternal and Infant Hygiene in the United States.* New York: Metropolitan Life Insurance Co., 1927.

39. Freeman, R. G. Fresh air in pediatric practice. *Trans. Am. Pediatr. Soc.* 28:7, 1916.

40. Freeman, R. G. The symptoms and treatment of thymus hypertrophy in infancy. *Trans. Am. Pediatr. Soc.* 35:116, 1923.

41. Friedlander, A. Whooping-Cough. In I. A. Abt (ed.), *Pediatrics,* Vol. VI. Philadelphia: Saunders, 1925.

42. Gale, A. H. *Epidemic Diseases.* London: Penguin Books, 1959.

43. Gamble, J. L. Presentation of the Kober Medal to Dr. Edwards A. Park. *Trans. Assoc. Am. Physicians* 63:21, 1950.

44. Gamble, J. L. Acceptance of the Kober Medal Award. *Trans. Assoc. Am. Physicians* 64:36, 1951.

44a. Gamble, J. L. Early history of fluid replacement therapy. *Pediatrics* 11:554, 1953.

45. Gamble, J. L., Ross, S. G., and Tisdall, F. F. A study of acidosis due to ketone acids. *Trans. Am. Pediatr. Soc.* 34:289, 1922.

46. Gelston, C. F. On the etiology of hemorrhagic disease of the new-born. *Am. J. Dis. Child.* 22:351, 1921.

47. Gordon, H. H. Oscar Menderson Schloss. In B. S. Veeder (ed.), *Pediatric Profiles.* St. Louis: Mosby, 1957.

48. Griffith, J. P. C. The so-called thymus death, with an account of seven cases of sudden death in one family. *Trans. Am. Pediatr. Soc.* 21:128, 1909.

49. Griffith, J. P. C. The ability of mothers to nurse their children. *J.A.M.A.* 59:1874, 1912.

50. Griffith, J. P. C. History and recollections of the development of pediatrics in Philadelphia. *Pa. Med. J.* 39:597, 1936.

51. Grulee, C. G., and Bonar, B. E. *The Newborn Clinical Pediatrics,* vol. II. New York: Appleton, 1926.

52. Hammer, J. A. The new views as to the morphology of the thymus gland and their bearing on the function of the thymus. *Endocrinology* 5:543, 1921.

53. Harvey, A. McG. The first full-time academic department of pediatrics: The story of the Harriet Lane Home. *Johns Hopkins Med. J.* 137:27, 1975.

54. Heiman, H. Report of a case of typhoid fever in an infant of 8 months transmitted through the breast milk of the mother. *Trans. Am. Pediatr. Soc.* 31:170, 1919.

55. Helmholz, H. F. The longitudinal sinus as the place of preference in infancy for intravenous aspirations and injections, including transfusion. *Am. J. Dis. Child.* 10:194, 1915.

56. Hess, A. F. Infantile Scurvy (Barlow's Disease). In I. A. Abt (ed.), *Pediatrics, vol. 2.* Philadelphia: Saunders, 1923.

57. Hess. A. F. *Rickets, Including Osteomalacia and Tetany.* Philadelphia: Lea & Febiger, 1929.

58. Hess, J. H. *Premature and Congenitally Diseased Infants.* Philadelphia: Lea & Febiger, 1922.

59. Holt, L. E. Inanition fever in the newly born. *Arch. Pediatr.* 12:561, 1895.

60. Holt, L. E. Infant mortality, ancient and modern: An historical sketch. *Arch. Pediatr.* 30:885, 1913.

61. Holt, L. E. and Howland, J. *The Diseases of Infancy and Childhood* (7th ed.). New York: Appleton, 1917.

62. Holt, L. E. American pediatrics: A retrospect and a forecast. *Trans. Am. Pediatr. Soc.* 35:9, 1923.

63. Howland, J. The symptoms of status lymphaticus in infants and young children. *Trans. Am. Pediatr. Soc.* 19:51, 1907.

64. Howland, J., and Marriott, W. McK. Indications for treatment of severe diarrhea in infancy. *Trans. Am. Pediatr. Soc.* 27:201, 1915.

65. Howland, J., and Marriott, W. McK. Acidosis oc-

curring with diarrhea. *Am. J. Dis. Child.* 11:309, 1916.

66. Howland, J., and Marriott, W. McK. A discussion of acidosis with special reference to that occurring in diseases of children. *Bull. Johns Hopkins Hosp.* 27:63, 1916.

67. Howland, J., and Marriott, W. McK. Observations upon the calcium content of the blood in infantile tetany and upon the effect of treatment by calcium. *Q. J. Med.* 11:289, 1918.

68. Howland, J., and Kramer, B. Calcium and phosphorus in the serum in relation to rickets. *Am. J. Dis. Child.* 22:105, 1921.

69. Howland, J., and Kramer, B. Factors concerned in the calcification of bone. *Trans. Am. Pediatr. Soc.* 34:204, 1922.

70. Jacobi, A. Discussion of vaginitis. In H. Koplik, Hospitals for the care of infants and children and the methods of prevention of infection. *Trans. Am. Pediatr. Soc.* 23:118, 1911.

70a. Jacobi, A. History of pediatrics in New York, II. *Arch. Pediatr.* 34:144, 1917.

71. Jeans, P. C. A review of the literature of syphilis in infancy and childhood. *Am. J. Dis. Child.* 20:55, 1920.

72. Klemperer, P. Icterus gravis of the new-born. *Am. J. Dis. Child.* 28:212, 1924.

73. Koplik, H. *The Diseases of Infancy and Childhood* (3rd ed.). Philadelphia: Lea & Febiger, 1910.

74. Koplik, H. Infant mortality in the first four weeks of life. *J.A.M.A.* 62:85, 1914.

75. Kramer, B., Tisdall, F. F., and Howland, J. Observations on infantile tetany. *Am. J. Dis. Child.* 22:431, 1921.

76. Kramer, B., and Howland, J. Factors which determine the concentration of calcium and of inorganic phosphorus in the blood serum of rats. *Bull. Johns Hopkins Hosp.* 33:313, 1922.

77. Ladd, M. The results of substitute feeding in premature infants. *Trans. Am. Pediatr. Soc.* 22:26, 1917.

78. LaFétra, L. E. The employment of salvarsan in infants and young children. *Trans. Am. Pediatr. Soc.* 24:183, 1912.

79. LaFétra, L. E. The hospital care of premature infants. *Trans. Am. Pediatr. Soc.* 28:90, 1916.

80. Latta, T. Letter to the Secretary of the Central Board of Health, London, affording a view of the rationale and results of his practice in the treatment of cholera by aqueous and saline injections. *Lancet* 2:274, 1831–1832.

81. Loeb, R. F. Presentation of the George M. Kober Medal to Dr. James L. Gamble. *Trans. Assoc. Am. Physicians* 64:29, 1951.

82. Lucas, W. P., et al. Blood studies in the new-born, morphological, chemical, coagulation, urobilin and bilirubin. *Am. J. Dis. Child.* 22:525, 1921.

83. Marriott, W. McK. The pathogenesis of certain nutritional disorders. *Trans. Am. Pediatr. Soc.* 31:34, 1919.

84. Marriott, W. McK. Some phases of the pathology of nutrition in infancy. *Harvey Lecture Series* 15:121, 1919–1920.

85. McCollum, E. V. An Adventure in Nutrition Investigation. In A. M. Beeuwkes, E. N. Todhunter, and E. S. Weigley (eds.), *Essay on History of Nutrition and Dietetics.* Chicago: American Dietetic Association, 1967.

86. O'Shaughnessy, W. B. Experiments on blood in cholera. *Lancet* 1:490, 1831–1832.

87. Osler, W. Sporadic Cretinism (Infantile and Juvenile Myxoedema). In W. A. Edwards (ed.), *Diseases of Children, Medical and Surgical.* Philadelphia: Lippincott, 1901, P. 359.

88. Paltauf, A. Ueber die Beziehungen der Thymus zum plötzlichen Tod. *Wien. Klin. Wochenschr.* 2:877, 1889; 3:172, 1890.

89. Parish, H. J. *A History of Immunization.* Edinburgh: Livingstone, 1965.

90. Park, E. A. Acceptance of the Kober Medal Award. *Trans. Assoc. Am. Physicians* 63:26, 1950.

91. Park, E. A. The Harriet Lane Home. In J. A. Askin, R. E. Cooke, and J. A. Haller, Jr. (eds.), *A Symposium on the Child.* Baltimore: Johns Hopkins Press, 1967.

92. Paul, J. R. *A History of Poliomyelitis.* New Haven: Yale University Press, 1971.

93. Peabody. F. W. A report of the Harvard Infantile Paralysis Commission on the diagnosis and treatment of acute cases of the disease during the year 1916. *Boston Med. Surg. J.* 176:637, 1917.

94. Platter, F. Quoted by John Ruhräh, *Pediatrics of the Past*, p. 239 New York: Hoeber, 1925.

95. Powers, G. F. Developments in pediatrics in the past quarter century. *Yale J. Biol. Med.* 12:1, 1939–1940.

96. Rachford, B. K. Maternal impressions: Report of a case. *Trans. Am. Pediatr. Soc.* 13:147, 1901.

97. Rachford, B. K. *Diseases of Children.* New York: Appleton, 1912.

98. Rachford, B. K. Epidemic vaginitis in children. *Trans. Am. Pediatr. Soc.* 28:162, 1916.

99. Ratner, A. B. A new apparatus and method for puncturing the superior longitudinal sinus in infants. *Am. J. Dis. Child.* 21:199, 1921.

100. Rotch, T. M. The position and work of the Amer-

ican Pediatric Society toward public questions. *Trans. Am. Pediatr. Soc.* 21:7, 1909.

101. Sauer, L. W. Whooping cough. *J.A.M.A.* 100:239, 1933.
102. Schloss, O. M. A case of allergy to common foods. *Am. J. Dis. Child.* 3:341, 1912.
103. Schloss, O. M. Intestinal intoxication in infants: the importance of impaired renal function. *Am. J. Dis. Child.* 15:165, 1918.
104. Schloss, O. M., and Harrington, H. Comparison of the carbon dioxid tension of the alveolar air and the hydrogen-ion concentration of the urine with the bicarbonate of the blood plasma. *Am. J. Dis. Child.* 17:85, 1919.
105. Schloss, O. M. and Stetson, R. E. The occurrence of acidosis with severe diarrhea. *Am. J. Dis. Child.* 13:218, 1917.
106. Schloss, O. M., and Worthen, T. W. The permeability of the gastro-enteric tract of infants to undigested protein. *Am. J. Dis. Child.* 11:342, 1916.
107. Schwarz, H. The treatment of poliomyelitis, prophylactic and curative. *Arch. Pediatr.* 33:859, 1916.
108. Schwarz, H., and Kohn, J. L. The infant of low birth weight; its growth and development. *Am. J. Dis. Child.* 21:296, 1921.
109. Sedgwick, J. P. A preliminary report of the study of breast feeding in Minneapolis. *Trans. Am. Pediatr. Soc.* 32:279, 1920.
110. Shermann, D. The premature infant. *N.Y. Med. J.* 82:272, 1905.
111. Sidbury, J. B. Transfusion through the umbilical vein in hemorrhage of the new-born. *Am. J. Dis. Child.* 25:290, 1923.
112. Siperstein, D. M. Intraperitoneal transfusion with citrated blood. *Am. J. Dis. Child.* 29:519, 1925.
113. Smith, C. H. The diagnosis of tuberculosis in childhood. *Trans. Am. Pediatr. Soc.* 33:246, 1921.
114. Smith, R. M. Medicine as a science: Pediatrics. *N. Engl. J. Med.* 244:176, 1951.
115. Strouse, S. Diabetes mellitus. In I. A. Abt (ed.), *Pediatrics*, vol. II. Philadelphia: Saunders, 1923.
116. Talbot, F. B. Periods in the life of the American Pediatric Society: Maturity. *Trans. Am. Pediatr. Soc.* 50:68, 1938.
117. Tannier, E. S. Des soins à donner aux enfants nés avant terme. *Bull. Acad. Méd. Paris* (2nd ser.) 14:944, 1885.
118. Van Ingen, P. Recent progress in infant welfare work. *Am. J. Dis. Child.* 7:471, 1914.
119. Van Slyke, D. D. A Survey of the History of the Acid-Base Field. In R. W. Winters (ed.), *The Body Fluids in Pediatrics*. Boston: Little, Brown, 1973.
120. Veeder, B. S., and Hempelmann, T. C. A febrile exanthem occurring in childhood (exanthem subitum). *Trans. Am. Pediatr. Soc.* 33:208, 1921.
121. Veeder, B. S., and Jeans, P. C. Hereditary Syphilis. In I. A. Abt (ed.), *Pediatrics*, vol. 5. Philadelphia: Saunders, 1923.
122. Weaver, G. H. Scarlet Fever. In I. A. Abt (ed.), *Pediatrics*, vol. 6. Philadelphia: Saunders, 1925.
123. Wertz, R. W., and Wertz, D. C. *Lying In: A History of Childbirth in America*. New York: Free Press, 1977.
124. Williams, J. W. The influence of treatment of syphilitic pregnant women upon the incidence of congenital syphilis. *Bull. Johns Hopkins Hosp.* 33:383, 1922.
125. Winters, J. E. Care and treatment of whooping cough patients. *Trans. Am. Pediatr. Soc.* 31:219, 1919.
126. Zahorsky, J. Roseola infantilis. *Pediatrics* (New York) 22:60, 1910.
127. Zahorsky, J. Roseola infantum. *J.A.M.A.* 61:1446, 1913.
128. Zahorsky, J. Herpetic sore thoat. *South Med. J.* 13:871, 1920.
129. Zahorsky, J. Herpangina. *Arch. Pediatr.* 41:181, 1924.

Antibiotics and Electrolytes

8

The past two and one-half decades have brought revolutionary changes in medicine. A number of us can remember clearly when a blood count was a highly scientific procedure and when the number of physical and chemical measurements designed to elucidate the manifestations of disease or even to be employed in research was limited, and viewed from the standpoint of the present-day superiority those methods were of questionable utility. So rapidly and yet so insidiously has the situation changed that it is difficult to trace even approximately the steps that have led up to the present position. One by one methods have been devised to supply data from physical and chemical analysis of body fluids and secretions or from biologic experiments; the application of these methods has served to produce an enormous literature the volume of which is ever increasing in almost geometric progression.

Oscar M. Schloss (1933)

As the second quarter of this century began, there were no sulfa drugs, no antibiotics, no steroids. Meningitis still killed 75 percent of its victims in many areas of our country. Viral respiratory diseases (called "the grippe") remained a mysterious and poorly understood part of pediatrics. Children's hospitals were widely scattered across the nation. However, most children stayed at home when sick because many parents had not shed their fears of hospitals, passed down to them from their parents and grandparents. Mothers often resorted to patent medicines or homeopathic drugs to treat their sick children; many such preparations were readily available without a prescription at almost any drugstore.

Less than five years later the country was plunged into an economic depression so serious that in 1932 New York City's Health Department found that 20 percent of the schoolchildren examined were suffering from malnutrition. In the Southern states there was an alarming increase in pellagra. Millions of families had no money to buy essential foods. In the mining counties of Ohio, West Virginia, Illinois, Kentucky, and Pennsylvania, the secretary of the American Friends Service Committee told a congressional committee, the proportion of malnourished children was sometimes over 90 percent.

During the years of the Depression there were fewer babies born. In 1931 the birthrate was 17.8 per 1,000 population, a decline of 5.8 percent from the 1930 rate and a 40 percent decline from the 1915 rate of 29.5. The birthrate in 1931 reached a new low for this country. All during the 1930's our birthrate remained under 20. By 1940 the rate had risen to 19.4 and by 1950 it had jumped to 24.1, an increase of 35.4 percent over the rate for 1931. Although the infant mortality rate did not increase during the Depression, there was much evidence that the health of many children was adversely affected. For example, hospitals and clinics in New York City reported a considerable increase in rickets among children.

And yet, with so inauspicious a beginning, no quarter of a century has ever seen so many spectacular advances in medicine as occurred between the years 1925 to 1950. Great leaps were made in medical therapy with the introduction of the sulfonamides in the mid-1930's and of antibiotics such as penicillin, streptomycin, chloramphenicol, and tetracyclines in the 1940's. In the late thirties several adrenocortical extracts were made available for clinical study and in the late 1940's the antimetabolites were introduced, especially for use in the treatment of children with acute lymphatic leukemia. The demonstration by Philip Levine (b. 1900)[60] and his colleagues in 1941 of the importance of Rh antigen isoimmunization in the pathogenesis of erythroblastosis fetalis led to increased interest in immunology and clinical genetics. In 1949 Linus Pauling (b. 1901),[71] with his recognition of a structural hemoglobin variant, clarified the molecular structure of hemoglobins; this study initiated the modern era of investigating diseases at the molecular level.

The vital statistics in this quarter-century showed a more precipitous decrease in the rates of infant and maternal mortality than in any other comparable period of time for which records are available. The infant mortality fell from 71.7 per 1,000 live births in 1925 to 29.2 in 1950, a decrease of almost 60 percent. During the same period the maternal mortality fell from 64.7 to 8.3 per 10,000 live births, a decrease of 87.2 percent. Our population increased by 33 percent and life expectancy rose from 59.7 years in 1930 to 68.2 years in 1950, an increase of more than 14 percent.

By 1925 almost every major city had a children's hospital and departments of pediatrics existed in all but a few of our medical schools. Pediatrics was fast moving into the biochemical and immunological era,

and an increasing emphasis was being placed on pediatric problems by the application of chemistry, physics, bacteriology, genetics, and immunology.

Despite the upheavals of World War II, which followed the severe economic depression, there were many significant pediatric advances. In a growing number of teaching hospitals, responsibility for the care of newborn infants, traditionally the concern of the obstetrical services as long as the mother stayed in the hospital, was being transferred to the pediatric service. Premature nurseries proliferated and technical improvements were made in the design of incubators, beginning with the one designed by Charles C. Chapple (1903–1979)[13] in 1938 (the forerunner of the Isolette), in which outside air was drawn in. Because the temperature and humidity were so well regulated, the infant could safely be unclothed. The hands and arms of attendants were introduced through portholes, bottles and diapers were inserted through airlocks, and because the internal pressure of the incubator was a bit higher than the outside, airborne infection from the room was less likely.

By 1940 about 60 percent of all white births were delivered in hospitals as compared to about 25 percent of all nonwhite births; but by 1950 the respective percentages were, for whites, 93 percent, and for nonwhites, 58 percent. This represented for whites a 55 percent increase, and for nonwhites, a 132 percent increase. The continued increase in the number of infants delivered in hospitals offered physicians a greatly expanding experience in the care of the neonate. By 1950 a few pediatricians were creating the field of neonatology in order to study the normal physiology of the newborn, as well as the pathophysiology of the disorders that have their onset in utero or during the neonatal period, so as to improve the medical care of the newborn infant.

During this period special pediatric clinics were established at the Harriet Lane Home by Edwards A. Park against some opposition. He organized for the first time in a children's hospital four special clinics: the tuberculosis clinic, directed by Miriam Brailey (b. 1900); the psychiatric clinic, headed by Leo Kanner (b. 1894); the cardiac clinic, first directed by Clifton B. Leech (b. 1895) for two years and then by Helen Taussig (b. 1898); the endocrine clinic, under the direction of Lawson Wilkins (1894–1963); and finally the epilepsy clinic, which was founded in

1926 and was headed for a short time by Wilkins and subsequently by Edward M. Bridge (b. 1901), Laslo Kajai (b. 1896), and in 1946 by Samuel Livingston (b. 1908).

The Founding of the American Academy of Pediatrics (1930)

A brief review of the fate of the Sheppard-Towner Act is in order at this point because of the vital role this act played in the founding of the American Academy of Pediatrics.

The Sheppard-Towner Act was signed into law in 1921 and was supposed to go out of existence in 1927 (p. 157). This was the first time in the nation's history that a federal formula grant program had been established in the field of health. But despite the act's noble intent, the hue and cry against its extension for an additional two years became vitriolic. Even before its enactment, professional opposition to it had been widespread. For example, the *Illinois Medical Journal* in 1921 in an editorial had this to say about the act: "The bill is a menace and represents another piece of destructive legislation sponsored by *endocrine perverts, derailed menopausics* and a lot of other men and women who have been bitten by that fatal parasite, the *upliftus putrifaciens,* in the guise of uplifters, all of whom are working overtime to devise means to destroy the country."

The Sheppard-Towner Act lapsed in 1929. Efforts to restore the program were introduced in each session of Congress after 1928 and eventually were included as Title V and Title VI of the Social Security Act of 1935.

The American Medical Association, it will be recalled, lobbied strongly against the original act and its continuation, labeling it "an imported socialistic scheme" (p. 157). A number of physicians, especially those who had been members of the Pediatric Section of the American Medical Association, broke away and formed the American Academy of Pediatrics in 1930. Organized pediatrics thus, according to Paul W. Beaven (1890–1974),[72] "made its bid for a share in the child welfare movement, in which its voice had been so small. Historically, this is the basis for the Academy's being." As with so many other developments in the child health movement, controversy concerning public responsibility for children was one factor leading to the creation of the American Academy of Pediatrics.

Marshall C. Pease (1890–1947),[72] has recounted the early history of the American Academy of Pediatrics much better than I could in his *History of the American Academy of Pediatrics* (1955). He wrote:

The story of the American Academy of Pediatrics in truth begins at a meeting of the Pediatric Section of the American Medical Association held in St. Louis in the Spring of 1922.

The Sheppard-Towner Act, a modest maternal and infant program, had recently been introduced into Congress and was brought before the Section for serious consideration. The discussion finally ended with a Resolution approving the Act. On the same day the House of Delegates of the American Medical Association passed a Resolution condemning the Sheppard-Towner Act. On the following morning the St. Louis papers appeared with banner headlines quoting the resolution in support of the Sheppard-Towner Act as passed by the Pediatric Section of the American Medical Association. Appended at the end of their articles in fine print was inserted the unfavorable resolution of the House of Delegates of the American Medical Association.

The fat was in the fire with a vengeance. Tempers rode high and were not restrained. A Committee of wrath was sent by the House of Delegates to reprimand the Pediatric Section. They were met with unrepentance and jeers. The House of Delegates in anger promptly passed a ruling to the effect that no Section of the American Medical Association would in the future adopt independently a resolution or in any other way as a group indicate approval or disapproval of matters having to do with policies involving the American Medical Association; and further that all Sections of the American Medical Association would confine their functions in the future strictly to those activities having to do with the social gathering of the members and to a presentation of a scientific program. . . .

In any event this ruling sterilizing the Pediatric Section of the American Medical Association made the American Academy of Pediatrics, or a similiar society, inevitable. . . .

On July 19, 1929 about 35 pediatricians met for dinner . . . in Portland, Oregon. . . . The discussion ranged far and wide, touching such topics as possible charter members, the prospective roll of a new pediatric society . . . and the initial steps necessary for the launching of new pediatric society.

On June 23-24, 1930, thirty-five pediatricians, meeting in the library of the Harper Hospital in De-

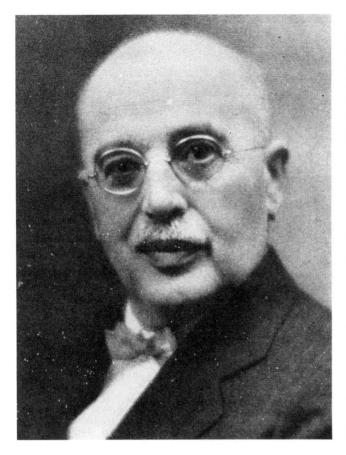

Figure 8–1. Isaac A. Abt, 1867–1955, first president of the American Academy of Pediatrics (1930–1931).

troit, drew up a constitution and by-laws and named the new society, the American Academy of Pediatrics. They elected Isaac A. Abt (Fig. 8–1) president, John Lovett Morse (Fig. 8–2) vice president, and Clifford G. Grulee (Fig. 8–3) treasurer, for the year 1930–1931. For administrative purposes the nation was divided into four regions, with the chairmen of the regions composing the executive board. Provision was made for a possible fifth region, to be composed of the Canadian provinces.

Fluid and Electrolyte Therapy

Special mention should be made of the 1914 report by Holt, Courtney, and Fales[50] on the chemical composition of diarrheal stools as compared with normal stools in infancy, because it contained this prophetic and significant comment:

The ratio of loss of salts to the intake is one of the most striking characteristics of loose, diarrheal stools and furnishes an important suggestion as to treatment. In attempting to supply this loss by hypodermoclysis it should be remembered that not only are water and sodium needed, but potassium and magnesium as well. With these facts in mind a better solution for the use in hypodermoclysis can certainly be devised than a normal saline or than Ringer's solution.

This paper, as Faber and McIntosh[36] have noted, laid the foundation "for the qualitative correction of mineral losses which had not been available before." The special value of potassium was not to be fully appreciated until James L. Gamble, Allan M. Butler (b. 1894), and Charles F. McKhann (b. 1898) in the early thirties, and especially Daniel C. Darrow (1895–1965) (Fig. 8–4) a little later had published their studies on mineral losses in diarrhea. The im-

Figure 8–2. John Lovett Morse (1865–1940), first vice president of the American Academy of Pediatrics (1930–1931).

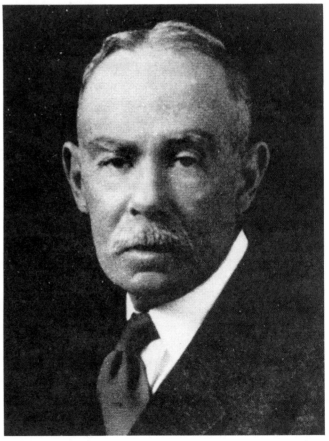

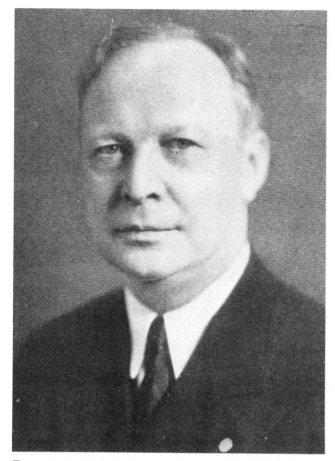

Figure 8–3. *Clifford Grosselle Grulee (1880–1962), first treasurer of the American Academy of Pediatrics.*

portance of magnesium in fluid and electrolyte therapy has been appreciated only within the last few years.

Despite Marriott's classical studies between 1916 and 1919 which shattered Finkelstein's concept of alimentary (intestinal) intoxication as being responsible for the clinical picture encountered in the depleting nutritional disorders of infants and children (p. 163), the term "intestinal intoxication" continued to be used by pediatricians as well known as Grover Powers until well into the 1930's. It will be recalled that Marriott, as early as 1915, had conclusively shown that the clinical picture noted in infants and children suffering from the dehydration caused by severe diarrhea could all be explained as the result of water loss and the accompanying acidosis and not by Finkelstein's theory of putative toxic substances, presumably formed in the intestine by improper food.

Grover Powers[73] in 1926 published a comprehen-

sive plan for the treatment of infants with diarrhea. This plan produced as satisfactory results as any other method for the next twenty years. For all practical purposes, according to Darrow,[44] writing in 1946 "no fundamental, new principle in the treatment of diarrhea has been introduced in the last twenty years [1926–1946]." The "fundamental, new principle," introduced by Clifton D. Govan (b. 1917) and Darrow[44] in 1946, was the addition of potassium chloride in the parenteral fluid used in the treatment of infants with severe diarrhea.

Powers's "comprehensive plan of treatment for the so-called intestinal intoxication of infants" was widely followed for twenty years or so after its publication in 1926. His therapeutic plan centered about four procedures: (a) The administration of fluids, (b) the transfusion of blood, (c) the withholding of food for a period of time, and (d) the administration of food at the end of the period of starvation in gradually increasing amounts.

The first procedure in his plan was to give the de-

Figure 8–4. *Daniel C. Darrow (1895–1965).*

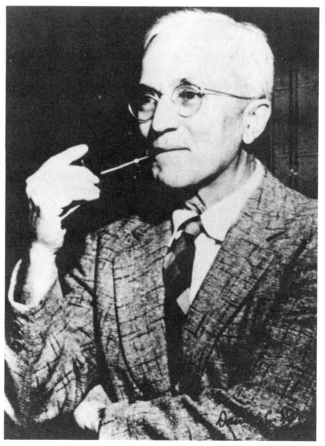

hydrated infant an injection of Ringer's solution intraperitoneally. Powers preferred the peritoneal route "even in very severe cases, because a larger quantity of fluid can be given intraperitoneally than intravenously and there is more gradual restoration of blood volume." The amount of fluid given intraperitoneally was determined by the capacity of the abdominal cavity to receive the fluid without distension; usually 150 to 350 ml of Ringer's solution was given at one time. Powers at this time (1926) considered the intraperitoneal route the "most satisfactory method of administering fluids to infants with intoxication."

After the patient had received parenteral fluid, a blood transfusion was given, varying in amount from 20 ml to 60 ml per kilogram of body weight. Blood transfusions were given intravenously and were repeated every twenty-four hours during the course of the first few days of the infant's hospitalization; usually three transfusions were given.

Following a period of starvation, varying from twelve hours as a minimum to a hundred and twenty hours as a maximum, food was then offered in the form of a dilute cooked cow's milk mixture. As the infant's condition improved, this milk mixture was gradually strengthened to equal 20 to 30 calories per ounce. The quandary Powers faced in regard to feeding these infants is well expressed in this sentence from his paper: "Torn between a desire to withhold food because of toxic symptoms and a compelling belief that food must be given because of the severity of the malnutrition and the feebleness of the child, I am sure that, to a large extent, one simply 'muddles along'." If Powers, a superb clinician, had to "muddle along," this was in no way a reflection on him, but reflected the "state of the art" of fluid and electrolyte therapy thirty to forty years ago.

If modern pediatricians were to review Powers's so-called comprehensive plan of treatment for dehydrated infants, two points would stand out. First routine serum electrolyte determinations were not obtained; the only blood chemistry levels reported were total protein, total nitrogen, and nonprotein nitrogen. Second, the mortality rate of 33 percent is exceedingly high by our present standards. However, Powers claimed that before his "comprehensive plan," the mortality from intestinal intoxication, when treated by enteral and parenteral fluids, intra-

venous injections of bicarbonate of sodium solution, and milk mixtures by mouth, was about 80 to 90 percent.

Darrow and Herman Yannet (b. 1904)[26] in 1934 described animal experiments in which 5 percent dextrose solution was injected into the peritoneal cavity of dogs with subsequent withdrawal five hours later, after it was thought that electrolyte equilibration had been established. They found that water absorption from the peritoneum had not taken place and that it now contained electrolytes in approximately the same concentration as in the extracellular fluid. These animals developed signs and symptoms of dehydration. The serum contained an increased concentration of protein and red cells, together with a decrease in electrolytes in both serum and cells—due, as they then thought, to a shift of water from extracellular to intracellular spaces.

These finding are now explained as follows: The rise in hematocrit and serum protein is the result not of a shift in water to the intracellular space, but of a shift of fluid from the intravascular to the intraperitoneal space as a consequence of the more rapid migration of sodium and chloride ions into intraperitoneal fluid than of glucose particles into the vascular compartments, thereby creating a transient osmotic gradient. Water then shifts into the intraperitoneal space as a consequence, thus reducing the intravascular volume and leading to a rise in hematocrit and serum protein. When the glucose is metabolized, then there is a shift of water in the cells if the excess water has not been excreted.

This study, according to Faber and McIntosh,[36] "had a profound influence on subsequent practices of fluid replacement." During the 1920's the intraperitoneal route was frequently used to replace fluids and electrolytes in dehydrated infants and children (p. 170).

Another noteworthy paper (1933) was that of Butler, McKhann, and Gamble[10] that described the intracellular fluid loss in diarrheal disease. The finding they considered most significant was "a loss of potassium which, relative to the loss of sodium, was greater than could be explained on the usual assumption that the body fluid lost in diarrheal disease is entirely extracellular." It was also "greater than could be explained as the result of destruction of protoplasm." They wrote that "the loss of potassium was taken to represent a reduction of intracellular fluid in the body" and that the results of the study are taken to support the use of potassium, as well as sodium in solutions designed to repair the effects of dehydration."

Darrow[24] in 1938, in another of his pioneer papers, discussed the metabolic disturbances observed in a patient with a severe burn treated by continuous soaking in a saline solution. This patient developed signs of dehydration and convulsions which Darrow considered analogous to water intoxication; he ascribed the clinical picture to mineral losses with a shift of water into the cells. The saline solution "was found to be not over one-third physiologic; the loss of extracellular electrolytes is explained by the diffusion of sodium and chloride from the areas denuded of skin by burns." He concluded "that loss of extracellular electrolyte rather than of water is the chief factor in so-called dehydration."

In 1942 Darrow and Herbert C. Miller, Jr. (b. 1907),[25] demonstrated that nearly half the potassium in skeletal muscle was replaced by almost equivalent amounts of sodium in experimental animals following feeding with a diet which contained low potassium and rather high sodium or with a normal diet accompanied by injections of desoxycorticosterone. Both procedures "led to metabolic alkalosis, moderately low heart potassium, and focal areas of cardiac necrosis replaced by round cells."

In 1945 Darrow[25] studied a three-year-old child with congenital alkalosis due to chloride-wasting diarrhea. By balance studies, he showed that the extracellular chloride deficit and bicarbonate excess were associated with a loss of potassium and a gain of sodium in the intracellular fluid. From this observation came two of his most important contributions to pediatrics: the livesaving use of potassium-containing fluid* and electrolyte infusions in patients suffering from potassium depletion—especially in infants with severe diarrhea—and the elucidation of the intimate relationship between extracellular acid-base equilibrium and the ionic composition of body cells.

In 1946 Darrow,[44] with the assistance of Govan at Johns Hopkins, extended his balance studies at Yale to infants with severe diarrhea admitted to the Harriet Lane Home in Baltimore. The administration of

* The solution he prepared, which came to be known as Darrow's solution, contained potassium 35 mEq/liter, sodium 122 mEq/liter, chloride 104 mEq/liter, and lactate 53 mEq/liter.

potassium chloride to these infants led to a striking decrease in mortality rate; seventeen of fifty-three patients treated without the addition of potassium chloride died (32 percent); with the addition of potassium chloride to the parenteral fluid solution only three of fifty patients died (6 percent).

Darrow and Govan found that the loss of body potassium was equivalent to about one-quarter of the estimated total body potassium in the most severe cases of diarrhea. They also demonstrated that this loss of potassium was not accounted for by "disintegration of the cells as a whole; that is, the deficit of potassium was not accompanied by a corresponding loss of nitrogen and intracellular phosphorus." And they further noted that during "the period of fasting when all fluids were given parenterally, retention of potassium unaccompanied by a positive balance of nitrogen and intracellular phosphorus was produced by the addition of potassium chloride to the solutions in general use for the replacement of body water and electrolyte." These findings formed the basis for Darrow's "new plan" in the treatment of dehydration in infants, which was the major advance in electrolyte replacement therapy during the second quarter of this century.

Up until Darrow's studies, fluid therapy was dominated by Gamble's concept of extracellular fluids. But by 1945 Darrow was able to describe a new frame of reference, largely from investigations on experimental animals, which visualized changes in both intracellular and extracellular fluids and which related changes in intracellular fluids to disturbances of acid-base equilibrium and hydration. What Marriott and Alexis F. Hartmann (1898–1964) had accomplished in emphasizing the importance in disease of plasma volume and extracellular acidosis, what Gamble and Butler had done for extracellular fluid, Darrow and his associates did for water and electrolytes inside the body cells.

In 1948 Darrow[25] demonstrated conclusively that metabolic alkalosis induced potassium deficiency and that potassium deficiency induced metabolic alkalosis. A few years later, largely due to studies by Robert E. Cooke (b. 1920),[21] this relation was found to depend on renal function. Darrrow[25] wrote in 1967:

First, the development of potassium deficiency is caused by a high output of potassium in the formation of an alkaline urine, and second, potassium deficiency alters renal function so that an acid urine is produced despite alkalosis. Apparently potassium deficiency leads to exchange of hydrogen for sodium reabsorbed in the distal tubules. The formation of an acid urine prevents reduction of serum bicarbonate in alkalosis and causes the development of metabolic alkalosis under certain circumstances.

By the early 1950's Darrow and his colleagues had a reasonably complete picture of the pathogenesis of metabolic alkalosis. Darrow's work showed not only that amounts of potassium adequate to replace large deficits of potassium were safe to give patients but also that striking benefits occurred. This was a major contribution to pediatrics because, until Darrow's studies, most pediatricians were afraid to include potassium in parenteral fluids because it was widely supposed that potassium might harm the patient's heart if an appreciable quantity were given parenterally.

Hematology

The first significant American contributions to pediatric hematology during this period were those of Thomas B. Cooley (1871–1945) and Pearl Lee (1871–1945),[22] beginning in 1925, when they presented a series of cases of "splenomegaly in children with anemia and peculiar changes in the bones" that they had salvaged from the conglomeration then known as von Jaksch's anemia, which was also called anemia pseudoleukemica infantum. These cases were later to be known as thalassemia, a term which covers a heterogeneous group of hereditary disorders that usually lead to the development of a hypochromic anemia. The type of thalassemia described by Cooley and Lee (A_2 thalassemia) has turned out to be a disturbance of beta-chain hemoglobin synthesis, which is the most common type of this disease. The description of their five cases in a one-page paper detailed the major clinical and laboratory findings of this disease.

All five presented the clinical syndrome ordinarily known as von Jaksch's disease or pseudoleukemic anemia. There was anemia, splenomegaly, and some enlargement of the liver, discoloration of the skin, and in some of the sclerae, without bile in the urine. The blood showed nor-

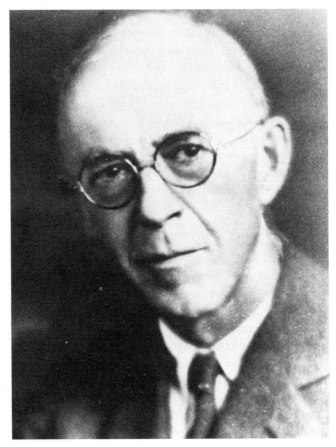

Figure 8–5. Thomas B. Cooley (1871–1945).

mal or increased resistance to hypotonic solutions. There was moderate leukocytosis in all, not of the leukemic type, nucleated red cells, chiefly normoblasts, and in two, many reticulated cells. In all of these cases the symptoms were noted by the parents as early as the eighth month, when they were apparently well advanced. Rickets was not probable in any, and in only one was there definite ground for believing that syphilis might be a contributing factor.

In addition to the splenomegaly and the blood picture. . . attention was called to a peculiar mongoloid appearance, caused by enlargement of the cranial and facial bones, combined with a skin discoloration. . . . Roentgen-ray examination of the skulls showed peculiar alterations of their structure, which the roentgenologist considered pathognomonic of this condition. The long bones also showed striking changes. . . .

Three of the patients died. . . .

Following Cooley's report, the terms thalassemia, Mediterranean anemia, and Cooley's anemia came to be applied to this disorder. Although Cooley made a number of additional contributions to pediatric hematology, the most important was his identification of the familial anemia that bears his name. He suspected its hereditary nature and was delighted when William N. Valentine (b. 1917) and James V. Neel (b. 1915)[86] demonstrated in 1944 its genetic origin and mode of inheritance. Cooley was similarly interested in sickle-cell anemia, another heritable disorder, at first supposed to occur only in children of African descent. He reported the first instance of sickle-cell disease in a Greek child; some years later Wolf W. Zuelzer (b. 1909)[91] found that this child had sickle-cell thalassemia. Cooley strongly urged the importance of genetics in medical education as a means of identifying hereditary factors in diseases.

In our present era of large well-equipped laboratories with the very latest in laboratory technology, it is worth noting that great discoveries in the past have been made in sparsely equipped laboratories. Zuelzer[91] noted that Cooley "had no formal training in hematology and very little technical help.... His equipment consisted of a monocular microscope of ancient vintage, a staining rack, a rather small card file, and—in an otherwise vacant upstairs room intended for the affairs of the Child Research Council of the American Academy of Pediatrics—a couch on which he took siestas and did much of his thinking." Cooley was one of the founders of the American Academy of Pediatrics and served as its president in 1934–1935. He also served as president of the American Pediatric Society in 1940–1941.

In 1949, by coincidence, two papers dealing with sickle-cell anemia appeared almost simultaneously. Each deserves the title of a classic contribution. The first was Linus C. Pauling and Harvey A. Itano's (b. 1920)[71] demonstration that sickle-cell anemia was a molecular disease; the second was Neel's study, solving at last the genetics of sickle-cell anemia and sickle-cell trait.

The story is told that William B. Castle (b. 1897) mentioned to Pauling that the red cell in deoxygenated blood from patients with sickle-cell anemia became sickled and then showed birefringence in polarized light. This prompted Pauling to suggest to Itano, a graduate student in Pauling's department, that he look into this problem since it could possibly represent a molecular abnormality of hemoglobin.[19] In 1949 they reported that this was the case and that the electrophoretic mobility and thus the basic structure of the hemoglobin of sickle-cell anemia was abnormal. They also showed that in patients with sickle-cell hemoglobin all the hemoglobin demonstrated an unusually slow rate of migration. But the parents of these children had both normal hemoglobin and the new, abnormal hemoglobin. In the same year studies by Neel clarified the genetic basis of sickle-cell anemia by showing that a single dose of sickle-cell gene resulted in sickle-cell trait without significant clinical symptoms, while a double dose of the gene resulted in sickle-cell anemia.

Between 1932 and 1942 George M. Guest (1898–1967), at the Children's Hospital Research Foundation in Cincinnati, performed a number of elaborate studies on the size and hemoglobin content of the erythrocytes in normal and anemic infants and children.[91] Guest in his studies showed that a fall of the mean corpuscular volume (MVC) and mean corpuscular hemoglobin (MCH) in the presence of seemingly adequate hemoglobin levels could be reversed or prevented by the administration of iron and was thus a sensitive indicator of an incipient deficiency state rather than a physiologic phenomenon. He concluded from these studies that iron deficiency anemia occurred more often among infants than had been previously realized and for this reason he advocated the use of prophylactic treatment. His earlier observations on glycolysis and the rise of inorganic phosphorus in stored blood coupled with his studies with Samuel Rapoport (b. 1912) on the role of the pH in the breakdown of diphosphoglycerate were, according to Zuelzer,[91] milestones in the understanding of red cell metabolism.

Two other pioneers in the evolution of pediatric hematology were William P. Lucas (1880–1960) and Hugh W. Josephs (b. 1892). Several of Lucas's papers dealt with quantitative studies of the blood of newborn infants, which he obtained from the superior longitudinal sinus. Included in his studies were hemoglobin determinations; erythrocyte, leukocyte, and platelet counts; nonprotein nitrogen, urea nitrogen, uric acid, creatinine, sugar, carbon dioxide, calcium, and bilirubin levels; as well as coagulation and prothrombin times.

Josephs, while a house officer on the Harriet Lane staff, developed an interest in the diseases of the blood and was soon recognized as an early contributor to pediatric hematology. Among his important contributions was his treatment of secondary anemia in infancy with iron and copper. In a study published in 1931 he found that copper, when given in addition to iron to anemic infants, accelerated the rise in hemoglobin.[55]

In 1928 Blackfan and Diamond[6] published a study on the monocyte in active tuberculosis. This was considered a pioneer study at that time. It showed that the ratio of monocytes to lymphocytes rose in advancing tuberculosis and decreased when the process was healing, and this ratio thus gave a prognostic clue of considerable value. Diamond (Fig. 8–6) emerged as the American pediatric hematologist par excellence, who became, according to Zuelzer,[91] "the mentor of a whole generation of pediatric hematologists now holding key positions in teaching institutions throughout the country."

Diamond, Blackfan, and James M. Baty (b. 1898)[28] in 1932 first recognized that hydrops fetalis, icterus gravis, and congenital anemia of the newborn—

Figure 8–6. Louis K. Diamond (b. 1902).

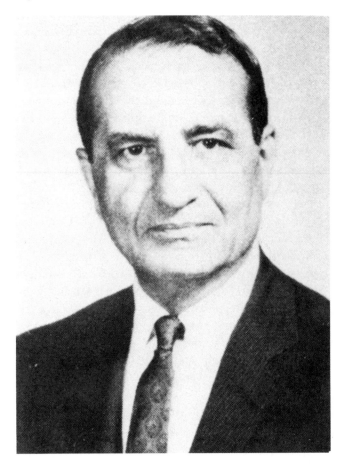

which had up to that time been considered three unrelated conditions—were in fact related and were all due to one basic mechanism, to which they applied the term erythroblastosis fetalis. This was a crucial step toward the understanding of hemolytic disease of the newborn. Philip Levine and Rufus Stetson (1886–1967)[59] demonstrated a serologic basis for materno-fetal blood group incompatibility in 1939. A year later, identification of the Rh system of antigens by the work of Landsteiner and Alexander S. Wiener (b. 1907)[58] and the observations of Levine and colleagues[60] on the mechanism and significance of materno-fetal blood group incompatibility set the stage for the explosion of knowledge of blood groups in man which occurred in the following two decades.

A little-chronicled item in the history of erythroblastosis fetalis is Ruth Darrow's[91] paper published in 1938. Zuelzer's[91] moving description of this paper follows:

In 1938, Ruth Darrow, a pathologist who had a deep personal interest in the subject, having experienced a series of stillbirths, sat down and reflected on the pathogenesis of what was then called erythroblastosis fetalis. Assembling all the then known facts, notably the sparing of the first child, the involvement of subsequent pregnancies after the birth of an afflicted baby, and the range of clinical and hematologic manifestations, she discussed all the current theories and concluded that the disease could only be explained as the result of maternal sensitization to an as yet unknown fetal antigen—a splendid example of the value of intelligent speculation.

Within three years Darrow's hypothesis was validated by Landsteiner and Wiener's report of the Rh factor.

An understanding of the basic mechanism of erythroblastosis fetalis led to an era of treatment during which exchange transfusion was developed and perfected. Alfred P. Hart,[46] a Canadian, in 1925 reported the first successful exchange transfusion on an infant with familial icterus gravis by "exsanguinating 300 cc of blood from the anterior fontanel and at the same time transfusing 335 cc of blood into the internal saphenous vein at the left ankle."

Twenty-one years after Hart's report, Wiener and Irving B. Wexler (b. 1911)[89] in 1946 successfully exchanged an infant by transfusing blood into the internal saphenous vein and removing blood from the right radial artery at the wrist. Harry Wallerstein (b. 1906)[87] in the same year successfully performed exchange transfusions on three infants with erythroblastosis fetalis by withdrawing blood from the sagittal sinus and administering blood by a superficial vein.

Diamond and co-workers,[30] beginning in November, 1946, were the first to introduce the technique of umbilical vein catheterization using a polyethylene catheter for alternate removal and administration of blood for exchange transfusion in erythroblastosis fetalis. This technique opened a new era for infants with this disease.

In 1938 Diamond and Blackfan[29] described a hitherto undefined blood dyscrasia which they termed "hypoplastic anemia." In contrast with aplastic anemia, failure of regeneration was limited to the red blood series. Treatment depended entirely on blood transfusions. In one of the cases "the child had been admitted fifty-five times in all. The total number of transfusions had reached one hundred and thirteen, and the amount of blood injected to date has been about 26,000 cc."

No historical review of American pediatric hematology, no matter how short, would be complete if Carl H. Smith's (1895–1971) name was not included. His book *Blood Diseases of Infancy and Childhood* was the first of its kind in the United States and it remains a major contribution to American pediatrics. In 1941 Smith[80] first described acute infectious lymphocytosis, an infection which was originally thought to be a variant of infectious mononucleosis. The characteristic finding noted by Smith was an absolute increase in the number of lymphocytes in the peripheral blood. The total white blood cell count was found to be generally greater than 40,000 per cubic millimeter. The lymphocyte percentage was high, in most cases being greater than 70 percent. Smith found the lymphocytes to be small in size and normal in appearance.

Attempts to identify a causative agent in this disease have thus far been inconclusive. The incubation period ranges from about twelve to twenty days. At times the condition is so mild as to escape attention and may be discovered incidentally by routine blood examinations. Fortunately, Smith and others found the disease to be self-limiting and no treatment was necessary.

Leukemia

Prior to 1948 occasional brief remissions were observed in children with leukemia following infection or blood transfusions, but only one child in ten lived for six months, one in a hundred for a year, and none as long as two years.[52] Today a child with acute lymphocytic leukemia who receives good treatment has an 80 to 90 percent chance of obtaining a "complete remission" of some duration with initial therapy and a 50 percent chance of surviving more than three years.[52]

The occurrence of what Sidney Farber (1903–1972) had interpreted as an "acceleration phenomenon" in the leukemic process, as seen in the marrow and viscera of children with acute leukemia treated by the injection of folic acid conjugates, suggested to him that folic acid antagonists might be of value in the treatment of patients with acute leukemia.

In 1948 Farber and his colleagues[41] reported the results of their clinical and hematologic studies on five children with acute lymphatic leukemia treated by the intravenous injection of aminopterin. They found that aminopterin had "a marked effect upon the leukemic bone marrow and upon the immature cells in the peripheral blood, and judging from the disappearance of enlargement of the spleen, liver and lymph nodes, when these organs were enlarged, very probably on leukemic deposits in the viscera as well."

These five children had temporary remissions of their disease. Farber[40,41] emphasized that "these remissions are temporary in character." He further stressed that there was "no evidence in this study that would justify the suggestion of the term 'cure' of acute leukemia in children." But he prophetically wrote: "A promising direction for further research concerning the nature and treatment of acute leukemia in children appears to have been established by the observations reported." He also noted that the toxicity of aminopterin "emphasized the need for less toxic compounds which it was hoped might be even more effective in their carcinolytic action." In 1937 a series of folic acid antagonists were made available. These included aminopterin, amethopterin, and amino-an-fol; the last two were considered to be less toxic than aminopterin.

The dramatic clinical results obtained by Farber and his co-workers with folic acid antagonists constituted a milestone in the history of chemotherapy.

Infectious Diseases

The Discovery of the Sulfonamides

As the fourth decade of the twentieth century began, the prospect of specific remedies for most of the infectious diseases of childhood seemed dim. It was true that diphtheria antitoxin had been successful and tetanus antitoxin somewhat less so. Also true was the availability of antipneumococcal serum, but its effectiveness was partially lessened by the need of typing pneumococci beforehand and by the cost of the specific serum. In spite of these successes, efforts to develop serums against other bacterial pathogens had been disappointing, and the partial success of antimeningococcal serum indicated how difficult it would be to match the type of serum and the microorganisms causing the disease in a particular child. There was also the annoying problem of adverse reactions, including fatal ones, even when carefully prepared serums were used.[32]

Until the 1930's attempts to synthesize drugs for the cure of bacterial diseases had been a failure, although Ehrlich, as has been noted (p. 180), had patented his synthetic preparation known as salvarsan in 1907 and other German investigators during the 1920's had developed additional synthetic compounds of value against malaria, such as pamaquine (Plasmoquin) and quinacrine (Atabrine).[32]

By the mid-thirties most investigators working in the field of infectious diseases had little hope that effective chemical agents would soon be synthesized for the treatment of bacterial infections. The impression, according to Harry F. Dowling (b. 1904),[32] "was that protozoa and treponemes could be attacked by chemicals without seriously injuring the host, whereas for some reason bacteria other than treponemes could not."

Fortunately, a few investigators refused to abandon the search for an effective synthetic drug against bacterial pathogens. Among them were a small group in the research laboratories of the I. G. Farbenindustrie in Germany. The director of this group, Gerhard Domagk (1895–1964),[31] set about testing azo dyes (manufactured by his company for use in the textile industry) by injecting selective dyes in mice that had been infected with streptococci. One of these dyes, later named Prontosil, cured mice that had been given lethal doses of hemolytic streptococci. This experiment, reported in February, 1935, was actually made three years earlier, and in the intervening time German clinicians had tried the remedy on a number of patients, one of whom was Domagk's daughter. To Domagk belongs the credit for the discovery of the chemotherapeutic value of Prontosil, for which he was awarded the Nobel Prize in Medicine in 1939.

In France in 1935, investigators discovered that in the tissues the azo linkage was split so that Prontosil yielded para-aminobenzenesulfonamide (sulfanilamide), which they correctly thought to be the chemotherapeutic moiety of the molecule. Ernest Fourneau (1872–1949), of the Pasteur Institute in Paris, then synthesized this compound; he and his colleagues in 1936 showed it to be as effective as Prontosil in curing experimental infections. The same year Leonard Colebrook (1883–1967) and others in England reported favorable clinical results with Prontosil and sulfanilamide in the treatment of puerperal sepsis and meningococcal infections. These reports stimulated enormous interest in the emerging field of bacterial chemotherapy; experimental and clinical articles soon followed in great number. American investigators also confirmed that sulfanilamide was the effective radical of the Prontosil molecule and that it exerted a bacteriostatic rather than bactericidal effect on microorganisms.

Although Prontosil was not commercially available in the United States until the latter part of 1936, A. Ashley Weech (1895–1977), the first pediatrician to use it experimentally in America, prescribed Prontosil on July 10, 1935, to treat a child with *Hemophilus influenzae* meningitis at Babies Hospital in New York.[4]

Beginning in 1937, when sulfanilamide came into general use, the mortality from several of the common contagious diseases fell precipitously. Numerous derivatives of sulfanilamide were soon synthesized. Sulfapyridine appeared in 1938, but it had two serious drawbacks: in therapeutic doses it frequently caused nausea and vomiting, and it tended to form crystals in the urine, leading to hematuria. Sulfathiazole was synthesized in 1939, and sulfadiazine in 1940.

In August, 1937, the *Journal of Pediatrics* published a special symposium on sulfanilamide therapy. This symposium contained brief reports on the results of sulfanilamide therapy in approximately three hundred and fifty patients from eleven American children's hospitals. All reported dramatic results. For example, Brennemann[9] wrote: "In two cases of erysipelas the result was so prompt as to be positively shocking." And A. Graeme Mitchell (1889–1941)[67] commented: "We cannot help but be favorably impressed by the effect of sulfanilamide and its derivatives in the treatment of streptococcic meningitis." The significance of Mitchell's comment was underscored by Francis F. Schwentker (1904–1954),[78] who reported that prior to the use of sulfanilamide, "none of 37 cases [of streptococcic meningitis] seen in the Johns Hopkins Hospital over a fifteen-year period recovered."

The Discovery of Penicillin and Other Antibiotics

In 1928 Sir Alexander Fleming (1881–1955), while studying staphylococcus variants in the laboratory of St. Mary's Hospital in London, accidentally discovered a mold that produced a substance that inhibited his cultures. Because the mold belonged to the genus *Penicillium*, Fleming named the antibacterial substance penicillin. Little was made of Fleming's discovery for nearly a decade until Howard W. Florey (1898–1968) and Ernest B. Chain (b. 1906) and colleagues demonstrated conclusively that penicillin yielded dramatic chemotherapeutic results in many bacterial illnesses.

Roger L. J. Kennedy (1897–1966)[48] in 1944 was one of the first pediatricians in this country to demonstrate the efficacy of penicillin in the treatment of infants and children suffering from various types of bacterial infections.* He treated fifty-four such patients, giving them a total daily dose of 20,000 to 40,000 units of either the sodium or calcium salt of penicillin. The results were so encouraging that he wrote: "A new chapter is being written in the chemotherapy of disease."

The ineffectiveness of penicillin in the treatment of infections due to gram-negative organisms led to a search for antibacterial agents effective against such bacteria. But unlike the serendipitous discovery of penicillin, the development of streptomycin was the result of a well-planned search for antibacterial substances. Streptomycin was introduced in 1944. The first of the tetracyclines, chlortetracycline, was introduced in 1948, and two years later, oxytetracycline became available. Chloramphenicol was introduced in 1948.

The period between 1930 and 1940 saw amazing progress in pediatrics, especially with the advent of the era of chemotherapy. For the first time many infectious diseases came under control as new and even more effective antibiotics were discovered.

Bacterial Diseases

DIPHTHERIA. With the increasing therapeutic use of diphtheria antitoxin, the mortality rate for American children under five years of age fell gradually but continuously from about 120 per 100,000 in 1900 to 7 per 100,000 in 1945. In Baltimore the decline was even more dramatic. The diphtheria rate in that city was 260 per 100,000 population in 1900, 124 per 100,000 in 1925, and 0.8 per 100,000 in 1951—a decrease of 99.7 percent.[51] In all the years prior to 1935, diphtheria caused more deaths than any of the other common contagious diseases.[20] The widespread use of specific toxin-antitoxin and then toxoid beginning about 1930 led to a marked decrease in both the morbidity and mortality of diphtheria. Diphtheria became one of the striking modern examples of the effect on a large population of specific therapy, since no doubt exists that the results in this period were attributable almost entirely to specific prophylactic vaccination.[20] Unfortunately, even in the mid-1940's almost 15,000 cases of diphtheria were reported annually with well over a thousand deaths yearly.

In the 1930's various workers attempted to immunize children against diphtheria or tetanus by the nasal route—spray or instillation of toxoid—as an alternative to the inconvenience of the injection needle.[69] The method was far from successful, even for reinforcing doses, since it gave no control over the amount of the antigen absorbed.

Treatment. Diphtheria antitoxin was administered as promptly as possible following skin or conjunctival test for sensitivity to horse serum. Also recommended was penicillin, but it was not effective enough to warrant its use without antitoxin in addition.

---

* I believe the first child to be treated with penicillin in this country was a seven-year-old girl reported by Wesley W. Spink.[82] She received her first dose of penicillin on July 11, 1942, "because of a severe staphylococcic bacteremia."

Prognosis. The case fatality rate in Baltimore between 1920 and 1949 remained remarkably constant, varying between 5 and 8 percent. Delay in administering antitoxin increased the danger of a fatal outcome. For example, children receiving antitoxin given during the first day of their illness had a mortality rate of only 0.27 percent. This rose to 11.39 percent if the antitoxin administration was delayed to the fourth day of the illness.[51]

PERTUSSIS. By 1935 whooping cough had displaced diphtheria as the chief cause of death among the common communicable diseases. The mortality rate in children under five years of age in 1930 was approximately 48 per 100,000; this rose to over 60 in 1934 and fell to less than 16 by 1945. The seriousness of pertussis, especially in infants less than a year old, is forcibly demonstrated by noting that in the United States Registration Area between 1940 and 1948, pertussis caused almost four times more deaths under one year of age than did measles, mumps, chickenpox, rubella, scarlet fever, diphtheria, and poliomyelitis combined.[51]

However, despite the dominant position of pertussis as a cause of death among infants, improvement in case fatality was evident between 1925 and 1950. For example, a twenty-five-year experience at the Herman Kiefer Hospital in Detroit showed that for the five-year period from 1925 to 1929, the case fatality for infants one year of age or less was 42.3 percent; this figure had fallen to 5.8 percent for the quinquennium 1945–1949, a decrease of 86.3 percent. The reasons for the decline in case fatality during this period were not entirely clear. Possible factors suggested were improved methods of therapy, changes in host resistance, altered infecting agent, or certain environmental factors that enhanced the host's resistance or limited the activity of the infecting agent.[43]

Leading exponents of pertussis vaccination in the United States during the 1930's were Louis W. Sauer (b. 1885)[76,77] and Pearl Kendrick (b. 1890).[56,57] Sauer during the 1930's began to use a vaccine prepared from freshly isolated, strongly hemolytic strains of the *Bordetella pertussis* as early as 1926 and in a paper published in 1933 claimed good active immunity in 300 children vaccinated between 1928 and 1933.[76]

Between 1933 and 1937 Sauer published a series of important papers on pertussis vaccination. In general, he recommended a total dosage of 75 to 100 billion organisms per milliliter of vaccine, prepared by scraping the growth from the medium rather than washing it off; he felt this huge total number of organisms was needed to obtain sufficient concentration of the essential immunizing substances.[77]

Kendrick insisted on the inclusion of a predesignated control group for each group of vaccinated children. Three clinical trials were carried out between 1938 and 1942. In the first study, 1,815 children between the ages of eight months and five years were vaccinated and 2,397 strictly comparable children served as controls. The vaccinated group received a total of 70 billion organisms, given in four injections. On the basis of person-years observations, the annual attack rates per 100 for the vaccinated and control groups were 2.3 and 15.1 respectively.[56] The disease was milder in the vaccinated group and no deaths occurred in either group. She concluded that there was a protective response to the pertussis vaccine under trial.

In her third trial, in 1943, Kendrick[57] reported favorable results when combined pertussis vaccine and diphtheria toxoid alum-precipitated were given as the second and third dose of the primary course. J. A. Bell[5] was the principal early advocate of alum-precipitated vaccine in this country. In 1941 he reported substantial protection in a carefully controlled trial among children of the general population in Norfolk, Virginia. In a later trial in 1948 he obtained satisfactory protection with an alum-precipitated mixture of pertussis vaccine and diphtheria toxoid. The attack rate in 407 children two to twenty-three months of age given two doses of the mixture was 12 percent, compared with 41 percent in 385 similar children given alum-precipitated diphtheria toxoid alone.

Harriet M. Felton (b. 1909) in 1945 reviewed the use of antisera, both human and rabbit, in prophylaxis and treatment of pertussis. Various preparations, especially human hyperimmune serum, were thought to be effective. However, most of the clinical data given were from uncontrolled studies. Joseph H. Lapin (b. 1900) also reported favorably in 1945 on specific treatment, although his results were not striking. He used the gamma globulin fraction of human hyperimmune serum, which was obtained from a pool of the sera of healthy adults who had

had whooping cough in the past and had subsequently received repeated doses of pertussis vaccine. Sauer in 1946 recommended human pertussis immune serum as a prophylactic measure for intimately exposed nonimmune infants and, as a therapeutic measure in larger doses, for infant and frail young pertussis patients.

In 1948 Randolph K. Byers (b. 1896) and Frederic C. Moll (b. 1915)[11] reported a hitherto unsuspected hazard of prophylaxis against pertussis, namely encephalopathy in fifteen infants and children who had received pertussis vaccine.

MENINGOCOCCAL MENINGITIS. The use of sulfonamides in the treatment of meningococcal meningitis, beginning in 1937, removed for the first time much of the dread of this disease and its sequelae. Serum therapy, introduced in 1908, was in common use until the beginning of the antibiotic era. Under favorable conditions and with the use of antimeningococcal serum therapy early in the infection, there was a modest reduction in the mortality from this disease. With the advent of sulfonamides there was a striking fall in mortality, infinitely greater than the reduction following the introduction of serum. For example, at the St. Louis Children's Hospital during the years 1912 to 1937, in 222 children under fifteen years of age admitted in various stages of meningococcal meningitis and treated by serum therapy, the case fatality was 40 percent, while in 135 children treated after 1937 with sulfonamides, the case fatality was only 5 percent, a decrease of 87.5 percent.[20] When penicillin became available in the early 1940's the fatality rate was reduced even further.

The value of the sulfonamides was proven by the fatality rates among military personnel during World War II. Among 14,504 American soldiers with meningococcal infection, only 3.8 percent died —far different from the 39 percent fatality rate of World War I.[32]

SCARLET FEVER. During the eleven-year period from 1926 until the beginning of 1937, the mortality from scarlet fever in this country ranged around 2,500 yearly with a general mortality rate of just above 2 per 100,000. It was during this period that specific antiscarlatinal serum was used in some cities, although it was never used on a wide scale. No striking effect on mortality from scarlet fever was evident until 1937, after which the total deaths fell precipitously due to the use of sulfonamides.[20]

Even more dramatic was the drop in total reported deaths due to erysipelas, which remained slightly above 2,000 between 1931 and 1936. Within five years after the introduction of the sulfonamides the total deaths fell to less than 350—a decrease of 83 percent.[20]

RHEUMATIC FEVER. Rheumatic fever—from 1925 to 1950—ranked first as cause of death in American children and adolescents five to nineteen years of age. It was the leading cause of heart disease below the age of forty. During this period it was estimated that in the large cities of the north temperate zone the incidence of rheumatic heart disease in persons between the ages of five and nineteen years ranged between 2 and 3.9 cases per 1,000. In the late twenties, Alvin Coburn[16] found that in one New York City hospital one-fourth of the beds were occupied by patients with active rheumatic fever or its aftermath during the spring, the peak season for the disease. According to studies in the schools of several large American cities in the 1930's, rheumatic heart disease was encountered in 2 to 4 per 1,000 children between the ages of six and nineteen.

The acceptance of Group A hemolytic streptococcus as the actual causative agent of rheumatic fever was hampered by the failure to delineate the mechanism by which the rheumatic state was initiated by this organism. The manner in which rheumatic fever developed following Group A hemolytic streptococcal infection was outlined in four phases by Coburn[16,17] in 1931. Phase I designated the preceding acute streptococcal infection with group A hemolytic streptococci. This was followed by a latent period of one to two weeks (usually about fourteen days) during which there was no clinical evidence of the disease (phase II). The period of active rheumatic fever, which varied from weeks to a year or two, was phase III; and, finally, phase IV was the period of rheumatic inactivity, which could be permanent or might last for only a few weeks with repetition of the entire cycle. The criteria introduced by T. Duckett Jones (1899–1954)[54] in 1944 brought order into the clinical classification.

Treatment. Salicylates were considered, as they had been for more than seventy-five years, the mainstay in the treatment of active rheumatic fever. But by the end of 1949 Philip Hench (1896–1965) and his associates found that cortisone had a dramatic antirheumatic effect.

Prophylaxis. Control of recurrences by sulfonamide prophylaxis was first demonstrated in this country by Alvin Coburn[16] in 1939. Treatment of acute streptococcal infections with penicillin was first shown to reduce recurrent attacks of rheumatic fever by Benedict Massell (b. 1906)[62] in 1951.

TUBERCULOSIS. With the advent of the antituberculosis drugs—streptomycin (1944), para-aminosalicylic acid (PAS) (1946), and isoniazid (1951)—the treatment of tuberculosis became far simpler than it had been previously. However, even before the advent of specific therapy with streptomycin, the statistical data from a survey in New York City between 1900 and 1925 demonstrated marked improvement in the control of tuberculosis, especially in children, suggesting that other public health measures had been responsible.[33]

Prior to the discovery of effective antituberculosis chemotherapy, prophylaxis with BCG, the bacillus of Calmette and Guerin, was considered more seriously than at present, especially for tuberculin nonreactors who were likely to be in contact with tuberculosis—medical students, nurses, physicians, and other hospital personnel. BCG was also strongly recommended for uninfected children who, for one reason or another, could not be separated from a tuberculous adult.

Vaccination against tuberculosis was also carried out with the vole bacillus and also with heat-killed human tubercle bacilli.[51]

Virus Diseases

Although virology was still in its infancy during this period, several major contributions were reported. Some of these were the 1937 studies of Joseph Stokes, Jr. (1896–1972), proving that there was more than a single strain of influenza virus; the recovery of poliovirus from the stools of a patient with abortive poliomyelitis by James B. Trask and colleagues (1938); and Theodore C. Hempelmann's description of the then new St. Louis encephalitis (1935).[36]

COXSACKIE VIRUSES. In 1948 Gilbert J. Dalldorf (b. 1900) and his associate Grace M. Sickles (1898–1959)[23] investigated a number of small epidemics of what was thought to be poliomyelitis in upstate New York from which they had hoped to find evidence of mouse-adaptable poliovirus or any other viruses which might turn up from cases of poliomyelitis. From fecal suspensions obtained from two patients suspected of having paralytic poliomyelitis, they isolated what appeared to be a completely new virus with a number of unique features. This agent, though it caused paralysis of the limbs of suckling mice, could easily be differentiated from the Lansing strain of poliovirus and from several other neurotropic viruses, both by its serological reactions and by the pathological picture it produced. This new agent caused paralysis not by damaging the central nervous system but by causing widespread lesions in the skeletal muscles. Another striking feature was that only suckling mice one to seven days old were susceptible; animals more than a week of age were resistant to the infection.

Dalldorf and Sickles were unaware at first that they had uncovered a huge family of new viruses. The new agent was called "Coxsackie virus," since the first recognized human cases were residents of that New York village. Within a few years of Dalldorf and Sickles's discovery of Coxsackie virus, a number of other investigators had isolated related viruses from a number of different clinical diseases, some of which bore a resemblance to mild forms of poliomyelitis and some of which did not. Few of the illnesses were severe.

Coxsackie viruses were soon separated into two groups, A and B, on the basis of distribution of lesions produced in experimental animals. By 1976 there were twenty-three known viruses in Group A and six in Group B; the group assignment is based on different and specific lesions in mice. The Coxsackie viruses are included in the enteroviruses along with poliovirus and echovirus. In man, Coxsackie viruses have subsequently been found to be causally related to a number of diseases, including herpangina (Coxsackie A and B viruses); hand, foot, and mouth disease (Coxsackie A viruses); acute lymphoglandular pharyngitis (Coxsackie A virus); acute aseptic myocarditis of infants (Coxsackie B virus); a number of "new" viral exanthems (Coxsackie

A and B viruses); and nonspecific febrile illnesses, with or without rash (Coxsackie A and B viruses).

MEASLES. The actual number of deaths from measles in children under five years of age in the U.S. Registration Area fell from a peak figure of 6,771 in 1926 to 214 in 1945, a 97 percent decrease.[20] During this period approximately one-half of all deaths occurred in the first two years of life, with two-thirds under the age of five years; these proportions remained relatively constant during the period 1925 to 1945. The epidemic years were 1928, 1934, 1935, and 1941–1944, during which more than twice the number of cases were reported than at other times. The reported incidence during these epidemics exceeded 400,000 cases annually, and at times reached around 800,000, as compared with that of 200,000 in the intervening years.[20]

Since by far the most important cause of death in measles was pneumonia, it appeared that the decrease in the number of deaths due to measles between 1937 (when it was 2,140) and 1945 (when it was 214) was largely attributable to a diminished mortality from pneumonia that followed the introduction of sulfonamide drug therapy, beginning in 1937.

Passive prophylaxis against measles by the use of convalescent serum was first used in this country by William H. Park and Abraham Zingher in New York in 1918. McKhann[66] in 1933 recommended the use of placental extract (human immune globulin), in place of convalescent serum as a reliable source of antibodies against measles. The initial disadvantage of placental immune globulin was the high proportion of unpleasant febrile reactions which were caused by the early batches. Improvement in processing reduced the incidence of side effects.

Human immune serum globulin—the gamma globulin fraction of the appropriate antiserum, usually convalescent serum—was introduced by Edwin J. Cohn (1893–1953) and his colleagues[18] in 1944 and 1946. Measles antibody is present in high concentration in this fraction. Within a few years gamma globulin replaced all other products in the passive prophylaxis of measles.

POLIOMYELITIS. One of the great breakthroughs in the history of virology occurred in 1948 when John Enders (b. 1897) and his colleagues Thomas H. Wel-

ler (b. 1915) and Frederick C. Robbins (b. 1916)[35] succeeded in growing Lansing strain poliovirus in human embryonic non-nervous tissue. These investigators subsequently were able to cultivate strains of polioviruses representing each of the three serotypes in a variety of extraneural human tissues, both embryonic and other. Most significant of all was their extremely practical discovery that multiplication of polioviruses was accompanied by a characteristic change within the infected cells. The specific cellular injury was recognizable under the high power of the light microscope, and thus simple observation could detect whether or not viable and growing poliovirus existed in the culture. Channels were now opened that would eventually lead to making inactivated and attenuated poliovirus vaccines possible.

Little could be done for the patient with poliomyelitis who suffered from paralysis of the respiratory muscles prior to the lifesaving respirator invented by Philip Drinker in the late 1920's, the so-called "iron lung." The Drinker respirator consisted of a rigid cylinder into which a patient could be placed, and at short intervals negative and positive pressure could be alternately applied within the apparatus.

RUBELLA. Beginning in 1941 reports began to appear, at first from Australia, concerning the effects of maternal rubella in the early part of pregnancy. Norman McAlister Gregg (1892–1966), an Australian ophthalmologist, first revealed the teratogenicity of rubella by reporting that an unusually high number of infants with cataracts were being referred to him; he then discovered that their mothers had had rubella during an epidemic in Australia in 1940. Within the next few years the spectrum of anomalies produced by or attributed to rubella consisted of ocular, cardiovascular, aural, and mental defects.*

Several American reports of ocular and cardiac defects in infants following maternal rubella infection during the first trimester of pregnancy appeared between 1946 and 1950.

ERYTHEMA INFECTIOSUM. The first detailed clinical report of the occurrence of this pediatric disease in this country appeared in 1926. This was an epidemic

* Because Gregg's paper appeared in a journal not widely read in this country, and during World War II, almost a decade elapsed before the importance of his observations was appreciated.

of seventy-four cases of erythema infectiosum observed by Theodore P. Herrick (1893–1966)[49] between 1924 and 1926. Herrick reported no prodromal symptoms in his patients. The first symptom usually noted was a dusky flush which appeared on the cheeks and was so sharply marked off that parents would describe it as "a touch of erysipelas." This was followed by a generalized rash which was always more prominent on the buttocks than on the trunk. He acknowledged that his series of cases threw "little light on the etiology," although "occurrences of cases in the same room at school and the successive involvement of members of the same family can hardly leave any doubt of its infectious nature." The incubation period was estimated to be from four to fourteen days. Herrick did not think any treatment was indicated nor did he believe that anything was gained by "keeping the children in bed or by changing the routine in any way."

No additional American reports of erythema infectiosum appeared until 1947, when a description of an epidemic in Milwaukee from February until the middle of July, 1944, was published.[42] Twenty-two cases were observed; none of the patients was febrile. The white blood cell counts were all within normal limits and the erythrocyte sedimentation was also normal. The authors of this report assumed that the disease was spread by droplets, not by fomites or carriers. The youngest patient in their series was four years of age and the oldest twenty-four.

Nutrition and Nutritional Disorders

During this period important new vitamins had been identified and there was an increase in our knowledge of those already discovered. For example, in 1926 Joseph Goldberger (1874–1929) and colleagues reported the discovery of vitamin B$_2$ (riboflavin), which they identified as the antipellagra vitamin. Albert Szent-Györgyi (b. 1893) isolated vitamin C, ascorbic acid, in 1928. Robert R. Williams (1886–1965) synthesized vitamin B$_1$ in 1936, and Louis F. Fieser (1899–1977) synthesized vitamin K$_1$ in 1939.

Nutrition research had an important effect on pediatric practice in many ways. One long-term secular trend was the more rapid growth of infants and children. Body length is significantly greater than it was

at the beginning of the century, requiring a change in the pediatrician's concept of normal growth standards. Rickets, scurvy, and nutritional anemia, once so common, were quite rare by 1950. Infants with marasmus also once so common had practically disappeared by mid-century.

Cystic Fibrosis of the Pancreas

The differentiation of cystic fibrosis of the pancreas from the celiac syndrome was a major medical breakthrough of the second quarter of this century. Arthur H. Parmelee (1883–1961)[70] in 1935 published an account of two patients with what he termed "pancreatic steatorrhea." His two patients died of bronchopneumonia. An autopsy, performed on only one of the patients, showed fibrotic changes in the pancreas with cystic dilatations and fibrotic changes in the lungs with signs of chronic bronchitis. Parmelee noted the difference between his cases and celiac disease. A principal objective of his report was to indicate that cystic fibrosis of the pancreas was a disease entity "which has a symptomatology and a clinical course quite different from celiac disease as generally pictured."

Dorothy H. Andersen (1901–1963)[2] in 1938 published her classic paper on cystic fibrosis and its relation to celiac disease, in which she presented a detailed clinical and pathological analysis of the patients studied at Babies Hospital in New York as well as those culled from the literature. These cases offered overwhelming evidence of the frequency of cystic fibrosis of the pancreas and the relation of this lesion to the clinical manifestations of the disease. By her meticulous analysis she established cystic fibrosis of the pancreas as a completely different clinical and pathological entity from the celiac syndrome. Andersen believed that the high susceptibility to respiratory infections in these children was due to the epithelial metaplasia of the respiratory tract caused by vitamin A deficiency because of poor absorption of this vitamin.

Five years before Andersen's paper was published, Blackfan and S. B. Wolbach (1880–1954)[8] presented the findings of their study of the pathology of vitamin A deficiency in infants. In the course of this study they had acquired an appreciation of the separate significance of the pancreatic lesion:

Six of the 11 cases studied at post-mortem showed extensive pancreatic lesions, all identical and presumably representing a disease entity. At first we regarded the pancreatic changes as the result of vitamin A deficiency. As the same condition has been found scores of times without other evidences of vitamin A deficiency and since it is not constant even in severe vitamin A deficiency, we must consider the two as not necessarily connected. The pancreatic lesion referred to is characterized by dilatation of acini and ducts, by inspissated secretion, atrophy of the acini, lymphoid and leucocytic infiltration to some degree, and fibrosis. Our preliminary studies indicate that the pathogenesis of this striking pancreatic affection resides in the production of an abnormal secretion which inspissates and leads to distention and atrophy of ducts and acini. It is reasonable to assume that this pancreatic lesion, if extensive, may be responsible for the failure to utilize fats and hence vitamin A in the presence of an adequate intake.

Blackfan and Charles D. May[7] (b. 1908) in 1938 described "35 examples of a well defined pathologic lesion [in the pancreas], the existence of which was unsuspected during life" although the patients were under clinical observation in an excellent pediatric clinic. May[64] has aptly noted: "It is easy in retrospect to wonder at the earlier failure to recognize the features of cystic fibrosis of the pancreas which seem to separate this disease so sharply from the celiac affection. The lesson to be learned is that differences are as important as similarities when manifestations are being assigned to disease syndromes. The tendency is to force observations into current categories and to be insufficiently disturbed by features that do not fit well."

Andersen[3] in 1942 described a method of assaying trypsin in the duodenal secretions for routine use in diagnosis of cystic fibrosis, and in 1944 Farber[39] expanded the original concept of cystic fibrosis as essentially a pancreatic disease into a theory of generalized "mucoviscidosis."

By 1946 the use of penicillin and sulfonamides in the form of aerosol inhalation therapy provided a new approach to the treatment of intrapulmonary infections in patients with cystic fibrosis. Inhalation therapy with antibiotics was developed in the hope of improving the use of sulfonamides orally and of penicillin intramuscularly because they had been only partially successful.

Celiac Disease

This disease was far more commonly diagnosed in the 1930's and 1940's than at present. For example, more than a hundred and fifty articles on celiac disease had been published during the five-year period between 1933 and 1938. Its etiology was unknown. Some believed that tropical sprue, nontropical sprue, and celiac disease were identical. Others held that carbohydrates or fats were the culprits. A few believed that celiac disease was an avitaminosis or perhaps an endocrine disturbance. A chronic parenteral focus of infection was also considered.

At the Harriet Lane Home during the 1930's celiac disease was encountered about one in every fifteen hundred admissions and it was noted particularly among the well-to-do. The disease was rarely encountered before the end of the first year of life; it was most frequently seen during the second and third years. However, because of the difficulty in defining the celiac syndrome, figures as to its overall incidence were unsatisfactory. There was a tendency to include in this category any patient in whom intestinal intolerance persisted for even a short period following an infection.

The successful management of patients with celiac disease was said to have been accomplished by a variety of different dietary regimens which had little in common. Some pediatricians rigidly excluded fats from the diet, whereas others found that liberal quantities of fat could be given without harm. Cow's milk was held by some to be the principal dietary fault; others were equally certain that sugar and starch caused the trouble and not the milk. Sidney V. Haas (1870–1964),[45] especially, advocated the use of ripe bananas as the source of carbohydrates. He emphatically claimed that ripe bananas when added to a high-protein diet regularly cured celiac disease. In Haas's opinion the symptoms noted in celiac disease depended upon the inability of the patient to utilize the usual carbohydrates. For reasons he did not explain, the carbohydrates in bananas were well tolerated. Reports of the successful treatment of adult sprue with folic acid led to its use in celiac disease of childhood. But treatment of a number of affected children with folic acid had no effect on the steatorrhea or any other clinical or laboratory features of the disease.

May, Blackfan, and McCreary[63] in 1941 in a study

on the pathogenesis of celiac disease concluded that "it is some defect in the intestinal mucosa which accounts for the defective fat absorption in that disease," a conclusion subsequently confirmed years later by intestinal biopsies.

The Newborn Infant

As the year 1950 approached, it was clear that the high morbidity and mortality rates of infants of low birth weight were emerging as one of the great challenges to pediatrics.

All during the second quarter of this century the major cause of deaths in the first year of life was prematurity, which rose in New York City from 25.8 percent of the total infant deaths in 1929, to 31.5 percent in 1938, and to 41.7 percent in 1946.[51]

Pneumonia and bronchitis were the second most important causes of death during the first year of life in 1929 and 1938; but by 1946 these two conditions had fallen to fourth place, largely because of the advent of chemotherapy.

Interest in neonatal survival was heightened by the sobering statistics revealed in a paper by Stewart H. Clifford (b. 1900),[15] published in 1936, which showed that although the infant mortality rate in the state of Massachusetts had undergone a decline from about 132 per 1,000 in 1910 to a figure slightly over 50 in 1933, the mortality in young infants, particularly in those less than fourteen days, had scarcely decreased at all. Clifford noted that the death rate in the first two weeks of life in Massachusetts had remained at approximately 30 per 1,000 live births during the entire period from 1910 to 1934. As Clement A. Smith (b. 1901)[79] (Fig. 8–7) pointed out in 1946: "The perils which infants face during and immediately after birth are not especially those of infection; they are difficulties in the onset of respiration, handicaps brought about by congenital abnormalities, hazards of obstetrical accidents, and other situations the alleviation of which depends in great part upon an understanding of normal physiology." Smith's book *The Physiology of the Newborn Infant,* published in 1946, helped to define the newborn infant's ability to maintain extrauterine homeostasis and offered guidelines for practical application. This book remained unique in its field for many years and served as a valuable reference work for the emerging discipline of neonatology.

The 1930's and 1940's were fertile years for metabolic studies of the infant. Among the leaders in these studies were Fritz B. Talbot, Harry H. Gordon, Samuel Z. Levine (b. 1895), and Richard Day (b. 1905).

During this quarter century specific therapy had been discovered for many formerly serious diseases of infancy. Among these were the use of vitamin K, discovered in 1935, to prevent hemorrhagic disease of the newborn, the use of the sulfonamides (beginning in 1935) and penicillin (beginning in 1944) to treat infections, and the use of vitamins C and D to prevent scurvy and rickets.

Survival rates for premature infants weighing 1,000 grams or less improved dramatically. For example, Levine,[61] who had the overall supervision of the premature nursery at the New York Hospital–Cornell Medical Center for more than a quarter of a century, reported that in the first eight-year period, from 1932 to 1939, none of the fifty-three babies in the premature nursery weighing 1,000 grams or less

Figure 8–7. Clement A. Smith (b. 1901).

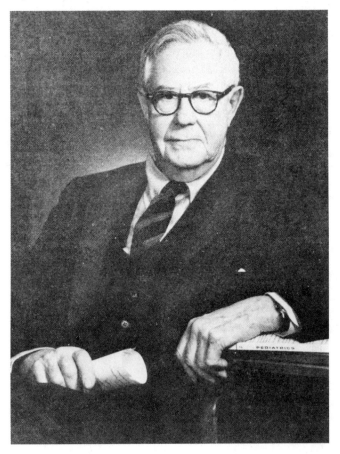

survived. This was an era of inadequate prenatal and maternal care, of routine oil baths and transfusions resulting in excessive handling of infants, of heat cradles and lamps, and the absence of good incubators.

With the introduction of better prenatal care and more gentle manipulation at delivery, the advent of antibiotic agents and better incubators, and a change from human milk to low-fat cow's milk mixtures, some of these premature infants began to survive. In the second eight-year period, from 1940 through 1947, 19 of 128 infants whose birth weights were 1,000 grams or less were saved, a survival rate of 14.8 percent. The survival rate for the third eight-year period, from 1948 through 1955, was 23.5 percent, representing the salvage of 54 of 230 infants weighing less than 1,000 grams at birth.

Day,[27] in a landmark paper published in 1943 on the regulation of body temperature in premature infants, confirmed that in "warm air the chief defect in the heat-regulating mechanism of the premature infant is an inadequacy of sweat production" and that "in cool air the total heat loss per unit area of skin appears to be greater than for adults." Day also found that "cool air provokes an increase in heat production and also in the amount of crying." Finally, he ascertained that "in cool air the chief handicaps from which the infant suffers are a large surface area in proportion to body weight and a feeble musculature; hence the sustained muscular movement necessary to raise heat production is more difficult for these feeble subjects than for adults." In sum, exposure to a cool environment causes caloric expenditure to increase in defense of body temperature.

Retrolental Fibroplasia

A dreaded retinopathy of prematurity was first reported by Theodore L. Terry (1899–1946)[84] in 1942, about two years after respiratory difficulties in immature infants began to be treated more aggressively with oxygen. Terry considered the condition a congenital anomaly of embryonic blood vessels in the vitreous persisting abnormally and subsequently undergoing a fibrous hyperplasia. He suggested that this fibrous overgrowth incorporated the retina in a mass behind the crystalline lens.

The association between oxygen exposure and this disease was not recognized until Dame Kate Campbell (b. 1899)[74] in Australia in 1951 reported that oxygen was the main causative factor of what was by this time called retrolental fibroplasia. However, a standard American pediatric textbook (Holt and McIntosh's *Pediatrics*) as late as 1953 stated that "the oxygen content of the incubator need not exceed 60 percent, although higher concentrations appear to do no harm."[51] By 1945, 12 percent of premature infants with a birth weight of 1,360 gm (3 pounds) or less were blind, and it has been estimated that by the time control of the disease was achieved, eight thousand infants had suffered this fate.[74]

Prior to 1940 the condition was virtually nonexistent. Within ten years, however, retrolental fibroplasia became the largest single cause of child blindness in the United States, greater than all other causes combined. After 1955, when a general restriction of oxygen usage was adopted (not to exceed 40 percent), the largely iatrogenic condition virtually disappeared, and only sporadic cases are now encountered. Immaturity was a major factor; most affected infants had a gestational age of less than 34 weeks. However, even meticulously careful monitoring of oxygen concentrations has not entirely eliminated the condition. Because of the increasing survival rate of smaller preterm infants there appears to be a resurgence of retrolental fibroplasia because such infants seem particularly susceptible to oxygen damage.

During the upsurge in incidence of retrolental fibroplasia between 1945 and 1950 the condition was paradoxically prevalent in the larger and better-equipped medical centers but spared the smaller rural hospitals. It is now apparent that the larger institutions were the first to utilize the more efficient incubators which permitted the delivery of a higher concentration of oxygen.

Between 1925 and 1950 human milk was the food of choice for all feeble or sick infants. Medicine droppers with rubber tips were widely used, and, according to Gordon, "infants were fed every 1 or 2 hours by patient nurses who could be expected to place in the infant's mouth human or cow's milk mixture at a rate not exceeding his ability to swallow. Most of these infants gained slowly because of inadequate caloric intake." This led to long hospital stays, which in the pre-antibiotic era increased the risk of exposure to hospital infections. Strict isolation measures were instituted as a prophylaxis against nosocomial infections. Mothers, and personnel from other parts of the hospital, were excluded. The use of intermittent gavage and the introduction of the indwelling nasogastric polyethylene tube about 1950 speeded weight gains of the premature infant.

By 1950 the possibility of danger to the newborn infant—especially the preterm infant—from an excess of cow's milk had become evident. The presence of relatively larger amounts of phosphorus in cow's milk in relation to the calcium content, coupled with the failure of the kidneys to excrete the larger amount of phosphorus, would lead to an accumulation of phosphorus in the plasma, while the resulting decrease in calcium content would lead to "transient" tetany of the newborn; this was explained on the basis of a temporary functional hypoparathyroidism. With the advent of artificial formulas that simulate breast milk, the incidence of "transient" neonatal tetany has markedly decreased.

Some New Pediatric Diseases

Infantile Cortical Hyperostosis

This was described in 1945 by John Caffey (1895–1978) and William A. Silverman (b. 1917)[12] and by Francis Scott Smyth (1895–1972)[81] the following year. It appeared to be a new disease because the symptoms were too vivid to have been ignored by physicians prior to 1945. This disease, which occurs in the first few months of life, is characterized by systemic disturbance and an acute inflammatory reaction in the periosteum. In affected infants there is hyerplasia of subperiosteal bone with overlying soft tissue swelling and at times a brawny discoloration of the skin. The mandible and clavicles are most frequently affected. A triad of irritability, soft tissue swelling, and cortical thickening of the underlying bone is typical. The cause remains unknown.

Hypervitaminosis A

This poisoning caused by excessive ingestion of vitamin A was first reported by Josephs in 1944 and by John A. Toomey (1889–1950) and Russell A. Mor-

issette (b. 1918)[51] in 1947. Almost all recorded cases have followed ingestion of excessive amounts of vitamin A concentrates for six months or longer, in the range of over 75,000 international units daily. Taken in excessive dosage over long periods, vitamin A is toxic. In certain respect hypervitaminosis A can simulate infantile cortical hyperostosis. In hypervitaminosis A the ulnas and one or more metatarsals, other than the first, have been the most frequently involved bones; the mandible and flat bones are rarely, if ever, affected.

Familial Autonomic Dysfunction

This syndrome was first described in 1949 by Conrad M. Riley (b. 1913), Richard Day, David McL. Greeley (b. 1912) and William S. Langford (b. 1906),[75] all of whom at that time were at Babies Hospital in New York City. In the ensuing years Riley and others described the postural hypotonia consistently observed in patients suffering from this syndrome.

Polyostotic Fibrous Dysplasia

This congenital disorder characterized by an association of skin pigmentation, precocious sexual development, and areas of osseous rarefaction was described separately by Fuller Albright (1900–1969) and by Donovan J. McCune (1902–1976) in 1937. Girls are far more frequently affected than boys and it is only in girls that the sexual precocity is observed.

Rickettsialpox (Kew Gardens Spotted Fever)

In May, 1946, an epidemic of an unusual "spotted fever" disease occurred in a housing development in Kew Gardens, Queens, New York.[83] The disease was soon recognized as a new entity caused by a previously unknown rickettsia, *Rickettsia akari*, and transmitted by the mouse mite, *Allodermanyssus sanguineus*. This mite is a rather rare species discovered and classified in Egypt in 1913. Although it had no medical history up to 1946, it had always been considered by parasitologists as a possible transmitter of disease. The link between *Allodermanyssus sanguineus* and rickettsialpox was largely due to the detective work of Charles Pomerantz, a New York

City exterminator, who found the mites on the bodies of some of the mice he had trapped in the housing development.

In the Kew Gardens epidemic the disease was mild. Infants of six months as well as adults up to seventy-two years of age were stricken. The onset was indefinite; the first indication of any abnormality was the discovery by the patient of an area of erythema about the size of a pea, slightly elevated and slightly tender, which resembled an insect bite. The initial lesion was followed in two to seven days by headache, fever, chills, and sweats. The patient's temperature varied from 100 to 104° F. Within one to three days after the onset of fever there appeared a punctate, pink macular rash over the abdomen, chest, and upper extremities. The rash faded in about six to eight days. Except for leukopenia, studies of blood, urine, or stool showed no characteristic changes.

New Discoveries in Some Established Pediatric Diseases

Acrodynia

On May 5, 1945, Josef Warkany (b. 1902) and Donald M. Hubbard,[88] using a delicate test for mercury, found for the first time that this heavy metal was present in large amounts in the urine of a child, aged fourteen months, who had a severe form of acrodynia. The initial test revealed a level of 360 μg of mercury per liter; two days later another specimen of urine contained 320 μg per liter. Since these were appreciable amounts of mercury, the determinations were repeated about three weeks and six weeks later, when amounts of 90 and 140 μg per liter were found. The source of mercury could not be established in that child.

Their observation was not reported until 1938, a year after Guido Fanconi (b. 1892)[38], in Switzerland, called attention to a group of symptoms exhibited by thirty-nine children who had received calomel as a vermifuge. The course of the disease in most of the children reported by Fanconi was benign. However, in a few cases the typical picture of acrodynia developed. Three years after publishing their first paper incriminating the importance of mercury in the etiology of acrodynia, Warkany and Hubbard reported

forty-one children from various parts of the United States suffering from acrodynia, in thirty-eight of whom, or 93 percent, mercury was found in the urine, whereas in 85 percent of control cases it was absent.

From the studies of Warkany and Hubbard and others, it now appears that most and perhaps all cases of acrodynia represent the clinical response to repeated ingestion or contact with mercury. It is now believed that many of the clinical features of acrodynia are due to potentiation of the tissue response to adrenalin by mercury, so that the whole sympathetic system is activated. The stress of previous illness or other environmental influences will enhance this sympathetic overactivity.

Coccidioidomycosis

Although coccidioidomycosis was first reported in Argentina in 1892, little mention was made of this mycosis in American pediatric literature until the late 1930's. Faber, Charles E. Smith, and E. C. Dickson[37] were the first to report the association of acute coccidioidomycosis with erythema nodosum. In this paper they also called attention to focal areas of intrathoracic calcification caused by coccidioidomycosis in nontuberculous children.

Histoplasmosis

In 1945 Amos Christie (b. 1902) and John C. Peterson (b. 1904)[14] demonstrated that not all focal shadows of calcification seen in chest films of children and adolescents are caused by tuberculosis. Their patients who had focal calcified shadows in the lungs were uniformly tuberculin-negative by skin test, and for the most part they reacted strongly to a test antigen made from Histoplasma capsulatum. Faber and McIntosh,[36] in discussing this paper, noted that "so strongly entrenched had been the belief in the tuberculous etiology of such shadows that the pediatric world was with difficulty dissuaded from its conviction that patients harboring them must be tuberculous and yet, somehow, 'anergic' to tuberculin."

Christie and others between 1930 and 1940 called attention to the fact that histoplasmosis, like tuberculosis and coccidioidomycosis, was a widespread infection with common benign and rare severe forms.

Endocrine Disturbances

During this period adrenal hemorrhage in the newborn was said to occur in one percent of infants dying at, or shortly after, birth.[53] Predisposing factors were thought to be the great vascularity and friability of the large adrenal cortex of the newborn, postnatal hypoprothrombinemia, asphyxia, premature birth, and possibly the presence of toxemia of pregnancy in the mother. The immediate cause was attributed to the trauma of a prolonged or difficult labor, especially with a breech presentation. The clinical picture was that of shock characterized by tachycardia, tachypnea, and cyanosis. The symptoms were often said to have been indistinguishable from those of a fulminant septicemia.[53]

In addition to the acute cases, which usually terminated fatally to be discovered at postmortem, it was thought that there was an even larger number with less marked evidences of insufficiency and in which recovery usually occurred even without specific therapy. Such instances were reported, especially, by Joseph C. Jaudon (b. 1904).

Cancer of the Thyroid

Benedict J. Duffy and Patrick J. Fitzgerald's (1950)[34] study on the association between radiation therapy in infancy and later occurrence of thyroid carcinoma was a major contribution to pediatrics because it incriminated irradiation to the neck and adjacent areas during infancy for such benign conditions as "enlarged" thymus (p. 192), hypertrophied tonsils and adenoids, hemangioma, and cervical adenitis. Such irradiation in infancy has been found to carry at least a 4 percent risk of thyroid cancer.

Congenital Adrenal Hyperplasia

Wilkins and his co-workers,[90] beginning in 1949, and F. C. Barrter and colleagues simultaneously recognized the suppressibility of excessive adrenal androgen production by cortisone in congenital adrenal hyperplasia. These observations opened up the understanding and successful treatment of this familial disorder.

New Publications

American Textbooks of Pediatrics, 1925 to 1950

Among the major new general pediatric reference textbooks published between 1925 and 1950 were these:

1926 John Lovett Morse, *Clinical Pediatrics*
1927 William Palmer Lucas, *The Modern Practice of Pediatrics*
1937 Joseph Brennemann (ed.), *Practice of Pediatrics* (4 vols. plus index)
1948 Clifford G. Grulee and R. Cannon Eley, *The Child in Health and Disease*

American Pediatric Journals, 1925 to 1950

Three new pediatric journals appeared during this period. The first, the *Journal of Pediatrics*, began publication on July 1, 1932. The second, the *Quarterly Review of Pediatrics*, was published from 1946 until 1962. Finally, the third and last, *Pediatrics*, the official journal of the American Academy of Pediatrics, began publication in January, 1948.

Between 1925 and 1950 the practice of pediatrics was drastically changed by several epoch-making discoveries, any one of which, in other times, would have been of major historical importance. But a twenty-five-year period that saw the introduction of sulfonamides, antibiotics, adrenocortical steroids, antimetabolites, and the elucidation of the pathophysiological aspects of fluid and electrolyte disorders seemed to those who lived through the period to be the golden age of pediatrics.

However, the next quarter-century would see even greater progress and with it would come a far broader appreciation of the scope of pediatric practice.

References

1. Albright, F., et al. Syndrome characterized by osteitis fibrosa disseminata, areas of pigmentation and endocrine dysfunction with precocious puberty in females: Report of 5 cases. *N. Engl. J. Med.* 216:727, 1937.
2. Andersen, D. H. Cystic fibrosis of the pancreas and

its relation to celiac disease: A clinical and pathological study. *Am. J. Dis. Child.* 56:344, 1938.

3. Andersen, D. H., and Early, M. V. Method of assaying trypsin suitable for routine use in diagnosis of congenital pancreatic deficiency. *Am. J. Dis. Child.* 63:891, 1942.

4. Ayoub, E. M. Introduction of Dr. A. Ashley Weech for the John Howland Award. *Pediatr. Res.* 12:229, 1978.

5. Bell, J. A. Pertussis immunization: Use of an alum-precipitated mixture of pertussis vaccine and diphtheria toxoid. *J.A.M.A.* 137:1009, 1276, 1948.

6. Blackfan, K. D., and Diamond, L. K. The monocyte in active tuberculosis: Supravital studies of the blood. *Am. J. Dis. Child.* 37:233, 1929.

7. Blackfan, K. D., and May, C. D. Inspissation of secretion, dilatation of the ducts and acini, atrophy and fibrosis of the pancreas in infants: A clinical note. *J. Pediatr.* 13:627, 1938.

8. Blackfan, K. D., and Wolbach, S. B. Vitamin A deficiency in infants: A clinical and pathological study: *J. Pediatr.* 3:679, 1933.

9. Brennemann, J. Report on sulfanilamide from the Children's Memorial Hospital of Chicago. *J. Pediatr.* 11:238, 1937.

10. Butler, A. M., McKhann, C. F., and Gamble, J. L. Intracellular fluid loss in diarrheal disease. *J. Pediatr.* 3:84, 1933.

11. Byers, R. K., and Moll, F. C. Encephalopathies following pertussis vaccine. *Pediatrics* 1:437, 1948.

12. Caffey, J., and Silverman, W. A. Infantile cortical hyperostosis: Preliminary report on a new syndrome. *Am. J. Roentgenol.* 54:1, 1945.

13. Chapple, C. C. A cabinet cubicle for infants, combining isolation with control of temperature and humidity. *J. Pediatr.* 16:215, 1940.

14. Christie, A., and Peterson, J. C. Pulmonary calcification in negative reactors to tuberculin. *Am. J. Public Health* 35:1131, 1945.

15. Clifford, S. W. A study of neonatal mortality. *J. Pediatr.* 8:367, 1936.

16. Coburn, A. F. *The Factor of Infection in the Rheumatic State.* Baltimore: Williams & Wilkins, 1931.

17. Coburn, A. F. The rheumatic fever problem. *Am. J. Dis. Child.* 70:339, 1945.

18. Cohn, E. J., et al. Chemical, clinical, and immunological studies on the products of human plasma fractionation. *J. Clin. Invest.* 23:417, 1944.

19. Comings, D. E. Sickle Cell Disease and Related Disorders. In W. J. Williams, E. Beutler, A. J. Erslev, and R. W. Rundles (eds.), *Hematology.* New York: McGraw-Hill, 1972.

20. Cooke, J. V. The effect of specific therapy on the common contagious diseases. *J. Pediatr.* 35:275, 1949.

21. Cooke, R. E., et al. The role of potassium in the prevention of alkalosis. *Am. J. Med.* 17:180, 1954.

22. Cooley, T. E., and Lee, P. A series of cases of splenomegaly in children with anemia and peculiar bone changes. *Trans. Am. Pediatr. Soc.* 37:29, 1925.

23. Dalldorf, G., and Sickles, G. M. An unidentified, filtrable agent isolated from the feces of children with paralysis. *Science* 108:61, 1948.

24. Darrow, D. C. Electrolyte deficit in a patient with severe burn treated by continuous tub. *Trans. Am. Pediatr. Soc.* 50:40, 1938.

25. Darrow, D. C. Association of alkalosis and potassium deficiency with cardiac necrosis. In J. A. Askin, R. E. Cooke, and J. A. Haller, Jr. (eds.), *A Symposium on the Child.* Baltimore: Johns Hopkins Press, 1967.

26. Darrow, D. C., and Yannet, H. Effect of changes in extracellular electrolyte on cellular electrolyte and water. *Trans. Am. Pediatr. Soc.* 46:62, 1934.

27. Day, R. Respiratory metabolism in infancy and in childhood, XXVII: Regulation of body temperature of premature infants. *Am. J. Dis. Child.* 63:376, 1943.

28. Diamond, L. K., Blackfan, K. D., and Baty, J. M. Erythroblastosis fetalis and its association with universal edema of the fetus, icterus gravis neonatorum, and anemia of the newborn. *J. Pediatr.* 1:269, 1932.

29. Diamond, L. K., and Blackfan, K. D. Hypoplastic anemia. *Am. J. Dis. Child.* 56:464, 1938.

30. Diamond, L. K., Allen,. F. H., and Thomas, W. O., Jr. Erythroblastosis fetalis, VII: Treatment with exchange transfusion. *N. Engl. J. Med.* 244:39, 1951.

31. Domagk, G. Ein Beitrag zur Chemotherapie der bakteriellen Infektionen. *Dtsch. Med. Wochenschr.* 61:250, 1935.

32. Dowling, H. E. *Fighting Infection: Conquests of the Twentieth Century.* Cambridge, Mass: Harvard University Press, 1977.

33. Drolet, G. J., and Lowell, A. M. *A Half Century's Progress against Tuberculosis in New York City, 1900 to 1950.* New York: New York Tuberculosis and Health Assn. 1952.

34. Duffy, B. J., Jr., and Fitzgerald, P. J. Cancer of the thyroid in children: A report of 28 cases. *J. Clin. Endocrinol.* 10:1296, 1950.

35. Enders, J. F., Weller, T. H., and Robbins, F. C. Cultivation of the Lansing strain of poliomyelitis virus in cultures of various human embryonic tissue. *Science* 109:85, 1949.

36. Faber, H. K., and McIntosh, R. *History of the American Pediatric Society, 1889–1965.* New York: McGraw-Hill, 1966.

37. Faber, H. K., Smith, C. E., and Dickson, E. C.

Acute coccidioidomycosis with erythema nodosum in children. *J. Pediatr.* 15:163, 1939.

38. Fanconi, G., and Botsztejn, A.   Die Feersche Krankheit (Akrodynie) und Quecksilbermedikation. *Helv. Paediatr. Acta* 3:264, 1948.

39. Farber, S.   Pathologic changes associated with pancreatic insufficiency in early life. *Arch. Pathol.* 37:238, 1944.

40. Farber, S.   Some observations on the effect of folic acid antagonists on acute leukemia and other forms of incurable cancer. *Blood* 4:160, 1949.

41. Farber, S., et al.   Temporary remissions in acute leukemia in children produced by folic acid antagonist 4-amino-pteroylglutamic acid (aminopterin). *New Engl. J. Med.* 238:787, 1948.

42. Fox, M. J., and Clark, J. M.   Erythema infectiosum. *Am. J. Dis. Child.* 73:453, 1947.

43. Gordon, J. E., and Hood, R. I.   Whooping cough and its epidemiological anomalies. *Am. J. Med. Sci.* 222:333, 1951.

44. Govan, C. D., Jr., and Darrow, D. C.   The use of potassium chloride in the treatment of the dehydration of diarrhea in infants. *J. Pediatr.* 28:541, 1946.

45. Haas, S. V.   Celiac disease and its ultimate prognosis. *J. Pediatr.* 13:390, 1938.

46. Hart, A. P.   Familial icterus gravis of the newborn and its treatment. *Can. Med. Assoc. J.* 15:1008, 1925.

47. Hedley, O. F.   Trends, geographical, and racial distribution of mortality from heart disease among persons 5–24 years of age in the United States during recent years (1922–1936). *Public Health Rep.* 54:2271, 1939.

48. Herrell, W. E., and Kennedy, R. L.   Penicillin: Its use in pediatrics. *J. Pediatr.* 25:505, 1944.

49. Herrick, T. P.   Erythema infectiosum. *Am. J. Dis. Child.* 31:486, 1926.

50. Holt, L. E., Courtney, A. M., and Fales, H. L.   The chemical composition of diarrheal as compared with normal stools in infants. *Am. J. Dis. Child.* 9:213, 1915.

51. Holt, L. E., and McIntosh, R.   *Pediatrics* (12th ed.) New York: Appleton-Century-Crofts, 1953.

52. Huguley, C. M., Jr.   Acute Lymphocytic Leukemia. In W. J. Williams, E. Beutler, A. J. Erslev, and R. W. Rundles (eds.), *Hematology*. New York: McGraw-Hill, 1972.

53. Jaudon, J. C.   Further observations concerning hypofunction of the adrenals during early life: "Salt and water" hormone deficiency. *J. Pediatr.* 32:641, 1948.

54. Jones, T. D.   The diagnosis of rheumatic fever. *J.A.M.A.* 126:481, 1944.

55. Josephs, H. W.   Anaemia of infancy and early childhood. *Medicine* 15:307, 1936.

56. Kendrick, P.   Secondary familial attack rates from pertussis in vaccinated and unvaccinated children. *Am. J. Hyg.* 32:89, 1940.

57. Kendrick, P.   A field study of alum-precipitated combined pertussis vaccine and diphtheria toxoid for active immunization. *Am. J. Hyg.* 38:193, 1943.

58. Landsteiner, K., and Wiener, A. S.   An agglutinable factor in human blood recognizable by immune sera for *Rhesus* blood. *Proc. Soc. Exp. Biol.* 43:223, 1940.

59. Levine, P., and Stetson, R.   An unusual case of intra-group agglutination. *J.A.M.A.* 113:126, 1939.

60. Levine, P., et al.   The role of iso-immunization in the pathogenesis of erythroblastosis fetalis. *Am. J. Obstet. Gynecol.* 42:925, 1941.

61. Levine, S. Z., and Dann, M.   Survival rates and weight gains in premature infants weighing 1,000 grams or less. *Ann. Paediatr. Fenn.* 3:185, 1957.

62. Massell, B. F., et al.   Prevention of rheumatic fever by prompt penicillin therapy of hemolytic streptococcic respiratory infections. *J.A.M.A.* 146:1469, 1951.

63. May, C. D., McCreary, J. F., and Blackfan, K. D.   Notes concerning the cause and treatment of celiac disease. *J. Pediatr.* 21:289, 1942.

64. May, C. D.   *Cystic Fibrosis of the Pancreas.* Springfield, Ill.: Thomas, 1943.

65. McCune, D. J., and Bruch, H.   Osteodystrophia fibrosa: Report of a case. *Am. J. Dis. Child.* 54:806, 1937.

66. McKhann, C. F., and Chu, F. T.   Use of placental extract in prevention and modification of measles. *Am. J. Dis. Child.* 45:475, 1933.

67. Mitchell, A. G., and Trachsler, W. H.   Report on the use of sulfanilamide and its derivatives at the Children's Hospital of Cincinnati. *J. Pediatr.* 11:183, 1937.

68. Neel, J. V.   The inheritance of sickle cell anemia. *Science* 110:64, 1949.

69. Parish, H. J.   *A History of Immunization.* Edinburgh: Livingstone, 1965.

70. Parmelee, A. H.   The pathology of steatorrhea. *Am. J. Dis. Child.* 50:1418, 1935.

71. Pauling, L. C., Itano, A. H., et al.   Sickle cell anemia, a molecular disease. *Science* 110:543, 1949.

72. Pease, M. C.   *History of the American Academy of Pediatrics.* Evanston, Ill.: American Academy of Pediatrics, 1952.

73. Powers, G. F.   A comprehensive plan of treatment for the so-called intestinal intoxication of infants. *Am. J. Dis. Child.* 32:232, 1926.

74. Reese, A. B.   Editorial: An epitaph for retrolental fibroplasia. *Am. J. Ophthalmol.* 40:267, 1955.

75. Riley, C. M., et al.   Central autonomic dysfunction

with defective lacrimation, I: Report of five cases. *Pediatrics* 3:468, 1949.

76. Sauer, L. Whooping cough: A study in immunization. *J.A.M.A.* 100:239, 1933.

77. Sauer, L. Municipal control of whooping cough. *J.A.M.A.* 109:487, 1937.

78. Schwentker, F. F., et al. Use of para-amino-benzene-sulphonamide or its derivatives in the treatment of β-hemolytic meningitis. *Bull. Johns Hopkins Hosp.* 60:297, 1937.

79. Smith, C. A. *The Physiology of the Newborn Infant.* Springfield, Ill.: Thomas, 1946.

80. Smith, C. H. Infectious lymphocytosis. *Am. J. Dis. Child.* 62:231, 1941.

81. Smyth, F. S., Potter, A., and Silverman, W. Periosteal reaction, fever and irritability in young infants: A new syndrome? *Am. J. Dis. Child.* 71:333, 1946.

82. Spink, W. W. *Infectious Diseases: Prevention and Treatment in the Nineteenth and Twentieth Centuries.* Minneapolis: University of Minnesota Press, 1978.

83. Sussman, L. N. Kew Gardens' spotted fever. *N.Y. Med.* 2(15):27, 1946.

84. Terry, T. L. Retrolental fibroplasia. *Am. J. Ophthalmol.* 25:203, 1942.

85. Trachsler, W. H., et al. Streptococcic meningitis. *J. Pediatr.* 11:248, 1937.

86. Valentine, W. N., and Neel, J. V. Hematologic and genetic study of the transmission of the thalassemia (Cooley's anemia: Mediterranean anemia). *Arch. Intern. Med.* 74:185, 1944.

87. Wallerstein, H. Treatment of severe erythroblastosis by simultaneous removal and replacement of the blood of the newborn infant. *Science* 103:583, 1946.

88. Warkany, J. and Hubbard, D. M. Mercury in the urine of children with acrodynia. *Lancet* 1:829, 1948.

89. Wiener, A. S., and Wexler, J. B. The use of heparin when performing exchange blood transfusions in newborn infants. *J. Lab. Clin. Med.* 31:1016, 1946.

90. Wilkins, L. *The Diagnosis and Treatment of Endocrine Disorders in Childhood and Adolescence.* Springfield, Ill. Thomas, 1950.

91. Zuelzer, W. W. Pediatric Hematology in Historic Perspective. In D. Nathan and F. Oski (eds.), *Hematology of Infancy and Childhood.* Philadelphia: Saunders, 1974.

9

The Changing Face of Pediatrics

The aim of pediatrics is to assist each boy and girl to reach maturity equipped physically, mentally, and socially to function as responsible members of society within limits approaching his or her own potential and to have had the opportunity of thoroughly enjoying the years of getting there.

Waldo E. Nelson (1972)

During the last twenty-eight years progress in pediatrics has been staggering. John Apley[2] has reminded us that it was not so long ago that pediatrics itself was just a modern trend in medicine. The past twenty years, particularly, have witnessed trends developing within that trend, such as preventive pediatrics, developmental pediatrics, fetology, adolescent medicine and gynecology, developmental pharmacology, and the epidemiology of congenital malformations.

The advances recorded during this period have been so numerous that only a few can be mentioned and even fewer will be discussed. The development of several new broad-spectrum antibiotics, of greater effectiveness in the treatment of childhood infectious diseases than the earlier drugs, the discovery of the therapeutic role of the corticosteroids in certain diseases, and the studies of bacterial genetics, especially in relation to the problems of resistance to antibiotics, are some of them. Unprecedented virological advances have been made, particularly following the developments by John F. Enders and colleagues of improved laboratory methods of growing viruses in tissue culture. The introduction of radioactive isotopes in clinical and physiologic studies have greatly enhanced the sophistication of pediatric practice.

The increased understanding of the cause of hemolytic disease of the newborn has greatly assisted its prevention, early recognition, and treatment. The development of the sweat test for cystic fibrosis has led to earlier detection of this disease. The use of new antimetabolites for the palliation of childhood cancers has given guarded hope that these ominous diseases might one day yield to cure. The increasing understanding of the physiology of respiration, especially in newborn infants, has greatly bettered their care and chances of survival. Since the introduction of the poliovirus vaccine by Jonas Salk and of Albert B. Sabin's orally administered attenuated strains, we have seen the previously dreaded epidemics of paralytic poliomyelitis disappear. Recently, an analogous approach has been made in active immunizations against measles. Studies of chromosome anomalies have expanded greatly; attention was first focused on the sex chromatin mass, through which a number of anomalies of sex development were clarified. Many metabolic defects caused by a congenitally conditioned deficiency of a specific intracellular enzyme system have been uncovered. Ogden C. Bruton's[9] discovery of a disease that he called agammaglobulinemia led to the finding of several additional immunodeficient diseases. Prenatal diagnosis by amniocentesis for a large number of chromosomal anomalies and metabolic diseases is now a reality. At present, in addition to hemolytic disease of the newborn and chromosomal disorders, nearly fifty genetic diseases are eligible for prenatal diagnosis because they are detectable by somatic cell culture.

Investigations of the pathogenesis of idiopathic respiratory distress syndrome (hyaline membrane disease) have leaned toward the important role that pulmonary surfactant might play in its origin. The cause—or causes—of sudden infant death syndrome continue to elude investigators studying this calamitous disease. Advances in human genetics have burgeoned. Genetic counseling services are available in every state of our country. The genetic control of the immune response to many antigens is currently an important area of experimental immunobiology.

Federal Support of Pediatric Research

Great impetus was given to pediatric research during this period by the creation of several funding agencies supported by the federal government. The National Science Foundation, an independent agency of the federal government, was established in 1950. Of enormous importance was the founding and expansion of the National Institutes of Health in Bethesda, Maryland, during these years because of their increasing support of scientific research in medical schools and universities. It was not until the National Institute of Child Health and Human Development (NICHD) was established in 1961 that a national center for basic research in child development existed. Legislation was passed in 1963 which authorized construction grants for research centers in which biological, medical, and behavioral research and training relating to mental retardation could be conducted. The NICHD remains the major federal agency that supports these centers.

Sudden Infant Death Syndrome (SIDS)

The syndrome (SIDS) is now recognized as a definite disease entity by a majority of investigators, both forensic and medical, despite a lack of agreement as to its precise definition, terminology, and causation. It is now the largest single cause of postneonatal infant mortality in the United States, accounting for approximately one-third of all deaths between one week and one year of age.[6] During the third and fourth months of life SIDS apparently accounts for more than half of all infant deaths. Nearly all studies reported to date have cited incidence figures in the range of 2 to 3 per 1,000 live births. If a mean figure of 2.5 per 1,000 live births is applied to our current estimated 3,313,000 live births in 1977, it is apparent that nearly 10,000 SIDS deaths occur yearly in the United States.[6]

After the growing disillusionment with the enlarged thymus theory and its final demise about 1950, a number of other causes of sudden death in infants were often cited during the 1940's and 1950's. Among these were immaturity, malformations, internal hemorrhage, infections, convulsions, asphyxia from sudden respiratory obstruction, and a large number of miscellaneous causes including immunologic dysfunction, nutritional problems, and metabolic diseases. Up to the present time more than seventy different theories have been proposed to explain SIDS; many have been refuted and discarded, while others have held sway for a time, only to be replaced by new theories.

J. Bruce Beckwith[6] considers that the "modern era" of SIDS research was initiated by the series of papers of Jacob Werne and Irene Garrow from the office of the chief medical examiner of the borough of Queens, New York, published between 1942 and 1953. These authors presented compelling evidence to disprove suffocation as the cause of sudden death in infants.

Initially, after SIDS had been delineated about 1960, it was generally accepted that the ususal victim of such a tragedy was a well-nourished and well-developed infant, usually two to four months of age, whose sudden and unexpected death was unexplained even after the performance of an autopsy. But by 1978, Marie A. Valdés-Dapena,[53] in reviewing all the morphologic, chemical, and functional differences between normal control groups of infants and individual infants who died suddenly, unexpectedly, and inexplicably, wrote:

It would now seem apparent that babies who die of crib death are not normal at the time of death and probably are never entirely normal. To put it another way, *as a group,* infants who ultimately die of crib death exhibit structural and functional abnormalities during life and at postmortem examination, which serve to indicate in some way, not as yet defined, they are physiologically defective. This is, of course, a revelation inasmuch as just a few years ago virtually everyone assumed that they were in no way abnormal.

To complicate further the issue of crib death or SIDS, Valdés-Dapena stresses that "there is not as yet one positive criterion that can be employed by the clinician to identify the future victim, nor is there yet one positive criterion that the pathologist can use to identify the subject at autopsy."

Battered Child Syndrome

At the 1961 annual meeting of the American Academy of Pediatrics, Henry C. Kempe conducted a symposium on the problem of child abuse. To direct attention to the seriousness of the problem he coined the term "battered child syndrome." This symposium was the catalyst for the enormous pres-ent-day interest in and concern for the physically abused child, whose plight has become one of the gravest current problems facing not only pediatricians but also society as a whole.

Although there had been scattered reports of child abuse in the medical literature over many centuries, it was not until John Caffey's[10] radiologic observations, published in 1946, that any sustained concern was directed toward the battered child. Caffey in his paper reported six infants who had multiple fractures of the long bones in association with subdural hematomas. Although Caffey suspected that the x-ray findings in the long bones were due to trauma, he did not at that time attempt to pinpoint the nature of the trauma. He wrote: "These skeletal complications of subdural hematoma may be unrecognized trauma, but it must be admitted that at present their exact pathogenesis is unknown."

Support for Caffey's observations of bone lesions with subdural hematomas was soon provided by other reports describing traumatic bone lesions with and without subdural hematomas. Harry Bakwin,[5] for example, in 1952 reported several cases of unusual traumatic reactions in bones, among which was at least one battered child. In 1953, in his report of three infants with skeletal trauma but without subdural hematomas, Frederick N. Silverman[47] insisted on a traumatic basis for the bone injuries of the type now known to occur in the battered child. In 1955 Paul V. Woolley, Jr., and William A. Evans[57] wrote that the skeletal lesions they noted on x-rays were the same whether or not a history of injury was obtained and the skeletal lesions "having the appearance of fracture—regardless of history for injury or the presence or absence of intracranial bleeding—are due to undesirable vectors of force." Caffey[11] reexamined his earlier observations in 1957 and at that time reached the conclusion that trauma, willfully inflicted by parents, may have caused the x-ray findings he had originally described in 1946. Similar conclusions were reached in several medical reports published during the late fifties. In each of these reports the authors strongly recommended the use of x-rays combined with careful case histories and descriptions of the circumstances surrounding the injuries as guides to uncover clues of possible parental abuse.

In 1962 Kempe[33] and several of his colleagues presented their findings of a study of child-abuse incidents reported by 71 hospitals and 77 district attorneys from many parts of the United States. Many of the children of the 302 hospital cases and 447 cases known to district attorneys had died or had been seriously injured; the authors left no doubt that physical abuse was a major cause of death and injury to infants and children. Many of the abusive parents were found to suffer from various types of personality disorders. Kempe's article discussed also the reluctance of physicians to believe in the possibility of parental abuse and their reluctance to take an investigative role.

Childhood Accidents

Although it had been apparent for some years that accidents led all causes of death in children from one to fifteen years of age, few pediatricians realized the seriousness of the problem until the American Academy of Pediatrics established its Accident Prevention Committee in 1952.[56] The committee began its work by surveying the academy's 3,000 members (there are now 20,621 members as of November 30, 1978) for information on the most common household factors associated with children's accidents. This survey revealed that 30 percent of all reported accidents were due to burns, a large proportion of which were associated with flammable clothing.

An unexpected finding of the academy's survey was that 50 percent of the reported accidents involved some type of poisoning. Analysis of the poisoning cases showed most were nonfatal and were caused by common household items such as cleaning agents, aspirin, and barbiturates.[56] Cases of childhood lead poisoning reported by pediatricians from cities such as Baltimore, Cincinnati, and St. Louis focused attention on peeling paint as a source. These findings helped to start the academy's project with the American Standards Association to develop the first standard for paint that would be safe to use on children's toys, furniture, and other surfaces likely to be exposed to children.

As a result of this study, Edward Press established the first poison control center in the world in Chicago in 1953.[56] And a few months later a poison control center was started at the Duke University Medical Center by Jay Arena.

Accidents and acts of violence have replaced microbes as the major threat to the lives of children and adolescents in contemporary American society. In 1976, 27.9 deaths per 100,000 population in children one through five years of age occurred as the result of all accidents. For this age group the accident rate is more than three times the rate of the next leading cause of death—congenital anomalies. Motor vehicle accidents alone account for more than one-third of all accidents. And for children five through fourteen years of age, the leading cause of death in 1976 was also accidents (16.9), primarily motor vehicle (8.5). For adolescents between the ages of fifteen and twenty, accidents (57.4), primarily motor vehicle (38.4), also accounted for the majority of deaths in this age group.

Some Recent Clinical Advances in Pediatrics

Immunology

In 1950, the thymus remained an enigmatic organ that was still being irradiated by some physicians for respiratory stridor, gamma globulin determination was still in the realm of research, organ transplantation was science fiction, the function of the lymphocyte remained a mystery, and immunodeficiency diseases were yet to be discovered.[50] Since then advances in immunology have burgeoned and with them has emerged a whole new specialty of pediatrics—clinical immunology. By 1978 American contributions to this new specialty have been of an enormous importance. The pediatric departments of the University of Minnesota and the Harvard Medical School, particularly, according to E. Richard Stiehm and Vincent Fulginiti,[50] have "under the leadership of Robert A. Good, Charles A. Janeway, and David Gitlin served as the training grounds for many contributors to immunology." Other American investigators who have been in the forefront in the study of the development and function of the immune system are Henry G. Kunkel, Max D. Cooper, Albert H. Coons, Fred S. Rosen, H. Hugh Fudenberg, and Paul G. Quie.

The classic paper, published in 1965 by Cooper, R. D. A. Peterson, and Good,[13] delineating the thymic and bursal lymphoid systems in the chicken, initiated the concept of the two component subpopulations of lymphocytes in immune function.

Experimental investigation of the cellular basis of immunity has established the thymus as a protagonist in the development of immunological capacity. Its essential function seems to be the differentiation and proliferation of primitive lymphoid cells entering it from the bone marrow. The cells that leave the thymus after this conditioning process, according to Good,[25] "represent a recirculating population of lymphoid cells responsible for cell-mediated immunities." These so-called thymus-dependent lymphocytes or T cells are not antibody-forming cells themselves. The T cells are responsible for delayed allergic reactions, for much of the immunity to certain solid tissue allografts, for the capacity to elicit graft-versus-host reactions, and, as Good[25] has demonstrated, they appear to be "major components of the body defense against facultative bacterial pyogenic pathogens, fungi, and certain viruses (e.g., the pox viruses)."

The antibody-forming lymphocytes, like T cells, originate in the bone marrow, and because of their more direct relationship to the bone marrow, they are called B cells. They are ultimately responsible for the synthesis and secretion of all forms of antibody and all circulating immunoglobulins. Through its antibody-secreting mechanism, the B cells, according to Good,[25,26] "represent a major line of defense against encapsulated, high-grade bacterial pyogenic pathogens—pneumococcus, Hemophilus influenzae, Streptococcus, meningococcus, and Pseudomonas aeruginosa. [B cells] also appear to be crucial to the defense against certain viruses such as poliovirus, the virus causing infectious hepatitis, and even the virus responsible for serum hepatitis."

AGAMMAGLOBULINEMIA (BRUTON'S INFANTILE X-LINKED AGAMMAGLOBULINEMIA). One of the milestones in the history of pediatric immunology was Bruton's[9] discovery in 1952 of a new disease in an eight-year-old boy at the Walter Reed Army Medical Center. This boy exhibited specific congenital protein deficiency involving the gamma globulin and an inability to respond to infectious diseases with sufficient antibodies. Bruton[9] called this new disease agammaglobulinemia. His case report pointed out many of the major findings of this disorder including male sex, early onset, recurrent major pyogenic in-

fections, and ineffectiveness of most forms of therapy. The relation of an inherited gamma globulin deficiency and recurrent infections with inadequate antibody titers has since been repeatedly confirmed, and a group of disease states, collectively referred to as the "antibody deficiency syndrome," has evolved from Bruton's original case report.

TRANSIENT HYPOGAMMAGLOBULINEMIA OF INFANCY. Gitlin and Janeway[23] in 1956 described patients with repeated infections between the ages of six and twenty-four months who had low serum concentrations of gamma globulin. In time, however, their gamma globulin levels returned to normal. Infants sustained a period of physiologic hypogammaglobulinemia between three and four months of age, at which time rates of synthesis of gamma G globulin began to rise rapidly as peripheral lymphoid tissue matured. A prolongation of physiologic hypogammaglobulinemia up to twenty-four months of age may occur.

CONGENITAL APLASIA OF THE THYMUS (DIGEORGE SYNDROME). This is the mirror image of the sex-linked infantile immunodeficiency. Angelo M. DiGeorge[16] in 1965 recognized a form of congenital hypoparathyroidism associated with infection and congenital absence of the thymus gland in three infants. These patients had hypocalcemic tetany in the neonatal period and then suffered recurrent infections. The last resulted from lymphopenia, failure of lymphocyte responsiveness and defective cellular immunity function. In addition, patients with this syndrome may have a right-sided aortic arch, cardiac defects, and abnormalities of the palate, ears, and face. Although these patients lack cellular immunity mechanisms, they retain the ability to synthesize humoral antibodies. The immune defect may be corrected by transplants of fetal thymus.

Hematology

RED-CELL ENZYME DEFICIENCIES. In 1956 Paul E. Carson and co-workers[12] described the first example of a congenital hemolytic anemia that was caused by a red-cell enzyme deficiency. This deficiency, glucose-6-phosphate dehydrogenase (G-6-PD), according to Frank A. Oski and James A. Stockman,[42] "now is recognized to affect at least 100 million individuals throughout the world and is believed to be the most common inherited disorder of metabolism." Since the discovery of G–6–PD deficiency, eighteen other steps in red cell metabolism have been delineated in which alterations of enzyme function have been discovered in association with a clinically recognizable hemolytic process.

In 1962 Ernest Beutler and co-workers[8] found the gene for G–6–PD deficiency to be sex-linked, and it has since served as an important genetic marker for population studies and for study of the mechanism of genetic inactivation of the X-chromosome. Studies of the gene for G–6–PD deficiency in heterozygous females formed one of the original bases in man for the now accepted Lyon hypotheses of X-inactivation.

In 1961, William N. Valentine, Kouichi R. Tanaka, and Shiro Miwa[54] demonstrated for the first time a severe deficiency of pyruvate kinase (PK) in the erythrocytes of three patients with hereditary hemolytic anemia. These findings were soon extended, and at present pyruvate kinase deficiency has been described in many parts of the world. In addition to G–6–PD and PK deficiencies, other enzyme deficiencies in the Emben-Meyerhof pathway, both glycolytic and nonglycolytic, have been described in association with hereditary hemolytic anemia.

CHRONIC GRANULOMATOUS DISEASE (CGD). Chronic granulomatous disease (CGD), an inherited defect of leukocyte bactericidal function, was first described concurrently in 1957 by Heinz Berendes, Robert A. Bridges, and Good[7] and by Benjamin H. Landing and Harry C. Shirkey,[37] and it was subsequently delineated as a distinct clinical syndrome, usually fatal during childhood, and usually inherited as a recessive sex-linked trait affecting the sons of asymptomatic mother carriers. Recently a few cases similar clinically to CGD have been described in young girls.

The basic defect in this disease is one of failure of the polymorphonuclear leukocytes and monocytes to kill certain bacteria after phagocytosis; among the bacteria not killed are Staphylococcus aureus, Serratia marcescens and Aerobacter aerogenes. It is essentially an inborn abnormality of phagocytic function. Robert L. Baehner and David G. Nathan[4] have shown that the extremely active system of respiratory enzymes in polymorphonuclear cells, which is stimulated by phagocytosis, is defective in these patients, and they developed a simple color reaction for testing this, using nitroblue tetrazolium (NBT) for this purpose.

INFECTIOUS MONONUCLEOSIS. Gertrude Henle, Werner Henle, and Volker Diehl[28] in 1968 reported the association of infectious mononucleosis with the development of antibodies to the Epstein-Barr virus, the cause of infectious mononucleosis. This virus belongs to the herpes group and has been termed the "herpes-like virus." It was originally observed in growing cultures derived from Burkitt lymphoma biopsies. The virus has also been uniformly demonstrated by electron microscopy in growing leukocyte cultures from patients with infectious mononucleosis and may persist for years in leukocytes following clinical disease.

Genetics

A landmark study in human genetics was Joe H. Tjio and Albert Levan's[52] paper, published in Sweden in 1956, which proved that the normal chromosome number of man is forty-six rather than forty-eight, which had previously been accepted as the normal diploid number. Some months later C. E. Ford and J. L. Hamerton,[21] in England, produced evidence that the germ cells in the testes of several men likewise possessed forty-six chromosomes.

At the beginning of 1959 Jérôme Lejeune and his colleagues[38] in Paris first discovered an extra small acrocentric chromosome in individuals with Down's syndrome. Since then, detectable abnormalities of chromosomes have been discovered at a truly astonishing rate. With the development of new techniques for chromosome study there followed an extensive revision of many of the concepts previously held in human genetics. Techniques were quickly developed for chromosome analysis of peripheral blood lymphocytes, bone marrow cells, and fibroblasts that could be applied to the study of infants and children with congenital malformations and disorders of sexual differentiation.

Antenatal Diagnosis

The recent development of amniocentesis for antenatal diagnosis represents a major breakthrough in the application of science to reduce human suffering.

In 1966 Mark W. Steele and W. Roy Breg[48] reported for the first time the successful karyotyping of human amniotic cells, and the next year Cecil B. Jacobson and Robert H. Barter[30] suggested the use of amniocentesis for the diagnosis and management of genetic defects.

Amniocentesis performed at about the fifteenth week of pregnancy now makes it possible, in many cases, to diagnose the presence of chromosomal abnormalities in the fetus, an ever-increasing number of genetically determined metabolic diseases by biochemical analysis performed on the amniotic fluid, and the presence of anencephaly and myelomeningocele by determining the level of alpha-fetoprotein in the amniotic fluid.

New Vaccines

POLIOMYELITIS VACCINE. In 1954, on the advice of a committee of experts under the chairmanship of Thomas Milton Rivers (1888–1962), of the Rockefeller Institute, The National Foundation for Infantile Paralysis introduced a nationwide trial of Salk vaccine in the United States.[44] The Salk vaccine is an inactivated poliovirus vaccine (IPV) consisting of the three poliovirus serotypes cultivated in monkey or in human cell cultures with special attenuated strains of virus. The director of the National Foundation's field trial was Thomas Francis, Jr. (1900–1969), of the University of Michigan. The vaccine evaluation program would finally involve 1,929,916 children in 211 areas of 44 states. These included the placebo controls and the observed controls.[44]

On April 12, 1955, at Ann Arbor, Michigan, on the tenth anniversary of the death of President Franklin D. Roosevelt, Francis gave an abbreviated report of the success of the Salk vaccine for the prevention of poliomyelitis. Although this was a preliminary report the results suggested that the vaccine was both effective and safe. The data in the abbreviated Francis report stated that the vaccine had been given to 200,745 children without producing any serious reactions or accidents.[44]

Fifteen days after the Ann Arbor meeting the alarming announcement was made that several children who had been vaccinated with the Salk vaccine had developed paralytic poliomyelitis because, as it was soon discovered, two recent production batches of vaccine contained residual living virus.[44] This tragedy was soon corrected by stricter regulations in the production of vaccine.

Oral live attenuated poliovaccine (OPV) was licensed for use in the United States in March, 1962, and extensive experience in this country and in many other countries has confirmed the safety and efficacy of all three types of attenuated oral poliovaccine. This vaccine was largely developed by Sabin between 1953 and 1955. By 1957, tests had been carried out by Sabin on 10,000 monkeys, 160 chimpanzees, and also 243 humans, starting with himself and his own family. Three significant advantages of this vaccine are that it induces local resistance to reinfection of the alimentary tract, it is antigenically potent (a single feeding produces a rapid immunologic response), and it is effective in aborting epidemics of poliomyelitis in progress. Controversy still persists, however, concerning the relative merits of IPV versus OPV. At present the almost universal belief is that the evidence supporting the many advantages of OPV far outweighs the minute risks involved.

Poliomyelitis is now such an infrequent disease that many physicians less than forty years of age have never encountered a case. During the five-year period (1951–1955) preceding the introduction of inactivated poliovirus vaccine (IPV), 79,112 cases of paralytic disease were reported in the United States. Between 1956 to 1960, when only inactivated vaccine was available, 21,401 cases were reported, with a consistent downward trend during the interval (7,911 cases in 1956, 2,218 cases in 1960). This was a reduction of approximately 75 percent between 1956 to 1960 compared to the quinquennium 1951 to 1955. Further reductions were noted from 1961 to the present, after the introduction of live attenuated oral poliomyelitis vaccines (OPV). Only 111 cases of paralytic poliomyelitis were reported between 1969 and 1974, and in 1976 only 8 paralytic cases were reported in the United States.[36]

From 1960 to 1975, IPV gradually declined in usage in the United States and eventually became unavailable in this country. One of the disadvantages of killed poliovirus vaccines is that antibody titers tend to drop below detectable levels in young children whose antibody status indicates no prior infection with poliomyelitis. The current estimate of risk of possible vaccine-associated paralytic disease in vaccines or their contacts is no more than one per 10 million doses.[45]

MEASLES VACCINE. Although active immunization against measles is a comparatively recent accomplishment, Francis Home (1719–1813),[29] of Edinburgh, in 1758 attempted active measles immunization. Cotton soaked with the fresh blood of patients in the eruptive stage was applied to scarified areas on the arms of persons with no previous history of this disease. In seven of fifteen subjects, mild attacks of measles developed after an incubation period of about nine days.

Enders and Thomas C. Peebles[18] in 1954 reported the isolation of the measles virus in human and rhesus monkey kidney tissue cultures and also the cytopathic changes produced within the infected cell. At the beginning of their study human or monkey epithelial cells were inoculated with blood or throat washings of patients with typical measles. They then studied quantitatively the propagation of the virus, estimated the antibodies, and investigated attenuated variant strains which might prove suitable for vaccines. Enders, as has been mentioned, had already made an outstanding contribution to virology by cultivating the poliovirus in various nonneural tissue cultures (p. 217).

Enders, Milan Milovanović, Anna Mitus, and Samuel L. Katz, beginning in 1957, continued studies of the measles virus by passage of the Edmonston strain more than fifty times in human tissue culture; they then were successful in adapting it to tissue cultures of chick embryos. By 1958 these investigators had been able to attenuate the virus for man. Katz, who had been Enders' principal collaborator in the measles studies, prepared vaccines of the attenuated strain in chick embryo tissue cultures. When the vaccine was given to children by the subcutaneous or intramuscular route, antibody titers developed that were comparable with those found in naturally occuring measles. Katz,[32] in the tradition established by Boylston and Waterhouse, was so confident of the vaccine's safety that his own children were among the first to receive this attenuated measles vaccine.

On March 21, 1963, a vaccine composed of live attenuated measles virus of the Edmonston B strain was licensed in the United States for the prevention of measles. This represented the culmination of nine years of investigation by Enders and his associates. Widespread use of this vaccine reduced the number of reported cases of measles in the United States from about 482,000 in 1962 to a low of 22,000 in 1968, but then the number rose again, reaching 71,000 in 1971. The reason for this was not that the vaccine was ineffective, but rather that the immunization program tended to falter, particularly in low-income groups.

Experience with the use of more than 80 million doses of vaccine (1977) has made it possible to assess with great care the complications resulting from the use of live, attenuated measles vaccine. The only major complication associated with measles vaccine has been encephalitis. Its incidence has been estimated to be about one per million, as compared to one per thousand for natural measles.[45] The incidence of vaccine-associated subacute sclerosing panencephalitis (SSPE) has been estimated by the Committee on Infectious Diseases of the American Academy of Pediatrics (1977) to be "one per one to two million doses of vaccine as compared to one per one hundred thousand cases of natural measles. Thus, the use of live, attenuated measles vaccine may reduce the likelihood of the occurrence of a central nervous complication by a 10- to 100-fold factor."[45]

RUBELLA VACCINE. A major epidemic of rubella occurred in the United States in 1964. This epidemic resulted in thousands of deformed infants born to mothers who had developed rubella during pregnancy, especially in the first trimester. The cost of hospitalization, medical care, rehabilitation, and special education of the multihandicapped survivors has been estimated to exceed a billion dollars.[36]

The cultivation of rubella virus in tissue culture was reported independently and simultaneously by two American groups in 1962. Thomas H. Weller and Franklin A. Neva[55] observed a cytopathic effect in human amnion cells. At about the same time, Paul D. Parkman and co-workers[43] isolated the virus in cultures of African green monkey kidney tissue.

Harry M. Meyer, Parkman, and Theodore C. Panos[40] in 1966 reported the development of rubella vaccine from virus attenuated by repeated passage in tissue culture. After four years of field trials, rubella vaccine was licensed in the United States in June, 1969. Since then, and up until 1977, more than 70 million children have received rubella vaccine; the safety of the vaccine has been well documented. About 5 percent of children vaccinated have developed transient joint manifestations.[45]

Some Newer Viral Diseases

Enteroviral Infections

Polioviruses, Coxsackie viruses, and echoviruses are grouped together and designated enteroviruses because of their many similarities and because their natural habitat is the human enteric tract. At present there appear to be sixty-seven members of the enterovirus family distributed as follows: polioviruses, three types (1 to 3); Coxsackie viruses, group A, twenty-three types; Coxsackie viruses, Group B, six types; echoviruses, thirty-one types.[36]

Only a few examples of recently discovered diseases caused by these viruses will be given.

COXSACKIE GROUP A VIRUS INFECTIONS. The Coxsackie viruses, groups A and B, have now been shown to be causally related to the following diseases or syndromes: herpangina (p. 184), epidemic pleurodynia, febrile illness with exanthem, respiratory illness, generalized disease of the newborn, aseptic meningitis, and occasionally, paralysis and encephalitis.

Coxsackie A–9 Virus. has been a common cause of aseptic meningitis as well as exanthematous lesions. The earliest documented report of an epidemic of Coxsackie A–9 infection in this country occurred in Boston in 1959 and was published by A. Martin Lerner and co-workers.[39]

Coxsackie A–10 Virus (Acute Lymphonodular Pharyngitis). Alex J. Steigman[49] in 1962 first reported Coxsackie virus A–10 as the cause of an outbreak, largely among children, of an illness characterized by fever, sore throat, headache, and distinctive yellow nodules on the uvula, anterior pillars, and posterior pharynx.

Coxsackie A–16 Virus and Hand, Foot, and Mouth Disease. Coxsackie A–16 virus infection, called the hand, foot, and mouth disease, has been reported frequently in the United States since 1963. It was first definitively described in Toronto during the summer of 1957 by C. R. Robinson, Frances W. Doane, and A. J. Rhodes.[46] Subsequent reports have

added Coxsackie A–5 and A–10 viruses as other etiologic agents.

COXSACKIE GROUP B VIRUS INFECTIONS. Bornholm Disease, or epidemic pleurodynia, first recognized clinically more than a century ago, is now known to result from infection with Coxsackie B viruses, although occasionally group A viruses may be implicated. John J. Finn, Weller, and Herbert R. Morgan[20] in 1949 were among the first American investigators to identify Coxsackie B virus as the etiologic agent of this disease.

Coxsackie B Myocarditis of Infancy. Coxsackie viruses B–3 and B–4 have been found to be associated with this serious condition. It may occur in epidemic form in newborn nurseries during a community outbreak, particularly in newborn infants. It is frequently associated with encephalitis. The first report of this entity in the United States was published in 1956 by Sidney Kibrick and Kurt Benirschke.[34] The neonatal form is the most common.

ECHOVIRUS INFECTIONS. The ECHO (enteric cytopathogenic human orphan) viruses, as the name was first written, were so called because they are found in the human gastrointestinal tract, produce cytopathic changes in cells grown on tissue culture, and originally were not linked to disease in man. By 1977 there were thirty-one serotypes of echovirus. These agents have been shown to be etiologic factors in a surprising number of clinical syndromes. From the standpoint of morbidity, aseptic meningitis appears to be the most important clinical expression of echovirus infection.[36]

Echovirus Type 6. Epidemics of aseptic meningitis caused by echovirus type 6 were first reported in this country in 1956 by David C. Davis and Joseph L. Melnick[15] and by David T. Karzon and colleagues.[31]

Echovirus Type 9. Exanthem and aseptic meningitis due to this virus was first described in London during the summer of 1954. Since that year echovirus type 9 has been a continued, frequent worldwide cause of both aseptic meningitis and exanthem. Exanthem has been noted in about 35 percent of all echo type 9 illnesses. The rash usually appears as a rubelliform eruption. Kibrick and Enders[35] were among the first in this country to describe an epidemic of this disease in Massachusetts in 1958.

Echoviruses types 4 and 6 have also been responsible for large epidemics of aseptic meningitis.

Echovirus Type 16 (Boston Exanthem). This was the first of the "newer exanthems" to be described and virologically confirmed. During the summer of 1951 Neva and colleagues[41] described an epidemic of exanthematous disease in Boston which on later virologic examination proved to be due to echovirus type 16. This disease became known as "Boston exanthem." In 1954 a similar epidemic occurred in Pittsburgh.

Echovirus Type 18. In a hospital outbreak of mild diarrhea, echo type 18 virus was detected for the first time by Heinz F. Eichenwald et al[17] in 1958 in fifteen of seventeen infants with diarrhea but in none of the patients without diarrhea in the same wards.

The Newborn

In no branch of pediatrics have there been more dramatic advances during the last quarter-century than in neonatology. Space constraints will limit discussion to just a few of these advances.

Apgar Score

In 1952 Virginia Apgar (1909–1974)[1] (Fig. 9–1) proposed a new method of evaluation of the newborn infant. She chose five signs for evaluating the newborn infant and gave each of them a value of 0, 1 or 2. A rating of 10 points describes "the best possible condition" of the infant one minute after birth "with two points each given for respiratory effort, reflex irritability, muscle tone, heart rate, and color."

This quantitative assessment of the newborn remains the simplest and best way to evaluate the condition of an infant at birth. The only criticism some have made of the Apgar score is that it gives the same weight to different variables, whether changes in heart rate or changes in color. But against this its universal adoption and continued use are evidence of practical utility. It remains an excellent pragmatic tool.

At present the Apgar score is usually made at one minute after birth and repeated at five minutes. The

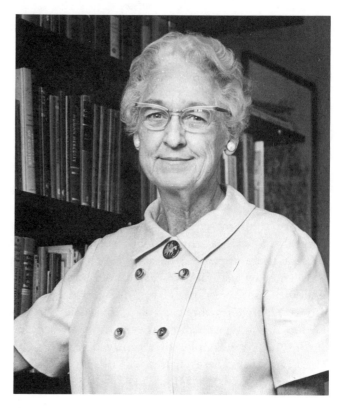

Figure 9–1. Virginia Apgar (1909–1974).

five-minute score has been shown to have some correlation with subsequent brain damage, while the one-minute score gives some index for the need for active resuscitation, correlates well with biochemical assessment of acidosis, and is inversely proportional to the neonatal death rate.

Phototherapy in Hyperbilirubinemia

Prevention of hyperbilirubinemia by phototherapy was first shown to be effective in 1958,[14] when it was demonstrated that exposure of premature infants to sunlight or blue fluorescent light produced a fall in serum bilirubin concentration. Subsequent reports from many centers have adequately documented the evidence that exposure of infants to sunlight or artificial blue light results in a decomposition of bilirubin to nontoxic dipyrroles. This technique provides a safe and simple method of preventing hyperbilirubinemia in many infants, especially the premature with nonhemolytic jaundice. Phototherapy, however, is usually too slow to treat adequately infants with hemolytic disease. However, phototherapy will modify the course of hyperbilirubinemia in

ABO and mild Rh hemolytic disease and will reduce, but not eliminate, the need for exchange transfusion.

Prevention of Erythroblastosis Fetalis

A major advance in neonatology was the development of a gamma globulin concentrate of anti-D Rh$_o$ (D) immune globulin (human) (RhoGAM), first reported in this country by Vincent J. Freda,[22] in 1963, for routine postpartum prophylaxis against sensitization of Rh-negative women.

When the nonsensitized mother receives an injection of this gamma globulin concentrate within seventy-two hours after delivery, abortion, or ectopic pregnancy, the fetal Rh-positive cells in her circulation become "coated" because of the interaction of the antibody and surface Rh antigen on the red blood cell; these red cells are thus "deformed" and removed rapidly from the circulation by the reticuloendothelial system of the mother. The Rh antigen is liberated from the "deformed" erythrocytes, and it is thought that in some way not yet explained, the injected anti-Rh immune globulin competes with antibody-forming tissues for the Rh antigen. Provided there is sufficient antibody present, a stable compound results which is not antigenic. This concept was originally demonstrated by Theobald Smith in 1910 (p. 171) with regard to toxin-antitoxin, namely that a passive antibody, when present in excess over an antigen, can block active immunization.

This discovery makes hemolytic disease of newborn infants a preventable disease. As recently as 1960, Rh disease claimed the lives of an estimated five to six thousand fetuses or newborns each year, but, by careful adherence to clinical and administrative guidelines, Rh disease can now be virtually eliminated.[22] Erythroblastosis fetalis thus became a disease whose cause was clearly determined (p. 210), its treatment successfully developed to a great extent (p. 211), and then its prevention found, all in a single generation.

Respiratory Distress Syndrome (RDS) (Hyaline Membrane Disease)

Respiratory distress syndrome (RDS) was first described as a specific pathological entity in 1953 under the name of hyaline membrane disease (HMD).* Prior to that date, infants who had signs and symptoms of this syndrome were diagnosed as having congenital atelectasis.

Between 1954 and 1958, RDS caused approximately twenty-five thousand neonatal deaths per year, representing 35 percent of all deaths in this age group. In addition, a substantial number of survivors had long-term neurologic sequelae. Between 1968 and 1973, the mortality from RDS was between ten and twelve thousand per year, representing 20 to 28 percent of all neonatal deaths and from 50 to 70 percent of all premature deaths. Not only has the mortality from RDS diminished within the last few years but the prognosis for intact neurologic survival has greatly improved as a result of important advances in perinatal medicine.[19] However, RDS still remains our most common cause of neonatal death. A conservative estimate is that in the United States, twelve thousand infants per year die from this disease. A recent study has strongly suggested that one-third of these cases could be prevented simply by avoiding iatrogenic prematurity, because RDS is a common condition of the premature infant and occurs rarely in the full-term infant. Of the various risk factors bearing on probability of survival from RDS, the best established is prematurity; the severity of this disease is strongly influenced by the degree of prematurity.

Most of the deaths due to RDS occur in the first seventy-two to ninety-six hours of life. Studies have shown that the fatality rate for RDS declines in a nearly exponential manner between the first and fourth twenty-four-hour periods. Almost 90 percent of deaths occur by the fourth day. From these data, it appears that the "natural" course of RDS (in the absence of assisted ventilation) is characterized by progressive deterioration in the first twenty-four to forty-eight hours, highest mortality in the first seventy-two hours, and a recovery period in survivors beginning at about seventy-two hours.

The single most important discovery in advancing our knowledge of the pathogenesis of RDS was reported in 1959 by Mary Ellen Avery and Jere Mead.[3]

---

* The term hyaline membrane disease (HMD), also referred to as respiratory distress syndrome (RDS), is now less favored than the latter term because there is considerable doubt whether the stainable membrane fully explains all the symptoms. Further, it is known that hyaline membrane may be formed in the course of other disorders, although its distribution is different. Nevertheless, the two terms are often used synonymously.

They observed that lungs of infants dying of this disorder, as well as lungs of immature newborns in general, were deficient in surface-active material (surfactant). In the years since 1959 many studies have been published to buttress the hypothesis that the symptoms of RDS reflect an underlying deficiency of pulmonary surfactant.

Louis Gluck and co-workers[24] beginning in 1971 introduced a method for the systematic evaluation of phospholipids in amniotic fluid to reflect the maturation of the fetal lung. There is a good correlation between surfactant levels in amniotic fluid and normal postnatal respiratory function. The major phospholipids in the amniotic fluid, lecithin and sphingomyelin, are now recognized as important components of the surfactant system of the lung and are found in fetal tracheal fluid. Following Gluck's study, many others during the past decade have demonstrated a continuity between fetal lung and amniotic fluid. During the course of pregnancy, the major surfactant compound, lecithin, tends to rise in concentration as pregnancy proceeds, while sphingomyelin plateaus and remains fairly constant throughout pregnancy. If one relates lecithin to sphingomyelin as a ratio (L/S), one can show maturation of lung associated with an L/S ratio of 2.0. By measurement of the ratio of lecithin to sphingomyelin (L/S) in the amniotic fluid the perinatologist is able to "diagnose" RDS antenatally.

Deficiency of surfactant leads to a decrease in lung compliance, alveolar instability, atelectasis, and possibly transudation into alveoli. The significance of surfactant compounds in maturation of the fetal lungs lies, according to Gluck,[24] in their function as the principal part of the alveolar lining layer that tends to stabilize the fine airspaces of the lung. The alveolus increases in diameter on inspiration and decreases on expiration. As the alveolar radius decreases, the wall tension tends to increase dramatically and, in the normal alveolus, the lining layer containing the surfactant phospholipids lowers the surface tension as this happens. Thus, it stabilizes the alveoli and prevents collapse. An inability to synthesize adequate amounts of the surfactant phospholipids is seen in a high proportion of premature births. Here the alveoli collapse each time the infant breathes out, resulting in the "idiopathic respiratory distress syndrome" (RDS). The progressive expiratory atelectasis results in consolidation of the lung with secondary problems of hypoxia, acidosis, shock, and death.

According to Gluck and Marie V. Kulovich,[24] we are emerging from an era of evaluation by "gestational age of the fetus and infant into a more realistic era in which we wish to know the 'functional maturity' of the fetus. The lung has proved to be a model organ for showing the phenomena of both functional maturity and fetal alarm to potential intrauterine catastrophe."

Abnormalities in the L/S ratio are seen with a wide variety of maternal, fetal, and placental conditions. When the L/S ratio is 2.0 or greater, there are essentially no deaths from RDS. However, when the L/S ratio is less than 2.0, a neonate may or may not develop RDS and die.

When a premature delivery is expected and the L/S ratio is less than 2.0, particular care is now given to the labor and delivery and adequate resuscitation measures are made ready. Even with an L/S ratio greater than 2.0, low Apgar scores contribute to an increased morbidity from RDS. It has been shown that the route of delivery (cesarean section versus vaginal) per se does not influence the incidence of RDS.

Regional Perinatal Services

In the late 1960's and early 1970's, reports began to appear in the pediatric and obstetrical literature describing improved outcomes in caring for high-risk pregnancies.

In nine hospitals throughout the United States and Canada, the introduction of regional neonatal intensive care units resulted in decreases in neonatal mortality from 25 to 42 percent. Encouraged by these decreases, the American Medical Association in 1971 urged the adoption of regionalized perinatal programs. Next, the National Foundation–March of Dimes established a joint committee on perinatal health services, which led to the publication of an extremely influential report, *Toward Improving the Outcome of Pregnancy* (1976). This report became the reference manual for regionalization. It set forth guidelines which any region could use in implementing a program and warned against duplication of effort, citing the "staggering cost" of providing comprehensive service to high-risk infants and mothers.

In 1972 the Robert Wood Johnson Foundation began planning for a national program to support regionalized perinatal care.

The salvage of premature infants has greatly improved because of centrally located intensive-care units to which high-risk prematures may be brought. The neonatologist is now aided by a variety of technological innovations and new biochemical testing procedures, such as amniocentesis, sonography, fetal monitoring, L/S ratio, continuous positive airway pressure (CPAP), and mechanical ventilation, which contributed to the significant decline in neonatal mortality from 20.5 per 1,000 live births in 1950 to 11.7 in 1975, a decrease of 43 percent.

Great advances have occurred in the management of infants of twenty-four to thirty weeks' gestation (usually 500 to 1,500 grams). For example, in 1978 a 900-gram infant born prematurely had a 42 percent chance of survival. Ten years earlier the chance of survival would have been nil. The limit of viability in 1978 appeared to be about 600 grams, corresponding to a gestational age of about twenty-four weeks.[51] Although these infants comprised only about 1.2 percent of the live-born infants, they account for 70 percent of all over-500-gram neonatal deaths and a significant proportion of later neurologic damage.

New Publications

American Textbooks of Pediatrics, 1950 to 1978

Among the new general pediatric reference textbooks were the following:

1968 Cooke, R. E. (ed.), *Biologic Basis of Pediatric Practice*

1978 Robert A. Hoekelman, Saul Blatman, Philip A. Brunell, Stanford B. Friedman, and Henry M. Seidel (eds.), *Principles of Pediatrics: Health Care of the Young*.

American Pediatric Journals, 1950 to 1978

The following new pediatric journals appeared during this period:

1954 *Pediatric Clinics of North America*
1962 *Clinical Pediatrics*

1967 *Pediatric Research*
1970 *Current Problems in Pediatrics*

The "New" Pediatric Morbidity

Pediatrics as a discipline began a century ago; its greatest concern for its first half-century was infant feeding. With the advent of clean milk, many pediatricians then directed their attention toward the deficiency and infectious diseases. By 1930 cod-liver oil and orange juice had largely conquered rickets and scurvy. With the discovery of the sulfonamides in the mid-1930's, and the antibiotics a bit later, many infectious diseases were also brought under control. Attention was then directed toward the inborn errors of metabolism, the diseases of immunodeficiency, those of a genetic nature, and the hazards associated with prematurity. Of course, none of these has been completely conquered, but continued effort and research have significantly brought many of them under at least partial control. But despite the many and impressive successes in the management of organic diseases, the pediatrician still faces an enormous number of challenges yet to be vanquished. This is so because the dimensions of child health care are expanding in all directions, and on all fronts.

As we begin the last quarter of the twentieth century a new pediatrics, or as some would call it, a new morbidity, has taken the place once occupied by many of the now manageable organic diseases that formerly made up almost all of pediatric practice. The obvious reason for this is that the health needs of children and adolescents are continually changing. Increasingly, pediatricians are asked to support parents and children in facing up to the psychological and environmental challenges of modern society. The problems of adaptation to life in our complex physical, cultural, and social environment grow more onerous with each passing year.

One of the most impressive changes in contemporary pediatric practice has been the increased demand for treatment of school-related problems and for the ever-expanding problems resulting from "social" diseases. Among these are divorce and its effect on parents and children, child abuse, venereal diseases, cigarette smoking, adolescent pregnancy, drug and alcohol abuse by children and adolescents, depression, alienation, homicide, and suicidal attempts.

Another vital development during this period was initiated by J. Roswell Gallagher in 1951 when he organized the first adolescents' unit in this country, located in Boston. The value of such a unit soon became apparent and before long many other comparable units were established both here and abroad.

The nature of pediatric practice in the future will depend largely on the fate of the American family. That the American family has been undergoing rapid and radical changes during the last quarter of a century is all too well documented. Among these are the increase in the number of working mothers, the increase in single-parent families, the increase in the number of children of unwed mothers, the increase in delinquency, the fragmentation of the extended family, the isolation of children from the world of work, and the decrease in the number of children being born.

The young pediatrician now beginning his or her career is faced with challenges of far greater complexity than those that past generations of pediatricians had to wrestle with. To even define these new problems, today's pediatricians will require knowledge far broader than that of microbes and biochemistry. They will also need a vivid imagination and the zest to analyze the forces and trends, both good and bad, buffeting and altering the social milieu. To measure the results of intervention will require far more than tidy biostatistical analyses.

References

1. Apgar, V. A proposal for a new method of evaluation of the newborn infant. *Anesth. Analg.* (Cleve.) 32:260, 1953.
2. Apley, J. (ed.) *Modern Trends in Paediatrics*, No. 3. London: Butterworth, 1970.
3. Avery, M. E., and Mead, J. Surface properties in relation to atelectasis and hyaline membrane disease. *Am. J. Dis. Child.* 97:517, 1959.
4. Baehner, R. L., and Nathan, D. G. Quantitative nitroblue tetrazolium test in chronic granulomatous disease. *New Engl. J. Med.* 278:971, 1968.
5. Bakwin, H. Roentgenologic changes in the bones following trauma in infants. *J. Newark Beth Israel Hosp.* 3:17, 1952.
6. Beckwith, J. B. *The Sudden Infant Death Syndrome.* Washington, D.C.: DHEW Publication No. (HSA) 75–5137, 1975.
7. Berendes, H., Bridges, R. A., and Good, R. A. A fatal granulomatosis of childhood. The clinical study of a new syndrome. *Minn. Med.* 40:309, 1957.
8. Beutler, E., Yeh, M., and Fairbanks, V. F. The normal human female as a mosaic of X-chromosome activity: Studies using the gene for G–6–PD deficiency as a marker. *Proc. Nat. Acad. Sci.* 48:9, 1962.
9. Bruton, O. Agammaglobulinemia. *Pediatrics* 9:722, 1952.
10. Caffey, J. Multiple fractures in the long bones of infants suffering from chronic subdural hematoma. *Am. J. Roentgenol.* 56:163, 1946.
11. Caffey, J. Some traumatic lesions in growing bones other than fractures and dislocations: Clinical and radiological features. *Br. J. Radiol.* 30:225, 1957.
12. Carson, P. E., et al. Enzymatic deficiency in primaquine-sensitive erythrocytes. *Science* 124:484, 1956.
13. Cooper, M. D., Peterson, R. D. A., and Good, R. A. Delineation of the thymic and bursal lymphoid systems in the chicken. *Nature* 205:143, 1965.
14. Cremer, R. J., Perryman, P. W., and Richards, D. H. Influence of light on the hyperbilirubinaemia of infants. *Lancet* 1:1094, 1958.
15. Davis, D. C., and Melnick, J. L. Association of ECHO virus type 6 with aseptic meningitis. *Proc. Soc. Exp. Biol. Med.* 92:839, 1956.
16. DiGeorge, A. M. Congenital Absence of the Thymus and Its Immunologic Consequences: Concurrence with Congenital Hypoparathyroidism. In R. A. Good and B. Bergsma (eds.), *Immunologic Deficiency Diseases in Man.* Birth Defects Original Article Ser., Vol. 4, No. 1. Baltimore: Williams & Wilkins, 1968.
17. Eichenwald, H. F., et al. Epidemic diarrhea in premature and older infants caused by ECHO virus type 18, *J.A.M.A.* 166:1563, 1958.
18. Enders, J., and Peebles, T. C. Propagation in tissue cultures of cytopathogenic agents from patients with measles. *Proc. Soc. Exp. Biol. Med.* 86:277, 1954.
19. Farrell, P. M., and Wood, R. E. Epidemiology of hyaline membrane disease in the United States: Analysis of national mortality statistics. *Pediatrics* 58:167, 1976.
20. Finn, J. J., Weller, T. H., and Morgan, H. R. Epidemic pleurodynia: Clinical and etiologic studies based on 114 cases. *Arch. Intern. Med.* 83:305, 1949.
21. Ford, C. E., and Hammerton, J. L. The chromosomes of man. *Nature* 178:1020, 1956.
22. Freda, V. J., et al. Rh Disease: How near the end? *Hosp. Pract.* 13:61, 1978.
23. Gitlin, D., and Janeway, C. A. Agammaglobuline-

mia: Congenital, acquired and transient forms. *Prog. Hematol.* 1:318, 1956.

24. Gluck, L., and Kulovich, M. V. The Evaluation of Functional Maturity in the Human Fetus. In L. Gluck (ed.), *Modern Perinatal Medicine.* Chicago: Year Book Medical Publishers, 1974.

25. Good, R. A. Crucial Experiments of Nature That have Guided Analysis of the Immunologic Apparatus. In E. R. Stiehm and V. A. Fulginiti (eds.), *Immunologic Disorders of Infants and Children.* Philadelphia: Saunders, 1973.

26. Good, R. A., Finstad, J., and Gatti, R. A. Bulwarks of the Bodily Defense. In S. Mudd (ed.), *Infectious Agents and Host Reactions.* Philadelphia: Saunders, 1970.

27. Gregg, N. M., et al. Occurrence of congenital defects in children following maternal rubella during pregnancy. *Med. J. Aust.* 2:122, 1945.

28. Henle, G., Henle, W., and Diehl, V. Relation of Burkitt's tumor-associated herpes-type virus to infectious mononucleosis. *Proc. Nat. Acad. Sci.* 59:94, 1968.

29. Home, F. *Medical Facts and Experiments.* London: Millar, 1759.

30. Jacobson, C. B., and Barter, R. H. Intrauterine diagnosis and management of genetic defects. *Am. J. Obstet. Gynecol.* 99:796, 1967.

31. Karzon, D. T., et al. Isolation of ECHO virus type 6 during outbreak of seasonal aseptic meningitis. *J.A.M.A.* 162:1298, 1956.

32. Katz, S., et al. Studies on an attenuated measles virus vaccine, VIII: General summary and evaluation of the results of vaccination. *New Engl. J. Med.* 263:180, 1960.

33. Kempe, C. H., et al. The battered-child syndrome. *J.A.M.A.* 181:17, 1962.

34. Kibrick, S., and Benirschke, K. Acute aseptic myocarditis and meningoencephalitis in the newborn child infected with Coxsackie virus group B, type 3. *New Engl. J. Med.* 255:883, 1956.

35. Kibrick, S., and Enders, J. F. Disease due to ECHO virus type 9 in Massachusetts. *New Engl. J. Med.* 259:482, 1958.

36. Krugman, S., Ward, R., and Katz, S. L. *Infectious Diseases of Children* (6th ed.). St. Louis: Mosby, 1977.

37. Landing, B. H., and Shirkey, H. C. A syndrome of recurrent infection and infiltration of viscera by pigmented lipid histiocytes. *Pediatrics* 20:431, 1957.

38. Lejeune, J., Turpin, R., and Gautier, M. Le mongolisme, premier exemple d'aberration autosomique humaine. *Ann. Genet.* (Paris) 1:141, 1959.

39. Lerner. A. M., et al. Infections due to Coxsackie virus group A, type 9, in Boston, 1959, with special reference to exanthems and pneumonia. *New Engl. J. Med.* 263: 1265, 1960.

40. Meyer, H. M., Jr., Parkman, P. D., and Panos, T. C. Attenuated rubella virus II: Production of an experimental live-virus vaccine and clinical trial. *New Engl. J. Med.* 275:575, 1966.

41. Neva, F. A., Feemster, R. F., and Gorback, I. J. Clinical and epidemiological features of an unusual epidemic exanthem. *J.A.M.A.* 155:544, 1954.

42. Oski, F. A., and Stockman, J. A. Congenital hemolytic anemias and red cell enzyme deficiencies. *Curr. Probl. Pediatr.* 4(2):3, 1973.

43. Parkman, P. D., Buescher, E. L., and Artenstein, M. S. Recovery of rubella virus from army recruits. *Proc. Soc. Exp. Biol. Med.* 111:225, 1962.

44. Parrish, H. J. *A History of Immunization.* Edinburgh: Livingstone, 1965.

45. *Report of the Committee on Infectious Diseases, American Academy of Pediatrics* (18th ed.), 1977.

46. Robinson, C. R., Doane, F. W., and Rhodes, A. J. Report of an outbreak of febrile illness with laryngeal lesions and exanthems, Toronto, summer 1957: Isolation of group A Coxsackie virus. *Can. Med. Assoc. J.* 79:615, 1957.

47. Silverman, F. N. The roentgen manifestations of unrecognized skeletal trauma in infants. *Am. J. Roentgenol.* 69:413, 1953.

48. Steele, M. W., and Breg, W. R., Jr. Chromosome analysis of human amniotic fluid cells. *Lancet* 1:383, 1966.

49. Steigman, A. J., Lipton, M. M., and Braspennickx, H. Acute lymphonodular pharyngitis: A newly described condition due to Coxsackie A virus. *J. Pediatr.* 61:331, 1962.

50. Stiehm, E. R., and Fulginiti, V. A. *Immunologic Disorders of Infants and Children.* Philadelphia: Saunders, 1973.

51. Taeusch, H. W., and Avery, M. E. Neonatal intensive care: "Incomplete solutions." *Harvard Med. Alum. Bull.* 53:27, 1978.

52. Tjio, J. H., and Levan, A. The chromosome number in man. *Hereditas* 42:1, 1956.

53. Valdés-Dapena, M. A. *Sudden Unexplained Infant Death, 1970 Through 1975.* Department of Health, Education and Welfare Publication No. (HSA) 78–5255, 1978.

54. Valentine, W. N., Tanaka, K. R., and Miwa, S. A specific erythrocyte glycolytic enzyme defect (pyruvate kinase) in three subjects with congenital nonspherocytic hemolytic anemia. *Trans. Assoc. Am. Physicians* 74:100, 1961.

55. Weller, T. H., and Neva, F. A. Propagation in tissue culture of cytopathic agents from patients with ru-

bella-like illness. *Proc. Soc. Exp. Biol. Med.* 111:215, 1962.

56. Wheatley, G. M. Childhood accidents 1952–72: An overview. *Pediatr. Ann.* 2:10, 1973.

57. Woolley, P. V., and Evans, W. A. Significance of skeletal lesions in infants resembling those of traumatic origin. *J.A.M.A.* 158:539, 1955.

From Complexity to Simplicity

10

Although the mechanics of infant feeding such as formulas, calories, vitamins and solid foods have become so simplified and well known that any detailed discussion of them seems unnecessary in this day and age, nevertheless certain problems still remain that occasionally challenge the physician in his feeding of infants.

Lee Forrest Hill (1967)

As the twentieth century began, the concept of the milk station, or infant consultation for the supervision of healthy infants, was still in the formative stages in this country. As has been noted, there were no public health nurses and there was not a single state or municipality with a special department of child hygiene or child welfare. Agitation for strict supervision of the production and distribution of milk had just begun, commercial pasteurization was hardly thought of, and the value of home sterilization of milk was just being timidly stressed. Chlorination of water had been instituted here and there in the United States only in the decade before the beginning of the twentieth century. Purchase of milk on a daily basis was not the common practice, and thus, with or without pasteurization, bacterial contamination of milk was a frequent occurrence. Wilburt C. Davison (1892–1972)[8] found that in America from 1881 to 1927, 791 outbreaks of milk-borne diseases had been reported, and from 1924 until 1932 inclusive, 394 additional milk-borne outbreaks had occurred.

The refrigerator is taken for granted today, but it was not until about 1910 that the kitchen icebox became commonplace in American homes. Without an icebox, storage of milk was not feasible and, when it was attempted, milk was usually stored on the outside windowsill.

Infant Feeding in Twentieth-Century America

Infants in 1900 whose mothers, for one reason or other, did not nurse them, were given either milk from some other woman (and this rarely) or a poorly devised concoction of which cow's milk was usually the basis. The milk was almost always dirty and unsterilized and was put into dirty bottles and fed through dirty nipples.

During the early 1900's American pediatricians were faced with several widely conflicting hypotheses about the causes of nutritional disturbances in feeding the infant. Philipp Biedert claimed that the difficulty of digesting casein was a prominent cause of infantile digestive disorder. Heinrich Finkelstein,[11] on the other hand, claimed that fats were injurious to the digestive tract, and Thomas Morgan Rotch's theory of percentage feeding was devised as a means of offsetting the putative harmfulness of proteids (proteins). Finkelstein also advanced the theory of an alimentary fever from sugar or salt; this led him to develop his protein milk, or *Eiweissmilch*. Finkelstein showed that proteins per se were not necessarily harmful, but his theory of salt-and-sugar fevers was opposed so strongly that he ultimately abandoned his dogmatic position concerning the supposed pyrogenic action of carbohydrates; he finally accepted Adalbert Czerny's view that fats were more harmful than casein in a bowel previously irritated by "sugar fermentation."

Pasteurization of Milk

As late as 1900 the predominant opinion of members of the American Pediatric Society was that raw milk was the best food for infant feeding if a clean supply was available. John Lovett Morse[37] had written that "a considerable number [of physicians] were willing to take chances with raw milk during certain seasons of the year and under certain conditions of dairy hygiene." Morse also commented that as late as 1912 many physicians still believed that infants did not thrive as well on pasteurized as they did on raw milk. The early meetings of the American Pediatric Society contained many reports about the pros and cons of raw as opposed to pasteurized milk. Infants fed raw milk were said to have far less chance of developing scurvy than those fed pasteur-

ized milk. There were even a few pediatricians as late as 1910 who were unwilling to accept the germ theory of disease. To this group, pasteurization appeared a waste of time.

In 1912 Morse, in questioning members of the American Pediatric Society, found that about one-half thought that "pasteurization of milk made no difference in digestibility; the others disagreed as to whether it made it more or less digestible. Rather more thought that babies did not thrive as well on pasteurized milk than thought they did. There was the same difference of opinion as to whether pasteurization predisposed to the development of the diseases of nutrition."

Incidentally, it is interesting to remember that at one time, at least in Boston, the pasteurization of milk by producers and distributors was a legal offense because the milk was not delivered in its natural state.

Caloric Feeding

John J. Thomas,[48] in a paper published in 1907, wrote: "I fail to find any references to the caloric value of foods in any American text or reference book on pediatrics with which I am acquainted." In the same year George W. Moorehouse[34] described a method for the calculation of calories in modified milk and Ernest Lackner[25] described to the Chicago Pediatric Society Otto Huebner's system of infant feeding based on calories. Huebner's contribution to the energy requirements of infants is basic to this day, along with similar studies by Francis G. Benedict, (1870–1957), Fritz Talbot, and John Howland. Grover Powers[38] had noted that "without knowledge of the energy requirement of the infant, no scientific program for his feeding can be laid down."

By 1917 the concept of caloric feeding had become universal in America. However, there was an occasional dissenter; for example, Morse[37] as late as 1935 wrote: "To me it [caloric feeding] still seems as irrational as it ever did to base any scheme or system of infant feeding solely on the caloric needs of babies or on the caloric values of food." L. Emmett Holt, Sr., and Howland[22] in 1917 described the caloric needs of infants as follows: "From numerous observations the nutritive needs of an infant of average size and weight in health have been shown to be 100 to 110 calories [daily] per kilo of body weight for the early months of the first year; gradually diminishing to 70 to 80 per kilo by the end of the year." These caloric intakes (1917) are somewhat less than those given (1974) by the Food and Nutrition Board of the National Academy of Sciences–National Research Council. The latter group recommended a daily caloric intake of 117 kcal/kg of body weight for full-term infants from birth to six months and 108 kcal/kg for those six months to one year. These figures allow for the recommended basal caloric requirement of 55 kcal/kg, for the growth requirement of approximately 35 kcal/kg, and for the normal ranges of activity of 10 to 25 kcal/kg.

Coprology

The preoccupation with infant's excreta by pediatricians from the turn of the century to the early twenties forms, as Alton Goldbloom[17] has written, "one of the most amusing chapters in the history of infant feeding." Goldbloom described this preoccupation:

It was the coprophilic era, or the era of divination by stool. Just as in the Middle Ages diagnoses were made by inspection of the urine . . . so in this era was far more attention paid to the stool than to the infant. . . . It was the ward nurse's duty to keep on hand a specimen of each child's stool. . . . [The few] surviving American paediatricians of that era remember the fetish that was made of the stools in those days. A young and progressive paediatrician travelling abroad would often bring home with him a complete set of moulages depicting in realistic—dare I say lifelike—form every variety of stool in every conceivable, real or imaginary, digestive derangement. Students were taught from these moulages and they were examined on them. The professor himself was, as you imagine, the expert. A familiar scene in the days of the old Boston Floating Hospital is typical of the practices of the day. It was the ward nurse's duty to keep on hand a specimen of each child's stool. In time for ward rounds, she had these specimens neatly done up in brown paper, with the infant's name in the upper right hand corner. These were placed in a basin in alphabetical order and it was the duty of the junior intern to hold this basin in his arms, at a safe distance from the professor and his assistants and visitors, and to come forward with the specimen whenever the bed of a given infant was approached. The professor carried a handful of wooden spatulas in his breast pocket, but I do not remember him ever using it for examining an infant's throat, it was used to smear the specimen of stool, to note its consistency, to search for curds . . . with

never a look at the infant, but only from this meticulous examination on which he would expatiate lengthily and eruditely, he would finally offer the suggestion for the next day's food. The order would be either increase or decrease the fat, the sugar or the protein by, usually, one quarter of 1%.

The visual study of infants' stools was considered as important in the beginning of this century as was the infant's temperature and pulse and respiratory rates. In fact, at the beginning of the century the temperature of the hospitalized infant in most American hospitals was taken only once a day and often just once every other day.

Curd Tension

In 1908 Thomas S. Southworth (1861–1940) and Oscar Schloss[46] demonstrated quite conclusively, as did other investigators, that there were two kinds of curds: small, soft curds derived from fat and large, hard curds the basis of which was coagulated casein. Joseph G. Brennemann (Fig. 10–1)[4,5] commented that "the whole matter might have passed off as of trivial significance if the dual nature of curds had not been so hotly contested by those who maintained that all curds were fat curds." By 1913 several papers had been published which demonstrated that even larger and harder curds were formed when fat-free milk was fed instead of whole milk, that hard curds could be produced and made to disappear by alternating raw and boiled milk feedings in a susceptible baby, and that these curds grew larger in the stomach for around two hours and harder and more impermeable the longer they existed anywhere.

Although William McK. Marriott[28] considered gastric acidity of paramount importance in the ease of digestibility of milk, nevertheless he recognized that the physical state of the curd was also an important factor and that acidification precipitated a fine casein curd. Brennemann,[5] on the other hand, contended that the physical state of the casein curd was the all-important factor and that the value of acids was due solely to the way in which they modified the curd. Human milk yields fine, soft, flocculent curds in the stomach, a physical state which permits full utilization with minimal intestinal losses. Cow's milk produces large, tough curds, described by

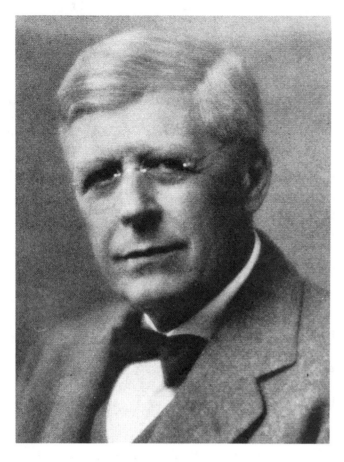

Figure 10–1. Joseph G. Brennemann (1872–1944).

Brennemann[4], characterized as being peculiarly solid. Partially digested, they may appear in the stools as protein curds, usually accompanied by fat curds, and thus may account for significant loss of nutrient material. As the importance of Brennemann's observations on the physical aspect of the curd became fully appreciated, it became routine to process the infant's milk formula by one of the methods effective in reducing curd tension; namely homogenization, evaporation, boiling, drying, or acidification. Pasteurization alone has little or no effect upon curd tension.

Choice of Carbohydrate in Infant Feeding

The sugars to be used in infant feeding gave pediatricians in the early part of this century a worrisome time. The cult of similarity, namely the effort to simulate human milk as nearly as possible, taught that the only sugar suitable for infant feeding was lactose, and this, despite its expense, was the sugar com-

monly used. Morse and Talbot,[35] for example, claimed that "there can be no doubt . . . that under normal conditions the preferable sugar for the well infant is lactose." Abraham Jacobi[23] never agreed and always used cane sugar in feeding infants. Milk sugar had nature as its advocate, but even this did not keep it from falling from grace at a later period.

One reason, perhaps, that lactose was never used universally (other than its price) was the fear on the part of some physicians that it was a dangerous substance, to be avoided. The probable reason for this fear lay in the teaching of Finkelstein and his school that lactose or acids caused by its fermentation produced inflammation of the alimentary tract and that the inflamed mucosa allowed undigested food components, including lactose itself, to be absorbed. So effective was his teaching that subsequent writers and investigators accepted his dicta without question. Finkelstein also continued to advance the concept of "sugar fever," which he said was more likely to be caused by lactose than by the other sugars, but this concept was never accepted by most American pediatricians. So-called fermentative diarrheas were rife, and all of these diagnosed by inspection of the stools were erroneously thought to be the result of fermentation of sugar in the gastrointestinal tract; therefore, nonfermentable sugars were recommended and preparations containing various proportions of dextrins and maltose were devised.

Jacobi[23] in 1901 in a paper entitled "Milk Sugar in Infant Feeding," and on many other occasions, decried its use and always stuck to cane sugar. Later, the dextrin-maltose preparations gradually crept in (about 1912–1915), although they had been long in use in Mellin's, Horlick's, and other proprietary infant foods.

In 1907 Charles G. Kerley (1863–1945)[24] described the dangers of cane sugar, using the term "cane sugar poisoning," which he claimed in some instances could be induced "by a few grains." In his series of seventy-eight cases he listed ten symptoms caused by cane sugar, among which, surprisingly, diarrhea does not appear.

Approach to Infant Feeding in Boston in 1916

Lewis Webb Hill (1889–1968),[21] who went on to become one of the pioneers of American pediatric allergy, in a book he wrote about infant feeding in

Butter-flour mixture never achieved the popularity in this country of Finkelstein's *Eiweissmilch,* nor was it ever marketed commercially by an American firm. However, it was used fairly widely in the 1920's in pediatric hospitals, including Babies Hospital in New York City.

Soybeans

John Ruhräh[40] (Fig. 10–2) in 1909 published the first paper on the use of soybeans in infant feeding; his was a pioneer contribution of considerable historical interest. He devised several preparations, including soybean milk, which he suggested might be used "as a substitute for milk in diarrhea, in intestinal and stomach disorders, and in diabetes mellitus." He went on to say that he "had hoped to be able to make a more complete clinical report . . . but . . . my first crop was eaten by rats and my second moulded in the pods owing to some unusual damp weather, and insects ate about two-thirds of my last crop." Two years later Ruhräh[41] published a second paper on the use of the soybean in summer diarrhea, and in cases in which milk disagrees with the infant. He also recommended soybean food for the child with diabetes because he claimed "the use of soybean tends to lessen the glycosuria."

By the early 1920's, Lewis Webb Hill was recommending the use of soybean milk in cases of infantile eczema. However, it was not until the 1950's that formulas with protein derived from soy flour were widely utilized in the United States as milk substitutes. Although more satisfactory than most other milk substitutes available at the time, parents often complained that soy flour formulas caused loose, malodorous stools, and excoriation of the diaper area. By the mid-1960's formulas with protein from water-soluble soy isolates had become so popular that they had almost replaced soy-flour formulas. Soy-isolate-based formulas are white in color, nearly odorless, and only rarely are reported to cause loose or malodorous stools.

Acidified Milks

Marriott,[26] as has been noted, advanced an explanation for the difference in the digestibility of human milk compared to cow's milk based upon the degree of acidity of the stomach contents after ingestion of

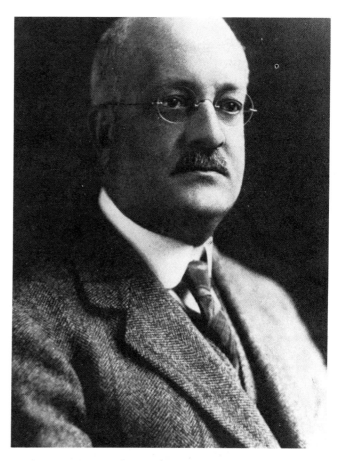

Figure 10–2. John Ruhräh (1872–1935).

either milk. For human milk, Marriott found the average pH to be 3.6. On the other hand, when equivalent amounts of undiluted cow's milk were fed, the gastric contents had an average pH of 5.3. The difference in the behavior of the two milks was believed due to the higher buffer content of cow's milk, which Marriott found to be three times that of human milk. He further reasoned that by adding sufficient lactic acid to neutralize its buffer content, cow's milk could be made as digestible as human milk and could be fed to infants in self-demand quantities in the same manner as breast-fed infants are allowed to take their fill from the breast.

Acidified milks, like buttermilk, have a bactericidal effect on bacteria in the gastrointestinal tract. They are also believed to exert their beneficial action through reduction of the buffering capacity of cow's milk. The high buffering capacity of unacidified cow's milk had long been blamed for promotion of bacterial growth, diminution in flow of pancreatic juice, and inhibition of gastric digestion. Acidified milks are well tolerated and are favored in the tropics, where the slight acidity can lessen the development of intestinal infection and consequent diarrhea.

The apparently beneficial effect of acidified milks in infants with diarrhea—reducing the number of stools and making them firmer in consistency—is now usually explained by the presence of unabsorbed calcium caseinate in the stools. The period of food intolerance which followed an acute nutritional disturbance was never shown to be actually shortened by this feeding, nor was the absorption of nutrients clearly improved. When the observation was made by Howland that patients with diarrhea did better when sugar was added to protein milk, it was difficult to maintain the concept that carbohydrate fermentation was the cause of diarrhea.

In the early 1920's Marriott and Leonard T. Davidson[27] discarded all previous methods of infant feeding and advised the use of whole cow's milk, boiled five minutes, with the addition of 1 dram (4 cc) of lactic acid U.S.P. to the pint, to which had been added one-tenth of its volume of corn syrup. They recommended this as a "routine infant food." Acidified milk was widely used from the mid-1920's until the mid-1930's and only gradually disappeared as evaporated milk and the commercially prepared formulas were developed as replacements.

Evaporated Milk

The idea of commercially preserving milk by evaporating much of the water and preserving with sugar (condensed milk) dates back to 1853 when Gail Borden (1801–1874) was granted patents in the United States and England for his vacuum-evaporation method, the principles of which still apply to modern methods of condensing milk.

The process of preserving unsweetened condensed (now known as evaporated) milk was introduced by John B. Myenberg in 1883, who sterilized the evaporated products by using steam under pressure; this method is still in use today. Such milk is made by evaporating about 60 percent of the water of ordinary milk, after which it is sterilized in the autoclave at a temperature of from 200° to 240° F. The heating gives rise to certain alterations in the chemical and physical properties of milk. The casein undergoes alteration, and the curd is much finer than in raw, pasteurized, or quickly boiled milk. However, it was not until 1927, when Marriott[26] in particular first recommended the use of unsweetened evaporated milk instead of ordinary cow's milk in the preparation of his lactic acid–milk formulas, that this milk was really considered acceptable for feeding infants. Marriott[29] pointed out that evaporated milk was already sterilized and heated sufficiently to insure the formation of very fine curds when lactic acid was added. Evaporated milk also had a lower buffer value than ordinary cow's milk because of the conversion of a part of the calcium and phosphate into the form of insoluble calcium phosphate. The fat was homogenized and, further, evaporated milk was inexpensive and easily obtainable.

His preferred method of preparing the lactic acid–evaporated milk formula was to mix the evaporated milk with an equal volume of an acid-sugar mixture. The formula was as follows:[28]

Acid-Sugar Solution

Corn syrup (brown)	90cc
Lactic acid U.S.P.	5cc
Water	to 250cc

The syrup was mixed with some water, the lactic acid added, and the whole made up to the final volume by mixing equal parts of evaporated milk and the acid-sugar solution.

Marriott recommended this formula for all healthy infants during the first six to eight months. The amount of sugar was decreased after cereal was given to the infant (usually not until the ninth month in 1927). Such formulas were far safer than those prepared from a questionable milk supply. Marriott[29] further claimed that "all evidence goes to show that the fat soluble vitamins A and D and the [water-soluble] B vitamins were not injured by the processes employed in the preparation of evaporated milk." Since vitamin C was destroyed, he recommended that "the formulas given be supplemented with orange juice daily." He also advised, especially during the winter months, the addition of "as much as one teaspoonful of cod-liver oil each day in addition to the milk mixtures."

Marriott and Ludwig Schoenthal,[29] in an experimental study published in 1929, found evaporated milk, without the addition of lactic acid, when fed to seven hundred and fifty-two young, well infants, resulted in an average gain in weight exactly equal to that of babies fed exclusively on breast milk or on formulas prepared from bottled pasteurized milk. They concluded:

> For a number of years past, unsweetened evaporated milk has been used in this clinic for the preparation of infant feeding formulas and good results have been obtained. Originally, this form of milk was used chiefly for the feeding of patients who were returning to homes in districts where the milk supply was of questionable purity or in the case of patients who were traveling or going to summer resorts. Later, the use of evaporated milk was extended to the poorer and more ignorant dispensary class of patients where it was felt that the mothers were not sufficiently intelligent to be trusted to sterilize formulas properly or did not have the facilities for the refrigeration of bottled milk. The results, even under adverse conditions, were so generally satisfactory that we have been led to make a much more extensive use of evaporated milk for the preparation of formulas for both well and sick infants of all classes.
>
> In the light of our experiences, it is difficult to understand why evaporated milk has not been more extensively used in infant feeding. It would appear that an uncritical prejudice has been the chief factor in the limitation of its use.

Evaporated milk during the 1930's and 1940's became the most widely accepted and versatile milk for infant formulas. By 1960 it was estimated that 80 percent of bottle-fed infants in the United States were fed either on evaporated milk or on some prepared milk feeding marketed in evaporated form. The former prejudices against "canned" milk had been overcome by the realization that, as Herman F. Meyer[33] noted in 1960, "the many qualities of this type of milk lend it safely to the most selective of infant digestive tracts."

In the early 1970's the number of American infants three months of age who received evaporated milk formulas had fallen to less than 5 percent; whereas approximately 70 percent of infants this age were fed commercially prepared milk formulas, although the cost of feeding the infant evaporated milk was at that time approximately half the cost of isocaloric amounts of commercially prepared formulas before the cost of vitamin and iron supplements are included.[30]

Dry Milk

The dried milks came along in the early 1920's. Some of them had all of the fat removed, some part of it, some very little. During the 1920's several studies showed that infants fed dried milk formulas did well, gaining five to six ounces per week during the first six months of life and about four and a half ounces per week during their second six months.

However, from France, in particular, reports published toward the end of the 1920's mentioned that unexplained fever would occur occasionally in infants receiving dried milk formulas, although the infants gained in weight and were otherwise without symptoms. The fever never appeared immediately after the infant was given a dried milk formula. There was a latent period varying from several days to months; if the infant had once previously been fed powdered milk, the fever would develop almost immediately on resumption of the same powdered milk, but not after the use of any other type of milk. The theory that there might be some toxic substance formed in the process of manufacture was not supported experimentally. Other hypotheses were that the fever was due to sensitization to some substance formed in the process of drying or that it was the result of insufficient water in the infant's diet. These adverse reports plus the highly favorable results obtained from feeding evaporated milk formulas greatly reduced the enthusiasm for dried milk.

Single-Formula Mixtures (Humanized Milks)

Partly as an outgrowth of the complexity of the percentage feeding method, the search for a single-formula food has always seemed alluring. As the years progressed, Rotch's method became increasingly more complicated and involved as new and so-called simpler methods of calculation appeared. Brennemann[4] recalled:

> Some of the articles seemed terrifyingly like treatises on mathematics or higher astronomy. . . . It all gradually became a headache to most of us and we could appreciate and share Jacobi's reaction when he said as early as 1906: "For many years it has been my intention never to participate again in any discussions on milk feeding [or] of fat feeding. . . ." The whole edifice [percentage feeding] finally collapsed because the superstructure was top heavy

and the foundation weak, and because really simpler ideas came into play.

At the meeting of the American Pediatric Society in May, 1915, Henry J. Gerstenberger (1881–1954)[14] (Fig. 10–3) first described an artificial milk or food that was "in all possible respects similar to human milk." Morse[37] recalled that all the members of the American Pediatric Society were given an opportunity to taste this preparation and that "fortunately, the assembly room was on the ground floor and had large, wide-open French windows." Gerstenberger imitated the fat of human milk by using a combination of various homogenized animal and vegetable fats. This mixture contained roughly 4.6 percent fat, 6.5 percent sugar, and 0.9 percent protein. Four years later (1919) Gerstenberger[15] described the successful use of this food in about three hundred cases and gave it the name "synthetic milk adapted." It will be recalled that the early nutritionists and chemists had tried to simulate human milk in their

Figure 10–3. Henry J. Gerstenberger (1881–1954).

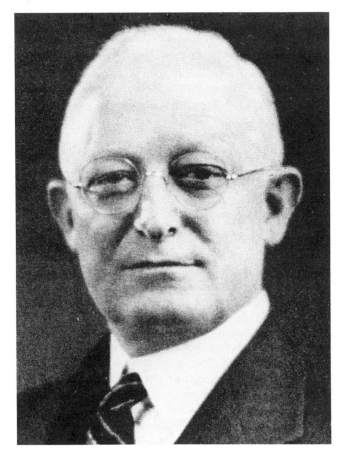

efforts to "humanize" milk preparations. As mentioned in Chapter 6, "Meigs's Mixture" was the counterpart of our present-day single all-inclusive foods for infants.

Even before Gerstenberger, the German physiologist Hans Friedenthal in 1910 had picked up the threads which led to the ideal set up by Biedert as early as 1869, namely an artificial milk similar in all its important characteristics to breast milk. Friedenthal gathered courage for another attempt at the solution of this important problem from the fact (for him at least) that the salt content and the physical and chemical characteristics of human milk had been entirely neglected by previous investigators, and also from his conviction that these were important, if not the most important, individual factors to be considered in the making of an artificial food similar to breast milk.

Others independently of Friedenthal also attempted to duplicate the composition of breast milk. They received their stimulus from Finkelstein's theory of the injuriousness of the whey of cow's milk. From this came, in addition to the "whey reduced milk" of Friedenthal (1910), the "whey adapted milk" of E. Schloss (1914), and finally the "synthetic milk adapted" of Gerstenberger (1915), bringing us closer to the modern era. Gerstenberger's preparation contained nonfat cow's milk, lactose, oleo oils, and vegetable oils. The percentage composition of fat, protein, and sugar was comparable to that of human milk and the caloric value was 20 kilocalories per ounce.

Some Current Trends in Infant Feeding Practices

Trends in Breast-Feeding

One of the major changes in infant feeding practices that has occurred during this century has been a decline in breast-feeding and a corresponding increase in artificial feeding, despite the well-documented advantages of the former practice. Noted with this trend is the feeding of solids to infants at an increasingly earlier age. The trend toward bottle-feeding has been accelerated, perhaps because some physicians are not convinced that there is a proven superiority of breast-feeding over formula-feeding.

About 46 percent of American women now nurse their infants in hospital, including those who also feed some supplemental formula.[30] Katherine Bain (b. 1897)[2] made the first nationwide survey of infant feeding practices in American hospital nurseries (1948); she found that 38 percent of the mothers left the hospital nursing their infants. Ten years later Meyer[32] surveyed the same hospitals and found that the percentage had fallen to 21 percent. Infants given the bottle alone at time of discharge rose from 35 percent in 1946 to 53 percent in 1956. By 1958, Eva J. Salber and colleagues[43] found that only 25 percent of seven-day-old infants in Boston were breast-fed. Recent data from Martinez and Nalezienski[30] indicate a resurgence in the incidence of breast-feeding after the infant's discharge from the hospital. In 1978, about 35 percent of infants at two months of age were breast-fed, and at five to six months of age about 20 percent were so fed.

It is of interest that social class seems to be an important variable influencing breast-feeding in this country and also quite probably in other developed countries. From 1920 until about the middle of the 1940's, breast-feeding was most common among the lower socioeconomic class of American mothers. But several studies performed within the past decade have indicated that breast-feeding is now less common among poor mothers than among the upper social classes in the United States. Salber and Manning Feinleib[44] in their study (1966) found that college students were most likely to breast-feed their infants, and another study in 1969 showed that physician-mothers were most likely to breast-feed their infants.[19a]

Why do so few American mothers nurse their infants? Is it because bottle-feeding has become so simple, safe, and almost uniformly successful that breast-feeding no longer seems worth the struggle?

Although some have claimed that there are no differences in morbidity and mortality rates between the breast-fed and the bottle-fed infant, a number of studies have shown that breast-feeding not only supplies nourishment but gives the infant immunologic protection against infections as well. In 1934 Clifford G. Grulee[18] and his co-workers found that breast-feeding insured almost complete freedom from gastrointestinal infections. Breast milk itself provides a continuing supply of antibody, documented particularly, as Sidney Sussman[47] has shown,

in respect to *Escherichia coli.* Toward the end of the nineteenth century and for the first decade of the present century the low mortality of breast-fed infants in the deadly epidemics of summer diarrhea was the more significant because breast-feeding was very much more common at that time. Of course, a similar comparison today would not produce such a difference because of the modifications and various safeguards which have made artificial feeding almost entirely free from bacterial contamination.

Breast milk is bacteriologically safe. The immune globulins and white cells of colostrum and early breast milk confer substantial immunity to bacteriologic infections, particularly enteritis, which is especially significant for infants at risk. There is some clinical evidence suggesting that immune substances in breast milk might provide protection from necrotizing enterocolitis.[45] Immunologic immaturity of the gut is considered to be a factor of possible importance in the pathogenesis of this ominous condition. However, the degree of protection offered by breast milk against necrotizing enterocolitis in the infant is not yet known.

Certain nutrient interactions may result in some advantages of human milk over formulas. The low protein content of breast milk may favor better absorption of small quantities of iron. The fat composition and sodium and phosphorus content may be desirable. However, these differences have not been entirely proven to be advantageous in terms of general health and long-term consequences.

Trends in Feeding of Milks and Formulas

Two distinct changes have occurred in the bottle-feeding of American infants between the years 1958 to 1978. These are a decrease in the number of two-month-old infants fed evaporated milk formulas, from approximately 45 percent in 1958 down to less than 5 percent today, and a concomitant increase in those receiving prepared milk formulas, rising from approximately 28 percent in 1958 to approximately 75 percent at present. Most of the prepared products are purchased in the form of concentrated liquids (133 kcal/100 ml) formulas. Powdered formulas are rarely fed at present, having fallen from about 50 percent of sales for commercially prepared formulas in 1950 to less than 5 percent at present. In the early

1950's most commercially prepared formulas were sold in the form of powder. Concentrated liquid formula marketed in 390 ml (13 fl oz) cans became available about 1950 and within ten years had captured a large share of the market. In 1968 ready-to-feed formula in one-quart cans was marketed, and it has become continually more popular.[30]

Commercially Prepared Formulas

Samuel Fomon[12] estimated in 1974 that "96% of all American infants [are] receiving commercially prepared milk-base formulas." Of infants for whom a milk-free formula was indicated, he estimated that "92 percent are receiving commercially prepared milk-free formulas."

After three months of age, fresh cow's milk (whole, "2 percent," or skim) accounts for an increasing percentage of infant feeding in the United States. In 1972, for example, at three months of age approximately 20 percent of American infants were fed cow's milk; by six months of age this figure had risen to approximately 65 percent. In 1975, approximately 47 percent of infants five to six months old were fed cow's milk.[30]

Solid Foods (Beikost)*

During the first quarter of this century infants were usually not offered solid food until they were about a year of age. But by 1925 Stafford McLean and Helen Fales[31] would write: "There is still much controversy regarding the age at which a varied dietary should be commenced. Many pediatrists still believe it inadvisable to introduce significant amounts of solids into the diet of the infant of less than one year of age. Many others are convinced that better results are obtained by giving part of the food requirements of infants after six months of age in solid form."

By the mid-1930's Brennemann suggested that six months was the proper age to introduce solid foods. He pointed out that "while there may still be considerable divergence of opinion as to what, when and how to feed babies, there has been a steady tendency to give more and to give earlier."

* Samuel Fomon is mainly responsible for the introduction of the German word Beikost for foods other than milk or formula; no equivalent word is available in the English language. Whether or not this term will be generally accepted by American physicians remains to be seen.

By 1953 Walter W. Sackett, Jr.,[42] reported that he offered infants solid foods on the second day of life on a six-hour schedule and that they were well tolerated. However, there is no proof that there is any nutritional or psychologic benefit in introducing solid foods so early in the infant's life. On the other hand, proof is lacking of actual harm.

One development which has made the feeding of vegetables and fruits easier for mothers was the beginning of the canned baby food industry in the late 1920's, playing a role in the promotion of earlier solid feeding. Widespread advertising and distribution of samples to physicians also hastened the acceptance of these new products by the American homemaker.

Suzanne F. Adams,[1] in her history of the use of vegetables in infant feeding (1959), followed the ages recommended for their introduction as indicated in successive editions of Holt's Diseases of Infancy and Childhood from 1897 until 1953. It was not until 1911 that green vegetables were recommended before thirty-six months of age. It is of interest that tomatoes were entirely forbidden until the eighth edition in 1922, and raw vegetables until the twelfth edition in 1953.

The age at which one should introduce solid foods into the infant's dietary regimen continues to be subject of controversy (albeit now far less passionate) in the pediatric community. The general tendency is toward their introduction at an increasingly earlier age. Also, peer pressures on the mother toward earlier and earlier introduction of solid foods may be so intense that she finds them impossible to withstand. Mothers are often led to believe that feeding of cereals will encourage the baby to sleep through the night.

A major objection to early feeding of solid foods is that the practice may encourage overfeeding, which may lead to infantile obesity. Because an adequate intake of all essential nutrients can be provided without solid foods, there seems to be no advantage in introducing such foods during the first three or four months of life.

What Do American Parents Now Feed Their Infants?

Both Fomon[13] and George A. Purvis[39] have recently published excellent articles on what American parents actually feed their infants. Both of these studies fully confirm the secular trend in infant feeding toward the decrease in breast-feeding and the earlier introduction of solid foods to supplement a milk diet. Purvis in his study (1973) was astonished at how many different foods were fed to infants thirteen months of age or younger. When he counted all the varieties of brand-name foods and home-made ones, he found that "this group of babies was being fed five hundred sixty-three different food items."

Data such as those obtained by Purvis were almost impossible for investigators to gather and digest until computers came along to help analyze the torrent of information from mothers that is necessary if one is to arrive at even a tentative opinion about how well babies really are fed. Even with computers, analyzing representative food samples, recording food intake, and computing the resulting volumes of data into accurate estimates of the nutrient intake is, as Purvis[39] comments, "not only tedious but beyond the capacity and patience of all but a few of the most dedicated investigators."

Fomon[13] in his study (1975) estimates the contemporary infant's total calorie intake and its distribution between milk formula and beikost, the relative prevalence of breast, formula, and milk feeding, the relative popularity of specific commercially prepared formulas, the percentage of calories consumed in the form of commercially prepared strained and junior foods, and "table" foods.

Results of an earlier survey (1954) conducted by mail questionnaire by Allan Butler and Irving J. Wolman (1905–1978)[6] pointed out that two-thirds of two thousand responding pediatricians twenty-four years ago routinely recommended introduction of solid foods before two months of age.

Helen Guthrie's[19] report (1966) revealed that all of the fifty-six bottle-fed infants in her study "had been introduced to solid foods by 9 weeks, 2 to 4 weeks prior to the age at which the American Academy of Pediatrics suggests that there is a rational basis from a nutritional and developmental point of view to begin supplementing the diet."

Just how accelerated the trend to introduce solid foods has been since the mid-1960's is not entirely clear. However, the weight of evidence indicates that almost all American infants currently are fed commercially prepared strained foods by six weeks of age, many before they are four weeks of age.

The data of Lloyd J. Filer, Jr., and Martinez[10] (1963) suggested that at that time an infant six months of age received approximately two-thirds of his caloric intake from milk and a third from solid foods. Fomon[13] has recently estimated (1975) that at present "many infants may receive considerably larger percentages of caloric intake from beikost [food other than milk or formula] at age six months." He also pointed out that "three categories of commercially prepared strained and junior foods (fruits, soups and dinners, and desserts) account for approximately 60% of sales." However, little information is available concerning percentage of sales accounted for by various categories on an age-specified basis.

During the first six months of life, Fomon[13] found that most of the solid foods given to American infants consist "of commercially prepared strained and junior foods. The three major manufacturers produce more than 400 varieties of strained and junior foods."

Table Foods

A subcommittee of the National Research Council in 1972 calculated that, for infants less than six months of age, approximately 13 percent by weight of solid foods was in the form of table foods; for infants six to twelve months of age, approximately 63 percent by weight of solid foods was in the form of table foods. Fomon[12] believes that for most American infants, table foods are likely to account for a relatively small percentage of calories until about 5 months of age. Between five and six months of age, table foods probably account for slightly less than one-third of the calories, between six and nine months of age for slightly less than half of the calories, and between nine and twelve months of age for more than two-thirds of the calories.

In the early years of our country, the successful practice of infant feeding consisted almost entirely in the use of human milk, either from the mother or from a wet nurse. Hand, or artificial, feeding until about a century ago was made up largely of animal milk, pap, panada, and broths, which rarely led to the development of a healthy child if they were the only sources of nutriment.

By the 1870's accurate analyses of both human and cow's milk stimulated the development of scientific infant feeding, to which American contributions were of extraordinary significance. The fight for clean, wholesome milk, spearheaded particularly by Coit, combined with the biochemical and clinical studies of milk by investigators such as Jacobi, Rotch, Holt, and Koplik during the early 1900's, finally made it feasible for bottle-fed infants to be reared successfully.

During this century infant feeding has become so simple and safe that we are liable to forget the long and dangerous road that has led to this accomplishment. We have emerged from a chaos of complexity to a chaos of simplicity. A review of even the highlights of the history of infant feeding in America will remind us of our enormous debt to those who preceded us.

References

1. Adams, S. F. Use of vegetables in infant feeding through the ages. *J. Am. Diet. Assoc.* 35:362, 1959.
2. Bain, K. The incidence of breast feeding in hospitals in the United States. *Pediatrics* 2:313, 1948.
3. Brennemann, J. Remarks on the feeding of the healthy infant. *J.A.M.A.* 51:101, 1908.
4. Brennemann, J. The care of infant's nutrition. *J.A.M.A.* 59:623, 1912.
5. Brennemann, J. The curd and buffer in infant feeding. *J.A.M.A.* 92:364, 1929.
6. Butler, A. M., and Wolman, I. J. Trends in the early feeding of supplementary foods to infants: An analysis and discussion based on a nationwide survey. *Q. Rev. Pediatr.* 9:63, 1954.
7. Czerny, A., and Kleinschmidt, H. Ueber eine Buttermehlnahrung für schwache Säuglinge. *Jahrb. Kinderheilkd.* 87:1, 1918.
8. Davison, W. C. Elimination of milk-borne disease. *Am. J. Dis. Child.* 49:72, 1935.
9. Denny, F. P. Human milk in the treatment of various infections. *Boston Med. Surg. J.* 160:161, 1909.
10. Filer, L. J., Jr., and Martinez, G. A. Intake of selected nutrients by infants in the United States: An evaluation of 4,000 representative six-month-olds. *Clin. Pediatr.* 3:633, 1964.
11. Finkelstein, H., and Meyer, L. F. Ueber "Eiweissmilch": Ein Beitrag zum Problem der künstlichen Ernährung. *Jahrb. Kinderheilkd.* 71:525, 1910.
12. Fomon, S. J. *Infant Nutrition* (2nd ed.). Philadelphia: Saunders, 1974.

13. Fomon, S. J. What are infants fed in the United States? *Pediatrics* 56:350, 1975.
14. Gerstenberger, H. J., et al. Studies in the adaptation of an artificial food to human milk. *Am. J. Dis. Child.* 10:249, 1915.
15. Gerstenberger, H. J., and Ruh, H. O. Studies in the adaptation of an artificial food to human milk, II: A report of three years' clinical experience with the feeding of S.M.A. (synthetic milk adapted). *Am. J. Dis. Child.* 17:1, 1919.
16. Gerstley, J. R. Infant nutrition, VII: Lactic acid milk—Has it solved the problem of infant nutrition? *Am. J. Dis. Child.* 45:538, 1933.
17. Goldbloom, A. The evolution of the concepts of infant feeding. *Arch. Dis. Child.* 29:385, 1954.
18. Grulee, C. G., et al. Breast and artificial feeding. *J.A.M.A.* 103:735, 1934.
19. Guthrie, H. A. Effect of early feeding of solid foods on nutritive intake of infant. *Pediatrics* 38:879, 1966.
19a. Harris, L. E., and Chan, J. C. M. Infant feeding practices. *Am. J. Dis. Child.* 117:483, 1969.
20. Hill, L. F. Infant feeding: Historical and current. *Pediatr. Clin. North Am.* 14:255, 1967.
21. Hill, L. W. *Lectures in Pediatrics.* Raleigh, N.C.: Edwards & Broughton, 1916.
22. Holt, L. E., and Howland, J. *Diseases of Infancy and Childhood* (7th ed.). New York: Appleton, 1917.
23. Jacobi, A. Milk-sugar in infant feeding. *Arch. Pediatr.* 18:801, 1901.
24. Kerley, C. G. Cane sugar in its relation to some of the diseases of children. *Trans. Am. Pediatr Soc.* 19:79, 1907.
25. Lackner, E. Heubner's system of infant feeding based on calories. *Arch. Pediatr.* 24:549, 1907.
26. Marriott, W. McK. Preparation of lactic acid milk mixtures for infant feeding. *J.A.M.A.* 89:862, 1927.
27. Marriott, W. McK., and Davidson, L. T. Acidified whole milk as a routine infant food. *J.A.M.A.* 81:2007, 1923.
28. Marriott, W. McK., and Jeans, P. C. *Infant Nutrition* (3rd ed.). St. Louis: Mosby, 1941.
29. Marriott, W. McK., and Schoenthal, L. An experimental study of the use of unsweetened evaporated milk for the preparation of infant feeding formulas. *Arch. Pediatr.* 46:135, 1929.
30. Martinez, G. A. and Nalezienski, J. P. The recent trend in breast-feeding. *Pediatrics* 64:686, 1979.
31. McLean, S., and Fales, H. L. *Scientific Nutrition in Infancy and Early Childhood.* Philadelphia: Lea & Febiger, 1925.
32. Meyer, H. F. Infant feeding practices in hospital maternity nurseries. *Pediatrics* 21:288, 1958.

33. Meyer, H. F. *Infant Foods and Feeding Practice.* Springfield, Ill.: Thomas, 1960.

34. Moorehouse, G. W. The determination of the caloric value of modified milk. *Arch. Pediatr.* 24:87, 1907.

35. Morse, J. L., and Talbot, F. B. *Diseases of Nutrition and Infant Feeding.* New York: Macmillan, 1915.

36. Morse, J. L. The history of pediatrics in Massachusetts. *N. Engl. J. Med.* 205:169, 1931.

37. Morse, J. L. Recollections and reflections of forty-five years of artificial feeding. *J. Pediatr.* 7:303, 1935.

38. Powers, G. Infant feeding: Historical background and modern practice. *J.A.M.A.* 105:753, 1935.

39. Purvis, G. A. What nutrients do our infants really get? *Nutr. Today* 8(5):28, 1973.

40. Ruhräh, J. The soy bean in infant feeding. *Arch. Pediatr.* 26:496, 1909.

41. Ruhräh, J. Further observations on the soy bean. *Trans. Am. Pediatr. Soc.* 23:386, 1911.

42. Sackett, W. W., Jr. Results of 3 years experience with a new concept of baby feeding. *South. Med. J.* 46:358, 1953.

43. Salber, E. J., et. al. Patterns of breast feeding, I: Factors affecting the frequency of breast feeding in the newborn period. *N. Engl. J. Med.* 259:707, 1958.

44. Salber, E. J., and Feinleib, M. Breast-feeding in Boston. *Pediatrics* 37:299, 1966.

45. Santulli, T. V., et al. Acute necrotizing enterocolitis in infancy. *Pediatrics* 55:376, 1975.

46. Southworth, T. S., and Schloss, O. M. The hard curds of infant stools: Their origin, nature and transformation. *Arch. Pediatr.* 26:241, 1909.

47. Sussman, S. The passive transfer of antibodies to *Escherichia coli* 0 111:B4 from mother to offspring. *Pediatrics* 27:308, 1961.

48. Thomas, J. J. The importance of the estimation of the caloric value of infant food. *Arch. Pediatr.* 24:81, 1907.

Indexes

Name Index

Abbott, Grace, 156
Abt, Isaac, 105, 109, 140, 142, 158, 191, 204
Adams, Samuel S., 102, 104, 110, 176
Adams, Suzanne, 256
Albright, Fuller, 222
Allerton, Isaac, 8
Allerton, Mary, 8
Allyn, John, 22
Andersen, Dorothy H., 218, 219
Anderson, Arthur F., 195
Andral, Gabriel, 90
Apgar, Virginia, 238, 240
Apley, John, 229
Arbuthnot, John, 49–50
Arena, Jay, 232
Armstrong, George, 51, 95
Ashmole, Elias, 13
Aspinwell, William, 84
Astruc, Jean, 64
Auenbrugger, Leopold, 72
Avery, Mary Ellen, 239
Ayers, Goody, 25

Bacon, Francis, 30
Baehner, Robert L., 234
Baginsky, Adolf, 102
Baillou, Guillaume de, 43
Bain, Katherine, 255
Baker, S. Josephine, 154, 157
Bakwin, Harry, 190–191, 231
Ballexserd, Jacques, 58
Banting, Sir Frederick, 194
Bard, Samuel, 38–40, 51, 83
  on diphtheria, 38–40
Barlow, Sir Thomas, 122
Barrter, F. C., 224
Barter, Robert H., 235
Bartlett, Josiah, 44

Baty, James M., 210
Bauer, Louis, 120
Beardsley, Hezekiah, 51, 84
Beaven, Paul W., 203
Beck, John Brodhead, 87, 92, 93, 94, 95
  on infanticide, 87
Beck, Theodoric R., 87
Beckwith, J. Bruce, 231
Bednar, Alois, 102
Behring, Emil von, 109, 110, 172
Bell, Joseph A., 214
Benedict, Francis G., 246
Benirschke, Kurt, 237
Bennett, John, 122
Berendes, Heinz, 234
Bergé, André, 112
Bergh, Henry, 100
Bernard, Claude, 101
Beutler, Ernest, 234
Biedert, Philipp, 102, 134, 246
Bigelow, Jacob, 93
Biggs, Hermann, 111
Billard, Charles M., 71
Blackfan, Kenneth, 161, 165, 169–170, 210, 211, 218–
  219, 220
Blake, Francis, 173
Bolduan, C. F., 106
Bonar, Barnet E., 190
Bond, Robert, 16
Booker, William D., 113
Boorstin, Daniel, 30
Borden, Gail, 252
Bordet, Jules Jean, 175
Bouchut, Eugène, 109
Bowditch, Henry I., 94
Bowditch, Henry I., 250
Bowditch, Henry P., 71
Boyd, Edith, 193

Boylston, Thomas, 32, 236
Boylston, Zabdiel, 32–33, 34, 52, 84, 236
  inoculates his son, 32
Bradford, William, 8, 21
Brailey, Miriam, 202
Breck, Samuel, 189n
  feeder, 189
Breg, W. Roy, 234
Brennemann, Joseph G., 174–175, 213, 247–248, 253, 256
Bretonneau, Pierre, 22, 83, 110
Bridenbaugh, Carl, 9
Bridge, Edward M., 203
Bridges, Robert A., 234
Bridgman, Laura, 89
Brieger, Gert H., 71
Brown, Dillon, 110, 128
Brown, John, 50
Browne, Sir Thomas, 117–118
Bruton, Ogden, 230, 233
Buchan, William, 46, 48, 49, 94, 133
  Domestic Medicine, 46
Buckingham, Edward M., 124
Budin, Pierre C., 156, 184, 187, 188
Butler, Allan M., 204, 206, 207, 257
Byers, Randolph K., 215

Cadogan, William, 46, 56, 58, 64, 100
Caffey, John, 222, 231
Caillé, August, 116, 123, 158
Caldwell, Charles, 50
Camerer, Wilhelm, 134, 139
Campbell, Dame Kate, 221
Cantani, Arnaldo, 114, 163
Carpenter, George, 128
Carr, Walter L., 189
Carson, Paul E., 233
Carter, Abby and Sophia, 88
Castle, William B., 209
Caulfield, Ernest, 22, 23, 31, 41, 56, 57
Caverly, Charles S., 181
Celsus, 11
Chadwick, Sir Edwin, 91
Chain, Ernest B., 213
Chalmers, Lionel, 40, 41, 43–44, 48, 49, 51, 62–63, 64
  on diphtheria, 40
  on infant feeding, 62–63
  on mumps, 43–44
  on whooping cough, 43
Chapin, Henry D., 119, 140
Chapple, Charles C., 202
  and the Isolette, 202
Chauncy, Charles, 11–12
Cheyne, John, 83
Chomel, August F., 90
Christie, Amos, 223
Christopher, Walter S., 158
Churchill, Frank S., 196
Clap, Roger, 26

Clarke, Sir Charles, 82
Clarke, Danielle, 17–18
Clayton, John, 23
Clerc, Laurent, 88
Clifford, Stewart H., 220
Coburn, Alvin, 174, 215–216
Cogswell, Alice, 88
Cohn, Edwin J., 217
Coit, Henry L., 141, 143, 144, 258
Colebrook, Leonard, 212
Condie, David F., 81–82, 84, 120
Cook, Paul, 190
Cooke, Jean V., 181
Cooke, Robert E., 207
Cooley, Thomas B., 208–209
Coons, Albert H., 232
Cooper, Max D., 232
Corvisart, Jean Nicholas, 72
Cotton, John, 33
Courtney, Angelia, 160
Cowie, David M., 194
Crandall, Floyd M., 116
Creighton, Charles, 41, 111
Cullen, William, 50
Culpeper, Nicholas, 31, 49, 58, 64
Czerny, Adalbert, 101, 134, 160, 192, 246, 250

Dale, Thomas, 36
Dalldorf, Gilbert J., 216
Dandy, Walter E., 170
Danforth, Samuel, 22, 25
Dare, Ananias, 7
Dare, Virginia, 7
Darrow, Daniel C., 204, 205, 207–208
Darrow, Ruth, 210
Davis, David C., 237
Davison, Wilburt C., 245
Day, Richard, 220, 221
Demos, John, 26, 55–56
Denny, Francis P., 249
Deventer, Hendrik van, 18
Dewees, William P., 69, 78–79, 83, 120, 132, 134
Diamond, Louis K., 171, 210, 211
Dick, George F., and Gladys R., 173–174
Dickens, Charles, 89
Dickinson, Jonathan, 37–38
Dickson, Ernest C., 223
Diehl, Volker, 234
DiGeorge, Angelo M., 233
Dittrick, Howard, 62
Dix, Dorothea, 90
Doane, Frances W., 237
Dochez, Alphonse R., 173
Domagk, Gerhard, 212
Douglass, William, 23, 30, 34–35, 37, 38, 40
  on colonial medical practice, 30
  describes scarlet fever, 40–41
  smallpox inoculation and, 34–35
Dowling, Harry F., 212

Drake, Daniel, 80
Draper, George, 183
Drinker, Cecil, 72
Drinker, Elizabeth S., 47–48, 49
Drinker, Henry, 47
Drinker, Philip, 217
Duffy, Benedict J., 224
Dufour, Leon, 156
Dunn, Charles H., 127
Dyer, Mary, 19

Eaton, Theophilus, 15
Eberle, John, 79–80, 84, 120
Edwards, William A., 125
Eggleston, Edward, 25
Ehrlich, Paul, 180, 181, 212
Eichenwald, Heinz F., 238
Elizabeth I, 5
Emerson, Haven, 182
Enders, John, 217, 229, 236, 237
Epstein, Alois, 102
Ericson, Thorstein, 7
Escherich, Theodor, 134, 142
Evans, William A., 231

Faber, Harold K., 117, 123, 124, 131, 162, 195, 204, 206, 223
Fagge, Charles H., 194
Fales, Helen, 160, 256
Fanconi, Guido, 223
Farber, Sidney, 211, 219
Feinleib, Manning, 255
Felton, Harriet M., 214
Fernald, Walter E., 90
Fieser, Louis F., 218
Filer, Lloyd J., 257
Finkelstein, Heinrich, 134, 161, 162, 163, 205, 246, 248, 250, 251
Finlayson, James, 127
Finn, John J., 237
Fitch, Jabez, 37
Fitzgerald, Patrick J., 224
Fleming, Sir Alexander, 213
Flexner, Simon, 116, 117, 142, 176, 177, 182
Flint, Austin, 103
Florey, Howard W., 213
Floyer, Sir John, 73
Folin, Otto, 164
Fomon, Samuel J., 256, 256n, 257
Ford, C. E., 234
Forsyth, David, 58
Fothergill, John, 40
Fourneau, Ernest, 212
Fournier, Jean, 119
Francis, Thomas, 235
Frankel, L. K., 185
Franklin, Benjamin, 25, 31, 36
Freda, Vincent J., 239
Freeman, Rowland G., 121

French, Daniel C., 88
Friedenthal, Hans, 254
Friedlander, Alfred, 193
Fruitnight, John H., 121, 122
Fudenberg, H. Hugh, 232
Fulginiti, Vincent A., 232
Fuller, Bridget Lee, 11, 18
Fuller, Samuel, 8, 11, 18, 20

Galen, 11, 24, 63
Gallagher, J. Roswell, 241
Gallaudet, Edward M., 88
Gallaudet, Thomas, 88
Gallaudet, Thomas H., 87–88
Gamble, James L., 161, 163–165, 192, 204, 206
Garrison, Fielding H., 73, 93
Garrod, Sir Archibald, 170
Garrow, Irene, 231
Gengou, Octave, 175
Gerarde, John, 14
Gerhard, William W., 90–91, 94
Gerhardt, Carl, 102, 125
Gerry, Elbridge T., 100
Gerstenberger, Henry J., 254
Gerstley, Jesse R., 250
Gibney, Virgil, 105
Gitlin, David, 232, 233
Glenny, Alexander T., 172
Glisson, Francis, 6
Gluck, Louis, 240
Goelet, Francis, 56
Goldberger, Joseph, 218
Goldbloom, Alton, 170, 247
Good, Robert A., 232, 233, 234
Gordon, Harry, 195, 220, 221
Govan, Clifton D., 205, 207
Graham, Sylvester, 72, 147
Greeley, David McL., 222
Gregg, Norman, 217
Greven, Philip J., 27
Griffith, J. P. Crozer, 115, 147, 179, 186, 193–194
Griscom, John H., 91
Grulee, Clifford G., 122, 186, 187, 189, 190, 255
Guéniot, Alexandre, 187
Guest, George M., 209
Guthrie, Helen, 257

Haas, Sidney V., 219
Hahnemann, Samuel, 72
Hales, Stephen, 57
Hall, Lyman, 44
Hamilton, Alexander, 57, 60
Hamilton, Robert, 43
Hammer, J. A., 193, 194
Hammerton, J. L., 234
Hammill, Samuel, 158
Hanway, Jonas, 57
Harrington, Helen, 162

Harris, Walter, 6, 23
  on pediatric practice, 6
Hart, Alfred P., 210
Hartley, Robert, 74, 141
Hartmann, Alexis, 207
Harvey, Governor, 10
Harvey, William, 6
Harvie, Dyonis, 7
Hata, Sahachiro, 180, 181
Haven, Henry C., 120
Hawkins, Jane, 19
Hayes, Rutherford B., 101
Heineke, Herman, 193
Helmholtz, Henry F., 170
Hemplemann, Theodore C., 183, 184, 216
Hench, Philip, 216
Henderson, Lawrence J., 164
Henle, Gertrude, 234
Henle, Werner, 234
Hennig, Carl, 102
Henoch, Eduard H., 84, 101, 102
Herrick, Theodore P., 218
Hess, Alfred F., 121, 168, 169
Hess, Julius H., 187, 188, 190
Heubner, Otto, 101, 134, 139, 246
Heubner, Robert J., 184
Higginson, Francis, 21, 25
Hill, Lee Forrest, 245, 250
Hill, Lewis Webb, 248–249, 251
Hippocrates, 11, 24, 63
Holmes, Oliver Wendell, 13, 17, 93, 94, 138
Holt, L. Emmett, Sr., 38, 79, 103, 104–105, 114, 115,
    119, 122, 127, 137, 140, 141, 146, 147, 158, 160,
    177, 178, 179, 181, 190, 193, 246, 258
Holyoke, Augustus, 51
Home, Francis, 236
Hoover, Herbert, 158
Hosack, David, and German measles, 90
Howe, Samuel G., 88–90
Howland, John, 38, 160–161, 162, 163, 164, 165, 166,
    167, 170, 193, 246, 252
Hubbard, Donald M., 223
Hubbard, Leverett, 51
Hull, John, 21–22, 43
Hutchinson, Anne, 19

Itano, Harvey A., 209

Jackson, James, 94, 113
Jacobi, Abraham, 39, 41, 86, 101, 102–103, 104, 105,
    108, 110, 115, 116, 119, 121, 127, 128, 138–139,
    144, 147, 151, 152, 157–158, 180, 196, 248, 250,
    258
Jacobson, Cecil B., 235
Janeway, Charles A., 232, 233
Janeway, Edward Gamaliel, 116
Janeway, Theodore C., 167
Jaudon, Joseph C., 224

Jeans, Philip C., 180, 181
Jefferson, Thomas, 26, 85, 92–93
Jenner, Edward, 36, 84
Jenner, Sir William, 120
Jennings, Charles G., 121
Jobling, James, 116, 117, 176, 177
Jones, T. Duckett, 215
Josephs, Hugh W., 209–210, 222
Josselyn, John, 23, 24

Kajai, Laslo, 203
Kanner, Leo, 202
Karzon, David, 237
Kassowitz, Max, 102, 119
Katz, Samuel L., 236
Keating, John M., 124–125
Keen, William W., 73
Kelley, Elizabeth, 156
Kempe, C. Henry, 231–232
Kendall, Amos, 88
Kendrick, Pearl, 214
Kennedy, Roger L. J., 213
Kerley, Charles G., 248
Kibrick, Sidney, 237
Killpatrick (Kirkpatrick), James, 36
Kircher, Athanasius, 35
Kitasato, Shibasaburo, 109
Klebs, Theodor, 109
Kleinschmidt, Hans, 250
Klemperer, Paul, 191
Koch, Robert, 70, 101, 111, 117, 118
Kohn, Jerome, 189
Koplik, Henry E., 122, 137, 138, 147, 168, 174, 180, 258
Kramer, Benjamin, 161, 165, 166, 167
Kuhn, Adam, 47–48
Kulovich, Marie, 240
Kunkel, Henry, 232

Lackner, Ernest, 246
Ladd, Maynard, 190
Laennec, René Théophile, 72
LaFétra, Linnaeus E., 141, 158, 181, 188–189
Lancefield, Rebecca, 174
Landing, Benjamin H., 234
Landsteiner, Karl, 171, 182, 210
Langford, William S., 222
Langstein, Leo, 187
Lapin, Joseph H., 214
Lathrop, Julia, 156
Latta, Thomas, 163
Laud, William, 11
Lee, Pearl, 208
Leech, Clifton B., 202
Leete, William, 15–16
Lejeune, Jérôme, 234
Lerner, A. Martin, 237
Levan, Albert, 234
Levine, Philip, 202, 210

Levine, Samuel Z., 220
Lewis, Paul A., 182
Liebig, Justus von, 144, 145
Lister, Lord, 118
"Little Mary Ellen," 100, 153
Livingston, Samuel, 203
Lobb, Theophilus, 46
Locke, John, 76
Lockridge, Kenneth A., 27
Loeb, Robert, 164
Loeffler, Friedrich, 109
Logan, George, 77–78, 113
Louis, Pierre C., 72, 73, 90
Lucas, William P., 209
Ludwig, Carl F., 101

Macaulay, Thomas, 21
Magendie, François, 144–145
Mann, Horace, 89, 96
Marfan, Bernard, 121
Marriott, William McK., 161, 162, 163, 165, 166, 205, 207, 247, 251
Marshall, John, 23, 40, 43
Martin, André, 109
Martinez, G. A., 257
Massell, Benedict, 216
Mather, Abigail, 20, 42
Mather, Cotton, 12, 15, 20, 22, 25, 27, 31–32, 40, 41–42, 45, 50, 52, 59, 64
Mather, Mrs. Cotton, 42
Mather, Eleazer, 42
Mather, Elizabeth, 64
Mather, Hannah, 20, 42
Mather, Increase, 33
  supports inoculation, 35
Mather, Increase (son), 40, 42, 50
Mather, Jerusha, 42
Mather, Katy, 40
Mather, Martha, 42
Mather, Samuel, 33, 42, 50
May, Charles D., 219, 220
McCollum, Elmer V., 167
McCreary, J. F., 219–220
McCune, Donovan J., 222
McIntosh, Rustin, 117, 123, 124, 131, 162, 195, 204, 206, 223
McKhann, Charles F., 204, 206, 217
McLean, Stafford, 256
Mead, Jere, 239
Medin, Karl O., 181
Meigs, Arthur V., 122, 134, 135–136, 141, 254
Meigs, Charles Delucena, 82, 83, 113, 134, 135
Meigs, John Forsyth, 82–83, 120, 134, 135
Melnick, Joseph L., 237
Metchnikoff, Elie, 180
Meyer, Harry M., 236
Meyer, Herman F., 137–138, 253, 255
Miller, Edward, 51

Miller, Herbert C., 207
Miller, Nickolay F., 187
Milovanović, Milan, 236
Minot, Francis, 104
Mitchell, A. Graeme, 213
Mittelberger, Gottlieb, 29
Mitus, Anna, 236
Miwa, Shiro, 234
Molière, 18
Moll, Frederic C., 215
Montagu, Lady Mary Wortley, 32
Moorehouse, George W., 246
Morgan, Herbert R., 237
Morison, Samuel Eliot, 6
Morissette, Russell, 222
Morse, John Lovett, 120–121, 137, 140, 158, 204, 246, 248, 249
Müller, Johannes, 101
Myenberg, John B., 252

Nathan, David, 234
Neel, James V., 209
Nelson, James, 56
Nelson, Waldo E., 229
Neva, Franklin A., 236
North, Elisha, 86–87, 116
Northrup, William P., 110, 122

O'Dwyer, Joseph, 109–110
O'Shaughnessy, William B., 163
Oski, Frank A., 233
Osler, Sir William, 39, 51, 90, 104, 108, 118, 126, 127, 179, 183, 194
Otto, John C., 84, 86
Otway, Lady, and cure for jaundice, 16n

Packard, Francis R., 41
Paltauf, Arnold, 192–193, 194
Panos, Theodore C., 236
Park, Edwards A., 127, 160, 161, 165, 166–167, 168, 202
Park, William H., 111, 172, 217
Parkman, Ebenezer, 55
Parkman, Paul D., 236
Parmelee, Arthur H., 218
Parry, John S., 120
Parsons, John P., 194
Pasteur, Louis, 35–36, 70, 101, 142
Paul, John R., 182–183
Pauling, Linus, 202, 209
Pavy, Frederick W., 133
Peabody, Francis W., 183
Pease, Marshall C., 203
Peebles, Thomas C., 236
Penhallow, Samuel, 40
Pepper, William, 82, 120
Perkins, Thomas H., 89
Peterson, John C., 223
Peterson, R. D. A., 232

Pirquet, Clemens von, 160, 172, 194, 195
Platter, Felix, 192
Pomerantz, Charles, 222–223
Popper, Erwin, 182
Portier, Paul, 110
Powers, Grover F., 142, 152, 161, 205–206
Press, Edward, 232
Priessnitz, Vincenz, 72
Prudden, T. Mitchell, 109
Purvis, George A., 256–257
Putnam, Charles, 104
Pynchon, John, 16

Quie, Paul G., 232
Quincke, Heinrich, 116

Rachford, Benjamin K., 152, 174
Radbill, Samuel X., 75, 79
Raleigh, Sir Walter, 6
Ramon, Gaston L., 111, 172
Rapoport, Samuel, 209
Ratner, Bret, 170–171
Reuss, August von, 184
Rhazes, 12
Rhodes, A. J., 237
Richet, Charles R., 110–111
Riley, Conrad M., 222
Ritter von Rittershain, Gottfried, 102
Rivers, Thomas M., 235
Robbins, Frederick C., 217
Robinson, C. R., 237
Roche, Mary, 36
Roentgen, Wilhelm C., 118
Rokitansky, Carl, 101
Roosevelt, Theodore, 235
Rosen, Fred S., 232
Rosén von Rosenstein, Nils, 250
Ross, S. Graham, 164
Rosseter, Mr., 25
Rotch, Thomas Morgan, 99, 102–103, 104, 113, 126–
    127, 128, 134, 136–138, 140, 141, 147, 158, 188,
    246, 253, 258
Rothstein, William, 70
Routh, Charles H., 132, 133
Roux, Pierre, 109, 180
Rowntree, Leonard G., 170
Rubner, Max, 134, 139
Ruhräh, John, 5, 251
Runge, Max, 184
Rush, Benjamin, 23, 41, 43, 57, 70, 86, 112, 113, 114
    on cholera infantum, 44–45
    and pediatrics, 44–45, 93
    on scarlet fever, 41

Sabin, Albert B., 230, 235
Sackett, Walter W., 256
St. Vincent de Paul, 75
Salber, Eva J., 255
Salk, Jonas, 230, 235

Sauer, Louis W., 176, 214
Schaudinn, Fritz R., 180
Schick, Béla, 172, 195
Schloss, E., 254
Schloss, Oscar, 161–162, 164, 165, 194–195, 201
Schlossmann, Arthur, 134
Schmidt, Martin B., 167
Schoenlein, Johann, 101
Schoenthal, Ludwig, 252
Schottmüller, Hugo, 173
Schwarz, Herman, 189
Schwentker, Francis F., 213
Sedgwick, Julius P., 186–187
Seibert, August, 110
Sewall, Samuel, 18–19, 20, 26, 56, 59, 60
Sewall, John, 56
Sewall, Mrs. Samuel, 56
Shattuck, George Cheyne, Jr., 94
Shattuck, Lemuel, 91, 100
Sherman, DeWitt, 189–190
Sherman, Lillian, 173
Shiga, Kiyoshi, 142
Shipley, Paul G., 167, 168
Shippen, William, Jr., 47–48
Shirkey, Harry C., 234
Shryock, Richard H., 29, 33
Sickles, Grace M., 216
Sidbury, James B., 171
Silverman, Frederick N., 231
Silverman, William A., 222
Simon, Johann, 83, 132, 134
Sims, J. Marion, 93
Siperstein, David M., 171
Skoda, Josef, 101
Skyrin, Elizabeth, 49
Smith, Carl H., 211
Smith, Charles E., 223
Smith, Charles Hendee, 177
Smith, Clement A., 220
Smith, H. L., 195
Smith, Hugh, 61–62
Smith, Job Lewis, 79, 81, 101, 103–104, 109, 112, 114,
    121, 124, 133, 147
Smith, Stephen, 91, 100, 101
Smith, Theobald, 118, 171, 172, 239
Smyth, Francis Scott, 222
Snorri, 7
Snow, Irving M., 121
Southworth, Thomas, 247
Soxhlet, Franz von, 142
Spink, Wesley W., 213n
Stafford, Edward, 13–14, 25
    "Receipts" for
        bloodie flix (flux), 13–14
        broken bone, 14
        falling sicknesse, 13
        jaunders (jaundice), 13
        panacea, 13
Standish, Lidia, 55

Stannard, David, 27
Starr, Louis, 105, 116, 122, 125–126
Steele, Mark W., 234
Steigman, Alex J., 237
Stetson, Rufus, 210
Stewart, James, 81
Stiehm, E. Richard, 232
Still, Sir George F., 61, 174, 183
Stillé, Alfred, 75, 94
Stockman, James A., 233
Stokes, Joseph, 216
Stone, Samuel, 16–17
Straus, Nathan, 144, 155
Sussman, Sidney, 255
Sydenham, Thomas, 6, 13, 23
Szent-Györgyi, Albert, 218

Talbot, Fritz B., 164, 165, 195, 220, 246, 248
Tallyrand, 44
Tanaka, Kouichi R., 234
Tarnier, Etienne, 187, 188
Taussig, Helen, 202
Terry, Theodore, 221
Thacher, Peter, 11
Thacher, Thomas, 11–13, 21, 26, 35
Thomas, John J., 246
Thompson, Samuel, 72
Thornton, Matthew, 44
Ticknor, Caleb, 133
Tisdall, Frederick F., 164, 165, 166
Tjio, Joe H., 234
Toomey, John A., 222
Trask, James D., 173, 216
Trollope, Anthony, 132
Trousseau, Armand, 110
Trudeau, Edward L., 118

Underwood, Michael, 6, 49, 59, 64, 65

Valdés-Dapeña, Marie, 231
Valentine, William N., 208, 234
Vallembert, Simon de, 63
Van Slyke, Donald D., 162
Vaughan, Victor C., 113
Veale, Henry R., 90
Veeder, Borden S., 181, 183, 184
Vieusseux, Gaspard, 116
Vinovskis, Maris A., 27
Virchow, Rudolf, 101

Wachenheim, F. L., 138
Wald, Lillian D., 154, 156
Wallerstein, Harry, 211

Waring, Joseph I., 36
Warkany, Josef, 223
Warren, John, 85
Waserman, Manfred J., 143
Wassermann, August von, 180
Waterhouse, Benjamin, 84–86, 236
Waterhouse, Benjamin (son), 84, 236
Waterhouse, Daniel, 84
Waterhouse, Mary, 84
Watson, William P., 127
Waxham, Frank E., 116
Webster, Noah, on epidemic and pestilential diseases, 107–108
Weech, A. Ashley, 212
Weichselbaum, Anton, 87
Weller, Thomas H., 217, 236, 237
Wentworth, Arthur H., 116–117
Werne, Jacob, 231
Wesley, John, 46–47, 48, 49
    Primitive Physick, 46
Wexler, Irving B., 210
White, John, 6
White, Peregrine, 8, 60
White, Susanna, 8
Whitefield, George, 75
Whytt, Robert, 90
Widal, Georges F., 179
Wiener, Alexander S., 210
Wilkins, Lawson, 202–203, 224
Willan, Robert, 90
Williams, Robert R., 218
Williams, J. Whitridge, 181
Willis, Thomas, 43
Winters, Joseph E., 121
Winthrop, Fitz-John, 22
Winthrop, John, Jr., 11, 13, 14–18, 22, 23, 25
    describes anencephaly, 19
    pediatric cases treated by, 15–18
    rubila, secret preparation of, 17
Winthrop, John, Sr., 9, 13, 14
    describes congenital syphilis, 14
Winthrop, Margaret, 17
Wolbach, S. Burt, 218–219
Wolcott, Oliver, 44
Wolman, Irving J., 257
Woolley, Paul V., 231
Wunderlich, Carl R., 72, 73, 86

Yannet, Herman, 206
Yersin, Alexandre E. J., 109

Zahorsky, John, 183, 184
Zingher, Abraham, 172, 217
Zuelzer, Wolf W., 209, 210

Subject Index

Academic pediatrics, beginnings of, 102–105
Accidents, childhood
  in eighteenth century, 47–48
  in seventeenth century, 20
  in twentieth century, 232
Acid-base studies, 161–163
Acidified milks, 251
Acidosis
  producing "alimentary intoxication", 161–163
  treatment of, 161, 162, 163, 205–208
Acrodynia, 223
Adolescents' unit, first, 241
Adrenal hemorrhage, in newborn, 224
Adrenocortical steroids, 224, 229
Adrenogenital syndrome, 224
Agammaglobulinemia, 233
Air, fresh, 81, 152
  as treatment
    in cholera infantum, 45, 82, 114, 126, 152
    in pneumonia, 179
    in tuberculosis, 118, 126
Alcohol
  and the fetus, 80
  in treatment of infants and children, 110, 126, 152, 178
  use of, by medical students, 85
Alimentary intoxication, 161. See also Acidosis
Alkalosis, and potassium deficiency, 207–208
Allergy, 194–195
  and infantile eczema, 195
Almanacs, 45–46
Almshouses, 74–75, 88
American Academy of Pediatrics, 232
  founding of, 203–204
American Association of Medical Milk Commissions, 143–144
American Association for Study and Prevention of Infant Mortality, 159

American Child Health Association, 159
American Child Hygiene Association, 159
American Friends Service Committee, 201
American Medical Association, 70–71, 203
  Section of Diseases of Children, 103, 104
  and the Sheppard-Towner Act, 157, 203
American Pediatric Society, 104, 110–111, 123–124, 157–158, 161, 164, 176, 246, 254
  first meeting of, 157–158
  report on antitoxin in treatment of diphtheria, 110–111
  report on infantile scurvy, 123–124
American Public Health Association, 100
American Society for the Prevention of Cruelty to Animals (ASPCA), 100
Amniotic fluid
  amniocentesis for analysis of, 230, 234–235
  sphingomyelin/lecithin ratio in, 240
Anemia
  congenital hypoplastic, 211
  Cooley's, 208–209
  of the newborn, 209–210
  sickle-cell, 209
Anencephaly, 19
Angina ulcusculosa. See Diphtheria
Antenatal diagnosis, 234–235
Antibiotics, development of, 224, 229
Antimetabolites, 202, 224, 230
Antitoxin. See Diphtheria antitoxin; Scarlet fever
Apgar score, 238, 240
Aphthae, 49, 79
Apprentices, 8–9, 10, 74
Artificial feeding. See Feeding, artificial
Asthma, 126
Atresia, anal, first mention of, 20

Babies Hospital, New York, 81, 105, 118, 160, 176, 212, 218
Bacillary dysentery, 142

Battered child syndrome, 100, 231–232, 241
  first American mention of, 15
  "Little Mary Ellen" case, 100, 153
BCG. See Tuberculosis
Bellevue Hospital, 103, 105, 106, 188
Bethesda Orphan House (Ga.), 75
Biochemical pediatric studies, 160–169
Birth defects, 20, 51, 83, 229
  in colonial America, 20, 51
  etiology of, 20
Birth rate, 27, 69, 201–202
Birth weight, average, 186
Births
  first child born in North America, 7
  first English-born child, 7
  midwives, 18–19, 157
Blind children, 88–89
Blisters, 40, 41, 80, 87, 92, 94, 128
Blood collecting, apparatus for, 169–170
Blood transfusions, 171
  by intraperitoneal injection, 171
  by umbilical vein, 171
Bloodletting in children, 40, 44, 46, 51, 79, 80, 81, 87,
    92, 93–94, 128
Boston Children's Hospital, 70, 165
Boston exanthem, 237–238
Boston Floating Hospital, 152, 249
Botanical (Thompsonian) system, 15, 72, 77
Breast-feeding, 55–58, 60, 78, 131–132, 254–255
  crusade for, 186–187
  decline in, 254–255
  and summer complaint, 249
  Trollope on, 132
Breast milk
  analyses of (Table 6-1), 132–133, 160
  composition of, 83
  for feeding feeble infants, 221–222
  influenced by maternal anxiety, 133
  qualities of, 255
  as therapeutic agent, 249
Brooklyn Jewish Hospital, 165
"Bubby-pot" baby feeder, 61
Bureau of Child Hygiene (New York City), 153–154
Burns, water and electrolyte metabolism in, 207
Butter-flour mixture, 250–251
Buttermilk, 250

Calomel, 47, 49, 51, 73, 78, 79, 80, 91, 92, 93, 94, 103,
    114, 116, 119
Carbohydrate, choice of in infant formulas, 248
Cathartics, 42, 91, 93, 128
Causes of diseases, theories of, 25, 70, 73. See also Theo-
    ries, medical
Celiac disease, 219–220
Cerebrospinal fever (cerebrospinal meningitis), 86, 87,
    116–117
  epidemics of, 116–117
  mortality from, 116

treatment of, 87, 116–117. See also Meningococcal
    meningitis
Certified milk, 143–144, 153
Charité (pediatric clinic), Berlin, 101
Child abuse. See Battered child syndrome
Child care, 10–11, 25–26, 100–101
  in colonial America, 10–11, 25–26
Child health problems, 100–101, 105–107
Child Hygiene Organization, 159
Child labor, 95–96, 158
Child mortality, 106
  causes of (Table 7-1), 159
Child welfare movement, 151–152, 157–158
Children, heroic treatment of, 43, 72, 79, 80, 91–95
Children's Hospital, Edinburgh, 70
Children's Hospital, Great Ormond Street, London, 70
Children's hospitals, 69–70, 81, 99, 101, 152, 164, 165,
    174, 180, 201, 202, 249. See also specific hospitals
Chloramphenicol, 202, 213
Cholera, 74, 81, 108, 163
  fluid and electrolyte treatment of, 113–114
Cholera infantum, 23, 44–45, 51, 74, 79, 80, 81, 82,
    106, 112–114, 147, 152, 249
  craving for salt in, 45, 80
  first description of, 44
  early history of, 113
  treatment of, 44–45, 113–114
Chorea, 174. See also Rheumatic fever
Chromosomes, human
  anomalies of, 230
  number of, 234
Chronic granulomatous disease (CGD), 234
Climatotherapy, 152. See also Air, fresh
Clothing, infant's, 26, 58
Coccidioidomycosis, 223
Cod-liver oil, 122, 166, 167, 168, 241, 252
College of Physicians and Surgeons, New York, 102, 103,
    105, 166, 167
Commonwealth Fund, 159
Congenital heart disease, 78, 82
Connecticut Asylum for the Education and Instruction of
    Deaf and Dumb Persons (1817), 75, 88
Consultation de Nourissons, 156
Convulsions, 47, 50, 80, 81, 82, 84, 95, 115
  in Cotton Mather's family, 50
  febrile, 127
Coprology, 247
Cortisone, 216
Coryza, 83
Coxsackie virus infections, 216–217, 237
  Coxsackie A-6 virus, 237
Cradles, infant, 60
Cretinism, 126, 194
  first mention of, 20
  treatment of, 126
Croup, 83–84. See also Diphtheria
Cupping, 81
Cynanche trachealis. See Diphtheria

Cystic fibrosis of the pancreas, 218–219
   sweat test for, 229
   treatment of, 219

Daffy's *Elixir Salutis*, 47
Dalby's carminative, 94, 94n
Deaf children, 87–88
Dehydration, 45, 113
   in cholera infantum, 45, 113
   first documented case of, 16
   fluid and electrolyte treatment of, 113–114
Dependent children
   care of, 74–76
   health problems of, 75–76. *See also* Apprentices; Orphans
Diabetes mellitus, 127, 194
Diarrheal diseases, 74, 82, 83, 94, 95, 115, 159, 238
   deaths from in 1850 (Table 5-4), 108
   deaths from in 1880 (Table 5-1), 107
   and Echovirus type, 18, 238
   fluid and electrolyte treatment of, 205–208, 252
   potassium loss in, 207–208
   varieties of, 79
Diatheses, 126
   concept of, 192
   types of, 192
Dick test, 173–174
DiGeorge syndrome, 233
Diphtheria, 22–23, 36–40, 51, 70, 80, 83–84, 91, 108–111, 127, 171–173, 213–214
   alternative names for, 22, 39n
   epidemics of, 22, 36–40, 108–109
   first American description of, 38
   intubation for, 109–110
   mortality from, 37, 109, 171, 213
   treatment of, 80, 109–111, 171, 213–214
Diphtheria antitoxin, use of, 151, 171–172, 213
Diphtheria toxin-antitoxin, use of, 151, 171–172
   catastrophes from, 171–172
Diphtheria toxoid, use of, 111, 172
Diphtheritic paralysis, 38
   description of, in *Diseases of Infancy and Childhood* (Holt and McIntosh, 1921), 38
Diseases. *See specific disease, e.g.,* Diphtheria; First American description of diseases
Division of Child Hygiene (New York City), 153–154
Domestic medicine, books on, 46–47
Down's syndrome, 234
Dry milk, 253
Dysentery, 8, 13–14, 23, 73. *See also* Cholera infantum; Diarrheal diseases

Echovirus infections, 237–238
Eczema, 195
Emetics, 40, 41, 79, 80, 87, 91, 92, 93, 95, 128
Encephalitis, St. Louis, 216
Encephalopathy, 215
Endocrine clinic, first, 202

Enteroviral infections, 237–238
Epidemic diseases, Colonial American contributions to, 31–32, 51–52
Epidemic meningitis. *See* Cerebrospinal fever (cerebrospinal meningitis); Meningococcal meningitis
Epilepsy, 13, 126, 164
   first pediatric clinic for, 203
   fluid and electrolyte studies of, 164
Epstein-Barr virus, 234
Erythema infectiosum, 217–218
Erythroblastosis fetalis, 229, 238–239
   exchange transfusion in, 210–211
   prevention of, 238–239
Exchange transfusion, 210–211

Familial autonomic dysfunction, 222
Family, changing aspects of, 242
Feeding, artificial, 57, 58–60, 80, 132, 133–134, 250–254
Feeding devices, 59, 60–61
Fever, treatment of, 76–77
First American description of diseases
   agammaglobulinemia, 233
   anal atresia, 20
   anencephaly, 19
   cerebrospinal fever, 86, 87
   child abuse, 20
   cholera infantum, 44
   chronic granulomatous disease, 234
   congenital hypoplastic anemia, 211
   congenital syphilis, 19
   cretinism, 20
   diphtheria, 36
   erythema infectiosum, 217
   herpangina, 184
   hypertrophy of pylorus, 51
   lymphocytosis, acute infectious, 211
   mumps, 43
   nursing bottle caries syndrome, 18
   poliomyelitis, 181
   roseola infantum, 183
   rubella, 90
   salaam spasms, 82
   scarlet fever, 40
   scurvy, 122
   tuberculous meningitis, 90–91
Fluid and electrolyte therapy, 113–114, 204, 208
   "comprehensive" treatment plan of, 205–206
   by intraperitoneal injection, 170–171
   by intravenous injection, 170–171
   by superior longitudinal sinus injection, 170–171
Foundlings, mortality of, 57, 76, 115
France, and infant welfare movement, 155–156
French medicine, influence of, on American medical practice, 71–72

Gamblegrams, 164
Genetics, recent advances in, 234–235

German pediatrics, influence on American practice, 101–102
Glomerulonephritis, 175
Glucose-6-phosphate dehydrogenase (G-6-PD) deficiency, 233–234
Godfrey's cordial, 94, 94n
Goutte de lait, 156
Governor-physicians
    Winthrop, John, Jr., 13–18
    Winthrop, John, Sr., 13–14
Granulomatous disease, chronic, 234
Growth, physical, 71–72, 218
Gum-lancing, 50, 76

Hand, foot, and mouth disease, 237
Harriet Lane Home, 160–161, 165, 166, 202, 207
Harvard Medical School, 103, 104, 165
Heart disease, congenital, 78, 82, 84
Hematology, 208–211
    recent advances in, 233–234. See also specific blood disease, e.g., Anemia
Hemolytic disease of the newborn. See Erythroblastosis fetalis
Hemophilia, 84, 86
Hemophilus influenzae meningitis, 212
Hemorrhagic disease of the newborn, 191–192, 220
    vitamin K in, 220
Henry Street Settlement for Nurses, 154
Herpangina, 184, 237
Histoplasmosis, 223
Homeopathy, 72
    homeopathic drugs, use of, 201
Hôpital des Enfants Malades (Paris), 69–70
Hospitals for children, suggested, 81
Humanized milks (single-formula mixtures), 253–254
Hyaline membrane disease (HMD). See Respiratory distress syndrome (RDS)
Hydatidiform mole, 19
Hydrocephalus, 81, 83
Hydropathy (hydrotherapy), 72
Hypertrophy of pylorus, first account of, 51
Hypervitaminosis A, 222
Hypodermoclysis, 113–114
Hypogammaglobulinemia of infancy, 233

Immigration to America, 5–10, 29–30, 105–106
Immunization, active
    against measles, 236
    against poliomyelitis, 235
    against rubella, 235
Immunology, 230
    recent advances in, 232–233
Inanition fever, 190–191
Incubators, 188, 189, 221
    Chapple (Isolette) incubator, 202
    Hess incubator (Fig. 8-17), 188
    history of, 188
    Rotch incubator (Fig. 7-16), 188

Infant
    newborn, 184–187, 220–222, 238–241
        Die Krankheiten der ersten Lebenstage, first book about, 184
        feeding of, 221–222
        percentage delivered in hospital, 184, 202
    premature, 187–190, 220–221, 240–241
        care of, 188–189, 240–241
        diagnosis of, 188–190
        feeding of, 189
        first hospital center for, 187
        history of, 187
        mortality of, 189–190, 220–221, 241
        prognosis of, 189, 220–221, 241
        treatment of, 188–190
Infant and child welfare movement, 151–155
    in France, 155–156
    health stations, 154–155
    in New York City, 153–155
Infant feeding, 26, 55–65, 80, 81, 128, 131–147, 184–187, 221–222, 246–258
    amount and frequency of, 140–141, 146–147
    calorimetric method, 102, 139–140, 246–247
    carbohydrate in, 248
    percentage method, 126, 136–138
    proprietary foods for, 146–147
    scientific methods in, 160
    starch and cereals in, 140
    trends in, 255–256. See also Breast-feeding; Feeding, artificial
Infant foods, proprietary, 144–146
    Liebig's mixture, 145
Infant milk depots, 144
Infant mortality, 26–27, 69, 73–74, 99–100, 101, 106, 131, 155, 184–186, 202, 220
    in nineteenth century, 69, 73–74, 99–100, 106, 114–115, 131
    in seventeenth century, 26–27
    in twentieth century, 151, 157, 159–160, 184–186, 202
Infant welfare stations, 154–155
Infanticide, 87. See also Beck, John Brodhead in Name Index
Infantile cortical hyperostosis, 222
Infantile spasms, 81
Inoculation. See Smallpox
Intoxication, alimentary, 161, 162, 163. See also Acidosis
Intraperitoneal injections, 170–171
Intravenous therapy, 114, 171
Intubation, 109–110
Ipecac, 41, 44, 73, 78, 80, 95
Isoniazid, 216
Issue, treatment by, 48, 48n

Jalap, 48, 93
Jamestown Colony, 7–8
    apprenticed servants in, 8
    diseases and starvation in, 7
Jaundice, 14, 16, 16n, 79, 95, 191

Jenner of America, 84–86
Johns Hopkins University School of Medicine, 126, 160, 167, 207, 213

Leeches, use of, in children, 79, 80, 81, 92, 94, 116
Leukemia, 126, 211
  antimetabolites in, 211
Lice, 29, 30
Life expectancy, 27
Little Mothers' League, 154
Lumbar puncture, 116–117
  first American report of, 116
Lymphocytosis, actue infectious, 211
Lymphoglandular pharyngitis, acute, (Coxsackie A-10), 237

Malaria, 73, 74, 106, 126
Malformations, congenital, 20, 83
Manchineel, poisoning from, 6
Massachusetts Bay Colony, 9
Massachusetts General Hospital, 164
Massachusetts School for Idiotic and Feeble-Minded Youth (Fernald School), 75, 90
Maternal impressions, 78, 80, 124, 152–153
  and nevi, 78
  Rachford on, 152–153
  Smith on, 124
Maternal mortality, 26, 202
  in relation to husband's income, 157
Maternity hospitals, 184, 202
  move to, 202
Mayflower, 8, 11, 60
Measles, 17, 21–22, 30, 41–42, 73, 79, 115–116, 217, 230, 236
  active immunization in, 236
  epidemics of, 22, 41–42, 115
  German. See Rubella
  in Mather family, 42
  passive immunization against, 217
  in Sewall family, 42
  treatment of, 115–116
Measles vaccine, 236
Medical Education, 10, 30, 70
  in eighteenth century, 30
  in nineteenth century, 70–71
  in seventeenth century, 10
Medical practice, 10–11, 24, 30–31, 72–73, 101–102
  in eighteenth century, 30–31
  in nineteenth century, 72–73
  in seventeenth century, 10–18, 24
Meningitis
  aseptic, and Echovirus, 237
  bacterial, 176–177. See also Hemophilus influenzae meningitis; Meningococcal meningitis; Streptococcal meningitis; Tuberculous meningitis
Meningococcal meningitis, 86–87, 116–117, 176–177
  epidemiology of, 86–87, 116, 176
  etiology of, 87

mortality of, 116, 176, 177, 215
serum treatment of, 116, 176–177
treatment of, 87, 116, 177, 215. See also Cerebrospinal fever (cerebrospinal meningitis)
Mentally retarded children, 89–90
Michael Reese Hospital, 187
Middle Atlantic colonies, 9–10
Midwives, 18–19, 157
Milk, 59–60, 61, 74, 83, 106, 134–135, 136–138, 141, 142–143, 144, 153–154, 241, 245, 246, 247–248
  adulteration of, 106
  analyses of, 59–60, 83, 134–135
  bacteriologic studies, of, 142–143
  "to boil or not to boil", 141
  dry, 253
  evaporated, 252–253
    use of, 253
  human. See Breast milk
  humanized, 253–254
  hygiene of, 74, 106, 153
  modification of, 59, 60–61, 135–139. See also Feeding, artificial
  pasteurization of, 142–143, 144, 246
  percentage feeding of, 136–138
  "swill milk", 74, 106, 141
Milk-borne diseases, 245
Milk laboratories, 126
Milk stations, 144, 154, 155
Mononucleosis, infectious, 211, 234
Morbidity, pediatric, new problems of, 241–242
Morbus caeruleus, 82
Mors thymica, 192
Mortality, childhood, 106, 159–160
  ten most common causes of childhood death 1896–1897, 1921–1922, (Table 7-1), 159. See also Infant mortality
Mortality trends, 159–160
Mumps, 43–44
  first American description of, 43–44
Myocarditis of infancy (Coxsackie B virus infection), 237

National Child Labor Committee, 156
National Education Association, 159
National Foundation for Infantile Paralysis, 235
National Institute of Child Health and Human Development (NICHD), 230
Neonatal mortality, 184–186
Nevi, and maternal impressions, 78
New England Asylum for the Education of the Blind, 75, 88–89
New Netherland, 10
New York City Division of Infant Hygiene, 154
New York City Health Department Bacteriological Laboratories, 109
New York City Milk Committee, 155
New York Founding Asylum, 132, 166
New York Institution for the Instruction of the Deaf and Dumb, 75

New York Medical College, 102, 103
New York Nursery and Child's Hospital, 81, 115
Newborn. *See* Infant, newborn
Newspapers, as source of pediatric information, 47, 56–57, 155
Nodules, rheumatic, 174–175. *See also* Rheumatic fever
Noma (cancrum oris), 82
Nosography, 84
Nursing bottle caries syndrome, first report of, 18
Nursing can (*Mammele*), 62. *See also* "Bubby-pot" baby feeder
Nutritional disorders, 218–220

Open air, benefit from. *See* Air, fresh
Ophthalmia, purulent, 75–76, 78, 81, 158
  in Philadelphia Almshouse, 75–76
Opium use of in children, 45, 51, 73, 87, 94–95, 114
  as *donum Dei*, 94
Orphanages, 74, 75, 78
  first American, 75
Orphans, 57

Panada, recipes for, 63
Pap, 60, 63
  papboat, 63–64
  pap spoon, 64
Para-aminosalicylic acid (PAS), 216
Pasteur Institute, 212
Pasteurization, 153, 246
Pastor-physicians, 11–13
  Fuller, Samuel, 11
  Mather, Cotton. *See* Mather, Cotton in *Name Index*
  Thacher, Thomas, 11–13
Pediatric clinics (specialty), 202–203
Pediatric journals, American. *See* Pediatrics, journals of, American
Pediatric morbidity, "new", 241–242
Pediatric publications, eighteenth century, 50–51. *See also* Pediatrics, journals of, American; Pediatrics, textbooks of, American
Pediatric research, federal support of, 230
Pediatric textbooks, American. *See* Pediatrics, textbooks of, American
Pediatrician, 70
Pediatrics
  academic, beginnings of, 102–105
  alternative words for, 70, 102
  child welfare movement and, 157–158
  eighteenth century publications on, 50–51
  hospitals. *See* Children's hospitals
  journals of, American
    1850–1900, 127–128
    1900–1925, 196
    1925–1950, 224
    1950–1978, 241
  social reform and, 158–160
  textbooks of, American
    1800–1850, 76–83

  1850–1900, 124–127
  1900–1925, 195
  1950–1978, 241
  organization of, 83–84
  word first used, 70
Pediatrists, 70
Pediatry. *See* Pediatrics
Pedology. *See* Pediatrics
Pellagra, 201
Penicillin, 202, 213, 214, 219
  discovery of, 213
  first American child treated with, 213n
Pennsylvania Hospital, 88
Percentage feeding, 126, 136–138, 246. *See also* Infant feeding
Perinatal services, regional, 240–241
Perkins Institution for the Blind, 89, 90
Pertussis. *See* Whooping cough
Philadelphia Almshouse, 75
Philadelphia Children's Hospital, 69
"Philopedos" (pseudonym for James Stewart), 81
Phototherapy in hyperbilirubinemia, 238
Pleurodynia, epidemic, 237
Plymouth Plantation, 8–9
Pneumonia, 70, 75, 91, 115, 126, 152, 178–179
  incidence of, 178
  mortality from, 178
Poisoning, 6, 48, 232
  from manchineel, 6
  from thorn-apple seeds, 48
Poliomyelitis, 181–183, 217, 230, 235
  constitutional factors in, 183
  epidemics of, 181–182
  mortality from, 181–182
  treatment of, with convalescent serum, 182–183
  vaccine immunization of, 235
Poliovirus, 216–217
Poliovirus vaccines, 230, 235
  clinical trials of, 235
  inactivated (Salk-type), 235
  and incidence of poliomyelitis, 235
  oral (live, Sabin-type), 235
Polyostotic fibrous dysplasia, 222
Poor Richard's Almanac for 1763, 45–46
Potassium
  metabolism of, in diarrheal diseases, 206–207
  use of, in intravenous therapy, 207–208
Premature infants. *See* Infant, premature
Protein milk (Eiweissmilch), 246, 250
Psychiatric clinic, first, 202
Pylorus, hypertrophy of, 5, 84
Pyruvate kinase deficiency, 234

Red-haired women, milk of, 132–133
Regional perinatal services, 240
Report of *The American Pediatric Society's Collective Investigation into the Use of Antitoxin in the Treatment of Diphtheria in Private Practice* (1896), 110–111

Respiratory distress syndrome (RDS), 230, 239–240
  lecithin/sphingomyelin ratio in amniotic fluid, 239–240
  mortality from, 239
  pathogenesis of, 239–240
Retrolental fibroplasia, 221–222
Rheumatic fever, 126, 174–175, 215–216
  clinical course of, 174, 215–216
  complications of, 126, 174, 215–216
  etiology of, 126, 174–175
  incidence of, 174, 215
  nodules in, 174–175
  prophylaxis of, 216
  treatment of, 126, 215–216
Rickets, 120–122, 127, 128, 165–168, 218, 220
  incidence of, 120–122, 218
  pathogenesis of, 167–168
  treatment of, 122, 168, 220
Rickettsialpox (Kew Gardens spotted fever), 222–223
Robert Wood Johnson Foundation, 240
Roseola infantum, 183–184
Rubella, 90, 217, 236
  first American description of, 90
  vaccine, 236
Rubila, 17
Russell Sage Foundation, 159

Sabin vaccine in poliomyelitis, 235
Salaam convulsion, first mention of, 82
Salk vaccine in poliomyelitis, 230, 235
Sanguis draconis (dragon's blood), 14n
Scarlet fever, 23, 40–41, 70, 81, 83, 89, 111–112, 126, 127, 173–174, 215
  antitoxin, 174
  clinical course of, 173
  etiology of, 112
  first documented American epidemic, 40
  immunization against, 174
  mortality from, 111–112
  treatment of, 41, 112, 215
Schick test, 172
School children
  health of, 201
  learning problems of, 241
Schools, first compulsory attendance statute, 96
Scrofula, 90, 117, 192
Scurvy, 8, 122–124, 127, 169, 220
  etiology of, 122–124
  first American description of, 8, 122
  report of special committee of the American Pediatric Society, 123–124
  treatment of, 169, 220
Section on Diseases of Children (A.M.A.), 103, 104
Seton, treatment by, 94
Sheppard-Towner Act, 157, 203
Sickle-cell anemia, 209
Signatures, doctrine of, 24–25
"Simulated milk adapted" (SMA), 254–255

Smallpox, 20–21, 30, 32–36, 45, 70, 73, 74, 95
  epidemics of, 20–21, 32–36, 106
  first mention of in the American English colonies, 21
  inoculation for, 32–36, 45
  mortality from, 21, 34
  vaccination for, 84–85
Social reform and pediatrics, 158–160
Société d'Allaitement Maternelle, 155
Société Protectrice de l'Enfance, 155
Society for the Prevention of Cruelty to Children (SPCC), 100, 153
Solid foods, 146–147, 256–257. *See also* Infant feeding
Soybean, in infant feeding, 251
Specialty pediatric clinics, emergence of, 202–203
Spirits, 9
Starch in infants' formulas, 140
Status thymicolymphaticus, 192–194. *See also* Sudden infant death syndrome; Thymus
Streptococcal diseases, 173–175. *See also* Glomerulonephritis; Rheumatic fever; Scarlet fever
Streptococcal meningitis, 176, 213
Streptomycin, 202, 213, 216
Sudden infant death syndrome, 193–194, 230–231
  first mention of, 20
  incidence of, 230
  thymus and, 192–193
Sulfonamides, 202, 215, 219, 224, 241
  discovery of, 212
  first use of in United States, 241
Summer complaint. *See* Cholera infantum
Supportive therapy, 169–171
  blood collecting, apparatus for, 169–170
Swaddling, 79
Swill milk, 74, 106, 141
Syphilis, congenital, 14, 118–120, 126, 180–181
  clinical course of, 119–120
  incidence of, 180–181
  mortality from, 119
  transmission of, 119–120, 181
  treatment of, 119–120

Table foods, age at which introduced, 257
Tartar emetic, 41, 45, 95
Teething, 45, 49–50, 76, 80, 94
  lancing gums in, 50, 76
Teratoma, 51
Terra sigillata (sealed earth), 14n
Tetanus, 50, 78
Tetany of the newborn, transient, 166, 222
Tetracyclines, 202, 213
Thalassemia, 208–209
Theories, medical, 15, 24, 35, 50–51, 92
  animalcular, 35
  germ, 70, 101
  humoral, 24, 73
  miasmatic, 107–108
  tension, 50, 73

Thermometry, 72–73, 86
Thomas Wilson Sanitarium, 142
Thrush. *See* Aphthae
Thymus, 192–194, 232–233
    and DiGeorge syndrome, 233
    irradiation of, 192, 194
    role of, in immunology, 233
    and status thymicolymphaticus, 192–194
    and sudden death, 192–194
Thyroid, cancer of, 224
Tinea capitis, 16, 48
Tobacco, use of, by Harvard medical students, 85
Tuberculin, 118
    treatment of tuberculosis with, 118
    tuberculin test, 177–178
Tuberculosis, 8, 74, 117–118, 126, 127, 152, 178, 202,
        210, 216
    first pediatric clinic for, 202
    incidence of, as determined by tuberculin testing (Fig.
        7-12), 177
    monocytes in, 210
    mortality from, 117
    treatment of, 117, 118, 152, 216
Tuberculous meningitis, 83, 90, 176
    first American description of, 90
Typhoid fever, 73, 74, 179
    incidence of, 179
    mortality from, 179
    treatment of, 179

United States Children's Bureau, establishment of, 156–
    157
Urban children, health hazards of, 73–74, 91, 105–
    106

Vaccination, 78, 84–85
    first compulsory law for, 85
    first performed in the United States, 84. *See also*
        Smallpox
Vegetables and infant feeding, 256
Venipuncture, 169–170
Virginia colonies, 6–8
    children in, 6
    first colony, 6
    Jamestown Colony, 7–8
    second (lost) colony, 7

Vital statistics, seventeenth century, 26–27. *See also* In-
    fant mortality; Maternal mortality; Neonatal mor-
    tality
Vitamin A deficiency, in cystic fibrosis, 219
Vitamin B_1, 218
Vitamin B_2, 218
Vitamin C, 169, 218, 252
Vitamin D, discovery of, 168
Vitamin K_1, 218–220
Vulvovaginitis, epidemic, 158, 179–180
    clinical course of, 179–180
    epidemics, 179–180
    history of, 179–180
    treatment of, 179–180

Walker-Gordon Milk Laboratory, 137
Wassermann test, 171, 181
Water therapy (hydrotherapy), 72
Weaning, 64–65, 147
    in eighteenth century, 64–65
    in seventeenth century, 64–65
    in nineteenth century, 147
Wet-nurses, 56–58, 81, 132–133
    advertisements for, 56
    hair color, importance of, 132–133
    rules for the selection of, 132–133
White House Conference on Children
    1909, 156
    1930, 158
Whooping cough, 23, 43, 81, 95, 114–115, 175, 176,
        214–215
    epidemics of, 23, 43
    mortality from, 114–115, 175, 214
    treatment of, 43, 115, 175–176
    vaccines for, 175–176, 214–215
Willard Parker Hospital, 112, 182
Wine
    for infants, 41, 45, 63
    for older children, 63, 87
Worm infestations, 45, 48–49, 83, 94

Yale University School of Medicine, 207
Yellow fever, 70, 73, 74

Zymotic diseases, 107
    deaths from—1850 census (Table 5-2), 108
    definition of, 107